Assessment in Mental Handicap

ASSESSMENT IN MENTAL HANDICAP

A Guide to Assessment Practices, Tests and Checklists

JAMES HOGG AND NORMA V. RAYNES

CROOM HELM
London & Sydney

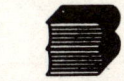

BROOKLINE BOOKS
Cambridge, Massachusetts

© 1987 James Hogg and Norma V. Raynes
Croom Helm Ltd, Provident House, Burrell Row,
Beckenham, Kent BR3 1AT

Croom Helm Australia, 44-50 Waterloo Road,
North Ryde, 2113, New South Wales

British Library Cataloguing in Publication Data

Assessment in mental handicap : a guide to
assessment practices, tests and checklists.
 1. Mentally handicapped — Testing
 I. Hogg, James, 1940– II. Raynes, Norma V.
 362.3'64   HV 3004
 ISBN 0-7099-3744-X
 ISBN 0-7099-3745-8 Pbk

Brookline Books, PO Box 1046
Cambridge, MA 02238

Library of Congress Cataloging-in-Publication Data

Assessment in mental handicap.

   Includes bibliographies and index.
   1. Mentally handicapped — Psychological testing.
2. Psychological tests. I. Hogg, J. (James)
II. Raynes, Norma V. (Norma Victoria) [DNLM:
1. Disability Evaluation. 2. Learning Disorders —
diagnosis. 3. Mental Retardation — diagnosis.
4. Psychological Tests. WM 304 A8457]
RC570.A757 1987   616.85'88075   86-26843
ISBN 0-914797-31-X
ISBN 0-914797-32-8 (soft)

Printed and bound in Great Britain by Mackays of Chatham Ltd, Kent

Contents

List of Contributors   vii

1   Assessing People with Mental Handicap: An Introduction
J. Hogg and N.V. Raynes   1

2   Psychometric Approaches
M. Berger and W. Yule   12

3   Early Development and Piagetian Tests
J. Hogg   45

4   Adaptive Behaviour Scales
N.V. Raynes   81

5   Behaviour Disturbance and its Assessment
I. Leudar and W.I. Fraser   107

6   Assessments of Physical Development, Hearing and Vision that can be used by Educational and Care Staff
J. Sebba   129

7   Criterion-referenced Tests
C. Kiernan   158

8   Direct Observation as an Assessment Tool in Functional Analysis and Treatment
G. Murphy   190

Appendix: Details of Cited Test Instruments   239

Author Index   276

Subject Index   284

Contributors

Dr Michael Berger
— Top Grade Clinical Psychologist, Department of Clinical Psychology, Lanesborough Wing, St George's Hospital, Blackshaw Road, London SW17 0QT
— Honorary Senior Lecturer, Departments of Psychology and Psychiatry, St George's Hospital Medical School, London SW17 0RE

Dr William I. Fraser
— Consultant Psychiatrist, Gogarburn Hospital, Glasgow Road, Edinburgh EH12 9BJ
— Part-time Senior Lecturer, Department of Psychiatry, University of Edinburgh, Morningside Drive, Edinburgh EH8 9YL
— Honorary Senior Lecturer, Department of Psychology, University of St Andrews, St Andrews KY16 9AJ

Dr James Hogg
— Reader and Deputy Director, Hester Adrian Research Centre, The University, Oxford Road, Manchester M13 9PL

Professor Chris Kiernan
— Director, Hester Adrian Research Centre, The University, Oxford Road, Manchester M13 9PL

Dr Ivan Leudar
— Lecturer, Department of Psychology, The University, Oxford Road, Manchester M13 9PL

CONTRIBUTORS

Dr Glynis Murphy
— Lecturer, Department of Child Psychiatry, Institute of Child Health, 30 Guildford Street, London WC1N 1EH

Dr Norma V. Raynes
— Senior Research Fellow, Department of Social Administration, Faculty of Economics and Social Studies, The University, Oxford Road, Manchester M13 9PL

Ms Judy Sebba
— Research Fellow, Hester Adrian Research Centre, The University, Oxford Road, Manchester M13 9PL
— Associate Director (Education), British Institute of Mental Handicap, Wolverhampton Road, Kidderminster, Worcs DY10 3PP

Dr William Yule
— Reader in Applied Child Psychology, Institute of Psychiatry, De Crespigny Park, Denmark Hill, London SE5 8AF
— Top Grade Clinical Psychologist, The Maudsley and Bethlem Royal Hospital Special Health Authority, Denmark Hill, London SE5 8AZ

1

Assessing People with Mental Handicap: An Introduction

J. Hogg and N.V. Raynes

It is now about 15 years since the publication of *The Psychological Assessment of Mental and Physical Handicaps* (edited by P.J. Mittler), a text that has remained throughout this period the authoritative account of the subject. In this period, however, we have seen far-reaching changes in virtually every aspect of society's approach to people with serious developmental disabilities, including those with a mental handicap. Legislation in England and Wales in 1970 made children and young people with mental handicap the responsibility of the education service. The impetus given to educational practice and social support arising from this change was accelerated by Warnock's report on special education in 1978 which in turn led to the 1981 Education Act. With respect to the life of adults with mental handicap, services have been geared increasingly to enabling them to live as normal a life as possible in the community, with the concomitant run down of the large institutions that for the past century have provided the main single alternative to such individuals living with their families. Similar developments have occurred in the United States. A Federal statute (Public Law 94–142) requires special education to be provided in the least restrictive environment for persons aged 3–21. This requirement has been interpreted to mean that education can be provided within ordinary schools. There is currently pressure on Congress to extend the provision of appropriate programming to children below the age of 3. The large institutions are also being run down. Residential alternatives to them present as wide a range as that in England, from individual tenancies unsupervised or minimally staffed to larger staffed facilities within rather than apart from local communities.

The implementation of these changes has had clear implications for the way in which those providing services meet their professional obligations. The emphasis on explicit intervention, whether for educational or training purposes, has brought the need for usable and technically acceptable assessment instruments to the fore, with respect to both determining the present status and competence of an individual and establishing the direction intervention should take. This has led to the development of a whole range of assessment instruments. These were not in existence at the time Mittler's (1970) text was published and nowhere are they described in a single volume. The impetus to bring together the papers assembled here came from enquiries regarding the availability of such a text from students and professionals involved in planning and providing services for people with a mental handicap.

Given the plethora of test and assessment instruments available to those working in the field of mental handicap, this volume sets out to meet two general aims. First, it is important to test-users to appreciate fully that different types of tests have quite distinct functions and hence, however suitable for that function, have limitations in other directions. A given test can be both used and abused. In Chapters 2 to 8 contributors write about the main groupings of tests, their functions, limitations and possible misuse. They also draw attention to the fact that assessment instruments have to meet certain technical requirements if we are to be confident in using them. While use of an assessment instrument can lead us to feel that we are meeting our professional aims in an objective fashion, in reality we can only achieve this end if the instrument we have chosen is both appropriate to those aims and theoretically and technically adequate. These chapters include sufficient theoretical and technical background to enable readers to inform themselves in these aspects of assessment instruments. The chapters also go some way to meeting the second aim of the volume, namely to describe some of the main assessment practices, tests and checklists that are available. To provide more explicit information, the second part of the book consists of a summary of each assessment procedure and provides information on its availability. Neither the chapters nor these summaries set out to be comprehensive. Authors have selected major or significant approaches that illustrate the nature and scope of given types of testing. However, on the basis of these chapters readers, if they wish, should be able to locate tests other than those described within the framework provided and evaluate their use and limitations in an informed way.

Before saying more about the book's framework, it is necessary to go beyond our brief sketch of legislation and attitudinal changes that have occurred from 1970 to 1986. First, though mental handicap is still regarded as pervasive in that a wide range of specific functions and competencies will be slow to, or will fail to, develop, any global characterisation of mental handicap is of little help in developing an educational curriculum or wide-ranging training programme. Thus, an understanding of mental handicap in terms of specific kinds of function, e.g. memory, attention, etc., and in terms of competence, e.g. use of public transport, ability to hold a spoon, is called for. This rejection of the usefulness of a global characterisation has also contributed to dissatisfaction with the very term 'mental handicap' with its suggestion of a generalised internal deficit. Further dissatisfaction with the term relates to the adjective 'mental' and leads to consideration of the second important trend over this period, the predominance of a behavioural approach to intervention. Here the term 'mental' loses any acceptability in describing the nature of the disability. A third, and related, trend has come with the rejection of handicap as being simply a property of a disabled individual. Disability is increasingly viewed as the outcome of an interaction between a person and the environment in which he or she lives. Appropriate alterations to this interaction can reduce the extent to which impairments handicap the person's day-to-day functioning and competence. These three changes in our view of mental handicap, from global to specific characterisation of the condition, from a view of *mental* deficiency to one of *behavioural* competence, and from emphasis on the person to person-environment interaction, have all contributed to the changing nature of assessment in the field of mental handicap and suggest a loose continuum along which the classes of assessment in this book can be ranged.

Four broad classes of approach to assessing people with mental handicap can be suggested: (1) norm-referenced; (2) assessment of adaptive behaviour; (3) criterion-referenced; (4) techniques of behavioural observation. These categories are by no means rigid as we will show, a given test perhaps sharing characteristics associated with more than one category. Nevertheless, the chapters in this book can be viewed from the perspective of (1) to (4).

NORM-REFERENCED TESTS

The main function of norm-referenced assessment is to discover how well an individual performs in relation to other people drawn from the same class of individuals. For example, with respect to a given ability, is this six-year-old child doing worse than, as well as, or better than, other six year olds? Both Berger and Yule (Chapter 2) and Kiernan (Chapter 7) discuss the general properties of such tests. *Psychometric norm-referenced tests* are considered in detail by Berger and Yule, who note that the origins of such tests lay in the attempt early in the century to identify children who were failing in the French school system in order to provide them with more suitable education. For many years such tests, directed to global measures of intelligence, were the main form of assessment for the identification of people with mental handicap — if indeed *any* attempt at formal assessment was undertaken. In addition to being global in their assessment, i.e. yielding, for example, a single Intelligence Quotient (IQ), psychometric assessment is concerned with evaluating *mental* functioning as Berger and Yule note: 'Psychological measurement depends on the outward expression in behaviour of otherwise inaccessible mental processes' (see p. 14). Ideally, therefore, choice of items for inclusion in the test reflects a theory of, or assumptions about, the nature of mental processes. While such processes will be sensitive to the influence of the environment, the concern is essentially with the individual's mental functioning and changes in this over time.

Though developments in assessment in mental handicap often reflect a reaction against psychometric approaches, Berger and Yule point to the enduring utility, despite acknowledged limitations, of intelligence testing '. . . we believe that it is best not to parade IQ tests as "measures of intelligence" because we do not as yet have compelling reasons to do so . . . What is important is the functional significance of IQ scores of different magnitudes, for instance that individuals with low IQs most commonly show limitations in many aspects of development' (see p. 21). They argue that such assessment has a place in an overall clinical evaluation through the interpretation of similarities and differences in test scores, their changes over time and the interpretation of profiles of ability. The limitation of psychometric tests as sources of programme material is emphasised by Kiernan (Chapter 7).

Norm-referenced developmental tests are also considered by Berger and Yule. Historically, these represent a downward extension of psychometric procedures to arrive at a Development Quotient (DQ) as against an IQ score. They share with intelligence testing the aim of arriving at global scores for major domains of development, e.g. mental versus motor development, though in some instances a more restricted area is entailed, such as language development. No theory of development typically underlies the choice of items which are included in such a scale. Their main function is to differentiate children at various Chronological Ages and their adequacy is judged in relation to their success in achieving this. The value of such tests should again be seen in relation to early clinical evaluation and their limitations as aids to intervention should be borne in mind (Chapter 7).

Partially norm-referenced tests refer here to a highly specific development in assessment in recent years. Norm-referenced developmental tests of the kind noted above emerged from the work of Gessell and his collaborators who described the course of child development as an essentially maturational occurrence. In contrast, Piaget has proposed that the development of intelligence is determined by the construction of intelligence through the child's interaction with the physical and social world. His theory has been specific with respect to both the mechanisms leading to such development and the organisation and structure of intelligence. Pioneering work by Inhelder and Woodward in which Piaget's theory was used as the basis for assessing people with mental handicap is described in Chapter 3 by Hogg. The main thrust to such assessment came with the development of Uzgiris and Hunt's *Ordinal Scales of Infant Development* published in 1975, followed by Dunst's formalisation of these scales in 1980. We have used the term 'partially non-referenced' because Uzgiris and Hunt explicitly did not attempt any referencing in their original instrument, i.e. they provided no age levels at which items on the various scales should be passed. Dunst, however, has provided mental age equivalents for such passes thus edging the scales towards norm referencing. The scales are nevertheless not psychometric in any strict sense of the term and differ from conventional psychometric assessment in being derived from an explicit theory of intelligence.

ASSESSING ADAPTIVE BEHAVIOUR

Social competence and its assessment has become a major focus of interest and concern in the field of mental handicap. Raynes in Chapter 4 notes that the term 'social competence' has given way to the more widely used term 'adaptive behaviour'. The development of instruments to assess social competence arose from inadequacies in IQ assessment and a need '. . . to find a basis for the overall functional classification of people with mental handicap' (see p. 81). This need for a functional classification reflects in part the move away from viewing mental handicap in terms of intellectual deficiency (with the dependence of this view on IQ testing) to mental handicap as reflecting diminished adaptive competence in everyday living. As Raynes points out, the number of adaptive behaviour instruments has proliferated as research and clinical demands have increased. Such instruments are typified by their assessment of several domains (e.g. self-feeding, personal hygiene, etc.) and avoid global statements about an individual. Raynes emphasises, though, that adaptive behaviour scales should not be seen as substitutes for psychometric procedures as their function differs. Indeed, the American Association on Mental Deficiency classification system of mental handicap employs both IQ and adaptive behaviour measures.

The function of adaptive behaviour scales has varied from general assessment of individuals with mental handicap in order to locate them in appropriate programmes and to monitor change, to prediction of successful adjustment to different kinds of community living. Whatever the heuristic value of the former aim to workers in this area, Raynes emphasises that prediction of community adjustment is limited and at present no better than that achieved with IQ as the predictor. It should also be noted that the two types of assessment are converging from a technical point of view as adaptive behaviour instruments themselves are norm referenced.

Behaviour disorders are a major concern in the field of mental handicap. They are regarded as potential barriers to the development of adaptive behaviour and community adjustment. The instruments described by Raynes in Chapter 4 frequently include sections concerned with behaviour problems and these are commented on in more detail in Chapter 5 by Leudar and Fraser. The concern with adaptive behaviour has led to an increasing emphasis on the environmental context in which the behaviour is assessed. Nowhere is this clearer than in the case of behaviour problems. Leudar and Fraser emphasise that such problems are not simply a property of the individual, but must also be considered in relation to the environment in which he or she lives. The fact presents problems of classification as a given piece of behaviour may be considered a problem or not depending on the context in which it occurs. This problem points towards the need for assessment to register behaviour *and* context as described in relation to observational techniques by Murphy in Chapter 8.

Leudar and Fraser point out that as with adaptive behaviour generally, it is necessary to consider the structure of behaviour problems and the factors influencing their organisation. Studies bearing on this important question are reviewed. Only in this chapter do contributors move into the specialised question of the relation between assessment and psychiatric diagnosis. In Chapter 6, Sebba describes a variety of procedures that can be employed by the nonspecialist, i.e. the individual who is not a physiotherapist, ophthalmologist, etc. The importance of such assessments is indicated by the evidence Sebba cites that the occurrence of physical and sensory impairments is greater among people with mental handicap than in the wider population. Given this state of affairs and the paucity of specialist services in general, then the opportunity to assess such impairments in an effective way is a considerable contribution to the overall assessment of adaptive functioning. It should be noted in passing that in many of the scales described by Raynes in Chapter 4, more limited recording of physical and sensory functioning is also provided for and that the techniques described by Sebba could well inform the completion of these sections of adaptive behaviour scales.

CRITERION-REFERENCED ASSESSMENT

The forms of assessment described up to this point will assist in providing information to make appropriate service provision for an individual. They will also identify areas of behaviour in which it would be desirable to enhance competence. It is criterion-referenced assessment, however, that addresses the issue of how we undertake assessments that point specifically to our teaching or training objectives. In Chapter 7, Kiernan notes that: 'Criterion-referenced tests can be defined as procedures in which items represent "achievements" which are of importance in the individual's adjustment to his or her environment or which reflect the outcome of teaching or training' (see p. 158). In contrast to norm-referenced assessment, criterion-referenced assessment is not concerned with comparing individuals. For this reason the basis for choosing items for the test is not related to how well they discriminate between individuals at different ages. Of more importance is the fact that the sequence of items are functionally related, i.e. that acquisition of a given behaviour is necessary for the acquisition of the next in the sequence and that both are included in the sequence of test items.

Criterion-referenced assessment shares with norm-referenced assessment the ideal that the form and content of the test have their basis in theory. They also have in common the fact that it is questionable that either type of assessment has yet yielded a test which is in reality rooted firmly in theory. As we have seen, Berger and

Yule do not believe that psychometric assessment is firmly grounded in any theory of intelligence. In the case of criterion-referenced assessment there are two distinct areas of theory that are required. As Kiernan points out, the authors of criterion-referenced tests make assumptions regarding the nature of community adjustment. What behaviours are critical to such adjustment and hence what is the place of the person with handicaps in society? Equally, the content of criterion-referenced tests should be based on a theory of development and skill acquisition.

In reality the theories of the nature of community adjustment are usually implicit while criterion-referenced tests draw from a whole range of theoretical and nontheoretical positions to draw up their list of items. Kiernan points to the dependence on Piagetian items of the sort explicitly included in the ordinal scales of development described by Hogg in Chapter 3. He also illustrates how specific developments in theory, specifically in the area of language and communication development, can and should be employed in developing criterion-referenced assessment. Criteria related to item selection and organisation are included among the seven Kiernan employs (see p. 167) in evaluating some of the best-known criterion-referenced assessment batteries, including the Portage checklists.

BEHAVIOURAL OBSERVATION

In line with the trends we have noted at the start of this chapter, criterion-referenced assessment is concerned with the evaluation of specific behaviours that become the targets for teaching and training. This in turn implies that the time and place in which the new learned abilities are shown becomes part of the evaluation of the programme. With this step, criterion-referenced assessment shades naturally into the gamut of observational procedures described in Chapter 8 by Murphy. As she points out, behavioural observation sets out to record directly and to monitor behaviour in everyday settings. In this the procedure goes beyond the use of checklists, whether in the form of adaptive behaviour scales or criterion-referenced tests. The approach has its origins in a range of disciplines including ethology, operant psychology, anthropology and sociology.

As Murphy points out, there is a natural continuity between behavioural observation and intervention, and indeed, evaluating the effects of teaching and training. The approach is an inherent part of behaviour modification without which such intervention would not be regarded as valid. Because of the variety of observational procedures available, Murphy presents greater detail on technical issues than is given in the other chapters. There is a good reason for this: The user of any of the assessment procedures described in Chapters 2 to 7 will receive the test or battery complete with all its strengths and weaknesses. Should the reader decide, however, to undertake a behavioural programme employing an observational procedure, he or she will have to *create* the observational strategy for that particular client in the circumstances pertaining. While Murphy's chapter illustrates the various options with respect to recording method, sampling procedure and so forth, the reader will have to make critical decisions leading to an essentially novel assessment meeting quite specific goals.

In all respects, behavioural observation as assessment stands in contrast to norm-referenced tests with which the book begins. Behavioural observation is concerned with specific rather than global functions; with the person as part of an ecological system rather than as a self-contained individual.

SOME TECHNICAL ASPECTS

We have shown above how four classes of assessment are contrasted and in what respects they have elements in common. We have also pointed out that any of these procedures should be considered from a technical standpoint. This the authors of the chapters do. Many of the core issues are dealt with in Chapter 2 by Berger and Yule where test standardisation (p. 15), measurement (p. 16), reliability (p. 20) and validity (p. 21) are considered. The question of reliability recurs throughout all chapters and in contrast to the extensive work undertaken by psychometricians over many decades, several major assessment instruments are found wanting in this respect. This is particularly the case with a number of widely used criterion-referenced tests as Kiernan points out in Chapter 7. At the other extreme from psychometric assessment, we find the issue of reliability central to Murphy's consideration of observational techniques. A vast literature has been developed on reliability in this area and adequate determination of reliability is an inherent part of the approach she describes. Sebba, in Chapter 6, draws attention to the problem of obtaining reliable assessments of visual, auditory and physical functioning in people with profound mental handicap, given the marked fluctuations in their general well-being from day to day.

ASSESSMENT IN CONTEXT

The importance of assessment to those providing services is reflected not only in the development of tests of the kind described in this volume, but also in the extent to which professionals have devised their own assessment procedures for individual schools, Adult Training/Social Education Centres, hospitals and residential establishments. Indeed, some of the instruments included in this book have their origins in such attempts to devise tailor-made methods of meeting local needs.

The state of assessment in the field of mental handicap is not so well advanced that such efforts should be decried, though hopefully we look to a future in which appropriate and sound tests will be available making the need for such individual initiatives less pressing. What must be urged, however, is that because an assessment device has been developed to meet local needs, and because it induces a feeling of familiarity and comfort in the service provider cum test designer, these facts do not mean it is an adequate or acceptable test by the criteria of good test construction. On the contrary, experience would suggest that there is a danger that in choice of items, their organisation, their scoring criteria and most other relevant factors, they will fall far below the standards of available tests. Where the need for use of an assessment instrument is felt by those providing services, we would urge that care is taken to define the exact purposes the assessment will serve. Then, detailed consideration should be given to existing tests that set out to meet the defined aim. Only when we are convinced that our aim cannot be met using standard available tests should we consider developing a new instrument which will inevitably absorb considerable resources if it is to be done properly.

It is hoped that the information provided in these chapters and the accompanying section describing the available tests cited (see Appendix) will contribute to our understanding of the variety of different forms of assessment which can be undertaken in both educational settings and in the wider context of services for both children and adults with mental handicap.

REFERENCE

Mittler, P.J. (ed.) (1970) *The Psychological Assessment of Mental and Physical Handicaps*, Methuen, London

2

Psychometric Approaches

M. Berger and W. Yule

INTRODUCTION

Tests are devices and procedures for measuring or quantifying psychological characteristics. They are the equivalent for psychologists of instruments for measuring blood pressure, electric current or length.

There are tests for quantifying a multitude of psychological characteristics. In this chapter we will discuss a sub-set of tests, those devised for measuring intelligence, educational attainment and language development. Other chapters will describe tests for different purposes.

TESTING AND INDIVIDUAL DIFFERENCES

If people were identical in all their characteristics, there would be little point in devising tests. While we share the human characteristics of being intelligent, sociable, emotional, active and so on, we also differ: individuals vary in height, abilities, the extent to which they are sociable, emotional and physically active, and in many other ways (see Berger 1985). Psychological tests are in the main developed to enable us to express individual differences quantitatively. Why we should want to do so is a question that might begin to be answered in one or several books, certainly not in a single chapter. Suffice it to say that measuring individual differences could contribute information that would help us to understand why people differ in the ways they do (an important question in relation to mental and physical handicap), as well as yielding information that is of immediate practical import, for instance, identifying individuals who have special needs, a topic we discuss below.

A BRIEF HISTORY OF TESTING

In the late nineteenth century, there was an interest in individual differences in abilities and other characteristics. Tests were used to study how well individuals could discriminate between different weights, sound frequencies or colours. Speed of reaction to sounds or lights or other stimuli were also studied extensively. Sensory acuity and speed were considered important because at the time, it was thought they were manifestations of intelligence. However, none of the tests of these functions showed strong relationships with what were considered to be other aspects of intelligence, such as academic performance, indexed by examination marks for instance.

In France at about the same time, Binet and Simon, who had been studying children's thinking, were asked to address themselves to the practical problem of identifying children who were not progressing in French state schools. The purpose of selection was to enable more appropriate education to be provided for them (see Anastasi 1982 for a more detailed account).

Prior to the advent of objective tests, the degree of retardation was assessed subjectively and, as it turned out, unreliably using a medical categorisation system and clinical judgements as ways of allocating people to these categories. The experimental tests of Galton and his contemporaries were found to be unsatisfactory for identifying different degrees of handicap. Tasks which involved 'higher mental processes' — problem solving, word definitions and the like — were found to be more suitable diagnostic tools.

In 1905, Binet and Simon published a scale or collection of tasks which are now regarded as the first intelligence tests. The scales consisted of a series of different items sampling a range of higher mental processes. The items were arranged in ascending order of difficulty and the total score — i.e. the number of correct solutions — was converted to a single index of intelligence, called 'Mental Age'. The difference between a child's mental and chronological ages was then used as an index of the degree of handicap.

The Binet-Simon test was received as a seemingly good solution to an important practical problem and was soon in widespread use and translated into several languages. The most popular American version of the test became known as the Stanford-Binet and was one of the main instruments used in the diagnosis of mental retardation.

As the years have passed it has become clear that this test is biased towards verbal skills so that it was possible that a person not generally retarded would be identified as such by this test if they had language difficulties. The latest version of the test continues to have many limitations and is not recommended for practical use (Kaufman and Reynolds 1983). It will not be considered in this chapter.

By the end of the 1914–18 war the use of psychological tests had begun to proliferate. Many new tests were introduced and testing became an important aspect of professional and applied psychology. Old tests continue to be revised and new tests appear from time to time.

Psychological testing, and the findings from psychological tests, particularly those relating to intelligence, have never been free from controversy. In the past decade or so there has for instance been legislation proscribing the use of tests in certain parts of the USA. There can be little doubt that tests have been misused and abused, and may well continue to be so. There are also grounds for believing that tests are misrepresented as possessing properties and powers they do not have. Despite these and other negative features of tests (topics we have discussed in greater detail elsewhere — Berger and Yule 1985), we have also argued that tests can make an important contribution to psychological assessment, and it is for this reason that we advocate their continued use. The remainder of this chapter will focus on some basic concepts in testing and will survey a number of tests encountered in the psychological assessment of handicap.

THE NATURE OF PSYCHOLOGICAL MEASUREMENT

Many psychological attributes and processes are not directly observable. We infer their existence from behaviour. We say that children can read (have the ability to read) when we observe them in the act of reading aloud passages not encountered before: we say they understand printed prose when they answer questions about the passages.

Psychological measurement depends on the outward expression in behaviour of otherwise inaccessible mental processes. These behaviours comprise people's actions and the accounts they give of their inner feelings and experiences. In order to initiate measurement, we have either to await the natural occurrence of the relevant behaviours or in some way provoke those behaviours believed to be manifestations of the psychological characteristics of interest. Hence, most psychological tests, particularly those discussed in this chapter, consist partly of tasks and questions specially contrived to provoke the expression of the attribute or process. Reading tests commonly consist of words or passages that the individual has to read; tests of language may require the person to describe the content of a picture to carry out a verbal instruction; and a test of intelligence might include problem-solving tasks and general knowledge questions. In sum, psychological tests are commonly 'provocative'.

THE ROLE OF THEORY

Given the enormous variety of human behaviour, how do we know which behaviours to provoke? In the main, the type of task selected is a function of the test designer's theory of intelligence. If it is believed that one of the ways in which intelligence shows itself is through verbal fluency, a test might include tasks requiring the testee to describe a picture or produce in one minute as many words beginning with 's' as possible. If intelligence is also thought to manifest itself in the ability to solve novel problems, the test would include such items. Hence, tests usually consist of sets of items, each set — called a sub-test — aimed at sampling different aspects of intelligence if it is an intelligence test, or of personality if a personality test, and so on. As will be seen later, the absence of a single generally accepted theory of intelligence has led to the development of a wide variety of tests of intelligence, each with somewhat different content.

STANDARDISATION

All measuring devices have rules about how they are to be used. This ensures that different people will use the procedure in the same way and helps ensure comparability of results. A clinical thermometer has to be placed in a particular location and left there for a fixed period before the temperature is read off. The temperature is not taken immediately after strenuous exercise nor is the person supposed to be sitting in a cold bath at the time. Likewise psychological tests usually have a set of rules governing their administration and scoring. When there are such rules, the test is said to be standardised.

MEASUREMENT

Age and ratio measures

How do psychological tests accomplish measurement? There are various answers to this question depending on the purpose of the test. One common way to do so is to assign an arbitrary score to a correct solution of each task contained in the test (e.g. 1 if the answer is correct, 0 if it is wrong), and then sum the total correct. This is usually called the raw score. The set of tasks is then administered according to the standard procedure to groups of people, each group perhaps different in age or some other characteristic, and the raw or total score for each person in every group is computed. It is then possible to derive some index of the overall performance of each group, for instance the average raw score. This set of raw scores, or some transformation of them, constitutes the test norms. For instance, ten year olds on average score 50, eleven year olds 65, and twelve year olds 80. If we then give the test to an eleven year old who scores 69, we can say their score is above the average of comparable individuals (i.e. the other eleven year olds). If the test purports to measure intelligence, the individual's score on the test could be interpreted as indicating that he or she is of above-average intelligence. If the score was below the age group average, the conclusion might be that the person is below average in intelligence. If the test was one that sampled language or reading skills, we would draw similar conclusions, only in these instances referring to linguistic functioning or reading competence, respectively.

Another way of expresssing test performance is through age-equivalent scores. In the above example, assume that the eleven year old obtained a total score of 79. This is very close to the average score of the twelve year olds. If the test were an intelligence test, we would say he or she has a Mental Age of twelve years; if it were a reading test, the child would be said to have a Reading Age of twelve.

Note that an eleven year old with any Age score of twelve is advanced in that characteristic whereas if the Age score obtained were at the nine-year level, he would be behind in the development of whatever functions were tapped by the test.

One way to express this relationship is via a Ratio Quotient, i.e. Test Age/Chronological Age (CA). The Ratio Intelligence Quotient (IQ) is one form of such score, where 'Test Age' is expressed as mental age:

$$[IQ = MA/CA \times 100]$$

the multiplication by 100 being introduced to eliminate decimals.

Ratio quotients and Age scores have certain limitations that make them somewhat unsatisfactory for indexing skills and are not used in contemporary tests. Nevertheless, Age scores such as Reading or Language Age are a useful way of communicating about an individual's current functioning. To be told that a five year old comprehends speech at the level of the average two to three year old provides immediately useful information that is not as readily conveyed by saying the child has a language quotient of 50.

Deviation scores

One of the problems with Age scores is the difficulty in devising items which 16 year olds pass easily but which the majority of 15 year olds fail. For a long time it seemed as if the upper level of mental age was 16 years and so when older people were tested, the highest ratio IQ that could be obtained by a 32 year old was 50! The limits of usefulness of the ratio IQ are then reached. It was manifestly silly to regard 'intelligence' as dropping rapidly after 16 years. Adults clearly differed in their ability to solve intelligence test items and, more importantly, in meeting the demands of everyday living. How would these differences be reflected in test scores?

The solution came with the use of Deviation scores which are technically more complex but more satisfactory measures than Ratio Quotients. In essence, deviation scores such as IQs express test performance in terms of the individual's 'total correct' or raw score from the average score obtained by individuals of the same age. Figure 2.1 illustrates this. Tests are constructed so that the scores obtained by a sample are normally distributed as shown. That means that most people get scores which cluster around the average or mean, and very few people get scores which are extremely above the average or extremely below. The curve of normal distribution has certain properties, one of which is that any point on the curve can be precisely located in terms of the distance from the mean. The distance is usually expressed in terms of 'standard deviations'. As can be seen, approximately 16 per cent of the population will have scores that are at or below one standard deviation below the mean and a further 16 per cent will have scores at or above one standard deviation above the mean. Approximately 2 per cent of the

Figure 2.1: The relationship between different methods of expresssing test scores

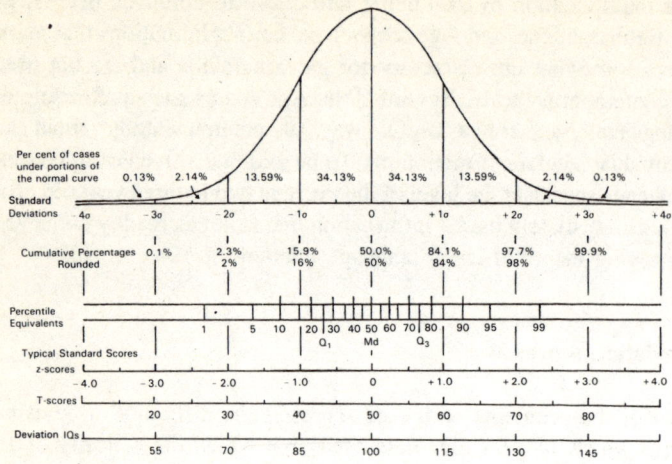

Adapted from Test Service Bulletin No. 48 of the Psychological Corporation, 1955.

population have scores at or below two standard deviations below the mean, and so on (see Figure 2.1).

There is a precise way of identifying where one person's score lies *in relation to the scores attained by the standardisation sample*. However, it is a clumsy way of giving the information. The three examples could, respectively be presented as -1 SD, $+1$ SD and -2 SD or as $-1z$, $+1z$ and $-2z$, usually say -1 standard deviation, etc. But this means that scores in between have to be expressed in clumsy fractions or decimals. The convention has arisen that the average score is given the value of 100 (stemming directly from the ratio of IQ) and the standard deviation is given the value of 15. Thus, the distribution of IQ scores is as shown in Figure 2.1. Fifty per cent of the population will have IQ scores in the range 90 to 110; 67 per cent will have IQs between 85 and 115; 95 per cent have IQs between 70 and 130.

No matter how the individual's score is expressed, note that all that is initially being said is that the test performance places the person at a particular point in relation to the scores obtained by the normative sample. To claim anything else requires a knowledge of the test measures or its validities, a topic we consider later.

In principle therefore, psychological measurement is similar to many other forms of measurement in that the number obtained from the measurement process is compared with some standard or criterion. To say for instance that someone has high blood presssure is only another way of saying that the individual's blood pressure is higher than is normally found in a large group of comparable individuals whose blood pressures have all been measured using a similar procedure under similar conditions. In practice, however, psychological measurement tends to be a somewhat more complex process as a consequence of the vagaries of people. For example, height or blood pressures do not normally change during the measurement procedures, but people learn how to solve problems more efficiently in the course of solving them: blocks of wood do not become less anxious while they are being measured whereas people do, and this can have a distorting effect on measurement. Hence, the development of psychological tests and their use in individual testing are more complex than might appear at first sight.

Precision

One of the assumptions of psychological testing is that the attribute of interest exists in quantitative form and that it has a particular magnitude. Psychological tests are then constructed to yield numbers such as 95 or 115, the numbers reflecting some correspondence with the magnitude of the attribute. However, it is important that these numbers are not invested with too much precision. For the most part, psychological measurement is crude. Whereas we can readily see the difference between a piece of wood that is 95 cm long and another that is 96 cm, psychologists would be hard put to discover any difference between two individuals, one with an IQ of 95, the other with an IQ of 96. Indeed, it would be difficult to tell the difference between individuals with IQs 95 and 105. All measurement, even in physics, entails some degree of error. In psychological testing, the degree of error is relatively large so that the numbers expressing the magnitude of the attribute may be much more or much less than the actual attribute, assuming we could even know its magnitude. In order to avoid misconstruing the precision of the numbers produced from psychological testing, it is probably more appropriate to refer to them as indices rather than measures. Other reasons for this will become apparent in the following paragraphs.

In the first instance, a test score reflects what the person was able to do at the time of testing, on the assumption that the test was scored correctly. In this sense, it is an index of the test performance. From this it follows that whatever influenced the performance could be reflected in the score. From both theory and research, it is likely that many influences affect test scores. For instance, if the person being tested was very anxious, or unwell, or tired, or misunderstood what was required, or if the test was incorrectly administered, the score would be different to the score that would have been obtained had these circumstances not prevailed.

One way of regarding test scores is to see them as made up of several components, apart from error. Thus, one part would be a function of the actual ability being tested, another would reflect the client's motivation, another understanding of what is required and so on. These and many other factors can influence performance at the time of testing and thus the test score. In the individual case, it is impossible to know just how much each is contributing, hence the caution about the precision of test scores.

Selecting tests: reliability

Decisions to use particular tests are commonly influenced by two major considerations. The first is whether the test is likely to yield reproducible results. There would be little point in using a test if the score depended on who administered it, or, if every time it was given, the testee produced widely variable results. A test that produces stable results despite reasonable variations in who administers it or when it is administered, tends to be called reliable. It is, however, increasingly recognised that tests found to be reliable in one set of circumstances may not be so under different circumstances. For instance, tests that function well when used by people trained to use them may produce variable results when used by untrained testers. Also, it is important to note that tests that are reliable do not guarantee reliable individual scores. The testee could have been very anxious at the time of testing or the tester could have made errors in calculating the score, and so on.

Selecting tests: validity

The second major consideration in the selection of a test is whether or not the results will be able to be interpreted in a way that is relevant to the purpose of testing. Whether or not it can be so interpreted is a function of what are called validity data. Validity is a general term that covers the meanings or interpretations of test scores, whether the test measures what it is supposed to measure. For instance, the question of whether or not an IQ test measures intelligence, or a reading test, reading, is established through theory and particularly research that examines the relations between test scores and other psychological variables or performance criteria. If someone was judged to be very articulate for their age and they then obtained a high score on a test of language facility, this relation would be taken as evidence in support of the test having validity as an index of language development.

It is helpful to distinguish between two types of interpretation that can be made from test data, statistical and psychological. The former is essentially a statement based on empirical relations. For instance, if as a result of carefully implemented research it is consistently found that individuals scoring 118 on test 'X' commonly succeed in obtaining a first degree at university, then one could interpret an individual's score in line with this empirical or statistical relation: i.e. a score less than 118 means, other things being equal, that the testee is unlikely to be successful in obtaining a degree. It should be noted that statistical interpretation of test scores are probabilistic rather than deterministic.

Psychological interpretation of test scores are of the type 'Test results indicate she is intelligent' or 'She is mentally retarded'. These sorts of interpretations pose special problems that can be illustrated as follows:

Statements about intelligence or mental retardation made on the basis of results from an IQ test, for instance, presuppose availability of a well-developed theory and supporting research that justify such interpretations. The problem is that there is no such generally accepted theory of intelligence nor is there a single test that is accepted by everyone as a good index of intelligence. Hence, we believe that it is best not to parade IQ tests as 'measures of intelligence' because we do not as yet have compelling grounds for doing so. While this may appear as a somewhat strange comment, the question of whether or not IQ tests measure intelligence is irrelevant in day-to-day practice. What is important is the functional significance of IQ scores of different magnitudes, for instance that individuals with low IQs most commonly show limitations in many aspects of their development. (See below for a more detailed presentation of the evidence.) It is this property of the IQ — its covariation with other aspects of development — that makes it an important index and not its status as a measure of intelligence.

In general, the utility of psychological tests derives not from their being indices of particular psychological attributes, but rather from the practical statements that they enable, the concurrent and predictive statements they allow to be made. It is the evidence of the practical utility of many tests that provides a justification for their continued use.

In summary, the scores from psychological tests should not be regarded as precise and it is probably better to regard them as indices rather than measures. Tests are selected for individual use because there is evidence that they tend to yield fairly consistent scores and that these scores can be interpreted in two ways that are of practical relevance.

NORM- AND CRITERION-REFERENCED TESTING

When the interest is in a person's abilities to perform particular tasks, two different types of questions can be asked: (1) Can he or she do the task and possibly, how well? (2) How does this performance compare with that of similar people? The former type of question assumes that there are clearly defined criteria against which the performance is judged. In assessing writing skills, one can check whether the individual is holding the pencil correctly and whether the letters are being formed in the correct way; or whether the individual can put on clothes unaided and do up the buttons. Provided the observer knows what to look for and the tasks or criteria are clearly defined, it is possible to obtain information about what the person can and cannot do in various areas of functioning. Tests for such purposes are essentially detailed guides for systematic observation. Their main purpose is to identify how close to a criterion performance an individual's present skills are. Such tests are called criterion referenced to distinguish them from tests whose main purpose is to discover how well the individual performs relative to comparable others. The latter type of test — where group data provide the norms for comparison — are called norm-referenced procedures. (For a fuller discussion of issues related to norm- and criterion-referenced testing and curriculum issues see Kiernan, Chapter 7.)

IQ AND DEVELOPMENTAL ASSESSMENT

The assessment of children below two years of age differs from that of older children. While the examiner may use some test material to see how the child responds, more commonly the tests tap a variety of spontaneous functions including reflexes, motor co-ordination, social responsiveness, early speech and language. Compared with testing older children, more emphasis is placed on discovering the infant's reactions to everyday stimuli. Passes and failures on test items are recorded and the total score is transformed into a standardised score, usually referred to as a *Development Quotient* (or DQ) to distinguish it from the IQ. A very low DQ alerts one to generally poor overall current functioning, but DQs in the normal range are not very good predictors of later IQs. It is not until the children are aged over two years that test scores show much relation to subsequent IQ scores (Madge and Tizard 1980; Vernon 1979). However, infants whose performance is very much below average on Developmental Assessment tend to remain below on subsequent tests.

The *Gesell Developmental Schedules* (Knobloch and Pasamanick 1974) and the very similar scales devised by Griffiths (1954) collate information on a wide range of behaviours — motor development, language, adaptive behaviour and personal-social behaviour. These scales provide good descriptions of current functioning. They detect severe mental handicap within the first year of life (Illingworth 1971), although the rate of misclassification remains high (Clarke and Clarke 1974).

The *Bayley Scales of Infant Development* (Bayley 1969) require the infant to interact more actively with test-like material provided by the examiner. There are two scales — the Mental Scale which tests such functions as perception, memory, problem-solving, early vocal communication, and the Motor Scale which indexes skill at sitting, standing and walking and gross and fine hand manipulation. The test is standardised on children aged two months to 30 months. The tests were intended to provide measures of current functioning rather than to predict later performance (Anastasi 1982).

Very low scores on the Bayley Scales do indicate poor current functioning and a high risk of continuing mental retardation. However, this expectation needs to be modified for infants with Down's Syndrome in the light of Carr's (1975) longitudinal study. Carr found that the prediction of later individual development was more accurate in the group of normal infants than in those with

Down's Syndrome. She points to the possibility that there is something unusual about the motor development of children with Down's Syndrome that makes it dangerous to generalise findings from studies of normal development to children with specific handicapping conditions. However, as a group, six-week-old Down's Syndrome children did score significantly lower than the normal controls, and the discriminative power of the test increased over the next few years.

What this means is that in general Down's Syndrome children are developmentally delayed, but they show large differences in the rates at which they develop. The earlier such a child is assessed, the more difficult it is to predict his or her later level of functioning. Early assessment is helpful in diagnosis and in describing current functioning; it is less helpful in making predictions.

IQ AND EDUCATIONAL ATTAINMENT

After the age of two years, IQ tests include many more verbal items. From age five onwards, IQ test scores correlate moderately highly, generally correlations of around +0.6, with scores on reading, spelling and mathematical achievement.

Academic performance depends on many other factors in addition to intelligence. In one study of a total school population (Rutter, Tizard and Whitmore 1970), it was found that there were as many children with measured IQs below 70 doing reasonably well in ordinary (mainstream) primary schools as there were children with IQs above 70 who were in a special school for slow learners. This was as it should be in a properly integrated educational system. The former children were coping with the educational demands of ordinary school, whereas the latter needed extra help. However, once one goes to IQs below 50, with rapidly increasing prevalence of physical and neurological handicaps, there is a closer relation between measured IQ and the identification of 'Special Educational Needs'.

ORDINAL SCALES

Traditional IQ tests are not very useful in leading directly to prescriptions for intervention. This is particularly true in the case of people who are severely mentally handicapped, where far too few such individuals have been studied during the standardisation of the test (Hogg and Mittler 1980). This objection has less force when considering ordinal scales of development discussed in Chapter 3 of this volume.

STABILITY AND CHANGE OF IQ SCORES

It is now widely accepted (Madge and Tizard 1980) that Developmental Quotients of children tested before expressive language is testable bear little relation to scores on later IQ tests. After the age of two, correlations begin to be higher and after the age of six years successive assessments seem more consistent. Correlational studies point to two general conclusions (Clarke and Clarke 1984): first, that measures of initial behaviour scarcely predicted later ordinal position within a group; and second, that the longer the period between assessments, the lower will be the correlation. Over a ten-year period, the correlation between two sets of IQ scores is usually around +0.5, although recent studies using the Wescher scales have produced correlations of 0.67 (Wilson 1983) and 0.86 (Yule, Gold and Busch 1982) with normal children, and of 0.92 (Tew and Laurence 1983) with a group of children with spina bifida.

High correlations tell us little about the stability of the level of individual children's IQ scores (Clarke and Clarke 1984). During childhood, IQ scores will change by 15 points or more in about one in three of the children (Vernon 1979; Madge and Tizard 1980; Hindley and Owen 1978). This applies to children with the IQs above 70.

What of the stability of scores of children with mental handicap? In general, the lower the IQ, the greater the stability though changes in IQ do occur (Madge and Tizard 1980). Goodman and Cameron (1978) obtained repeated estimates of IQ on 289 children who were retarded who were repeatedly tested after the age of 5 years. Among those children who originally scored 80 or above, the retest correlation was 0.32 for boys and 0.17 for girls; in the group scoring between 48 and 79, the retest correlation rose to 0.70; and for those scoring below 48, the retest correlation was 0.86. Similarly, Silverstein (1982) found correlations of around 0.85 on Stanford-Binet scores for 101 children classified as educable mentally retarded aged, initially, eleven years. Over all, less than 8 per cent of the sample altered their IQ scores by 10 or more points in either direction, confirming much greater stability in this group than among normal children.

GROUP TESTS

To cut down on time-consuming individual testing, group administered tests were introduced. There is a bewildering variety on the market (see Levy and Goldstein 1984; Buros 1978). Many of them may be useful as quick screening devices but many require that the child is able to read and/or manipulate a pencil. These requirements together with the need to keep children who are handicapped motivated and on task, make group tests, particularly of intelligence, unsuitable for diagnositic use with children who are mentally handicapped.

TESTING IN CLINICAL PRACTICE

In the main, clinical practice is concerned with individuals, their development and their problems. The tasks that face the clinicians in the first instance are those of identifying and describing, and then attempting to understand the problems that lead to referral. This process — clinical assessment — may involve the use of tests of the types described so far if it is thought they will yield useful information. Most commonly, clinicians gather their information via interviews and observation; they resort to tests for specific purposes, such as the provision of standard information on abilities. If it is suspected that a child is not developing appropriately, or that he or she is misbehaving because schoolwork is too hard or too easy, or that there may be an imbalance in abilities (e.g. language skill well below other skills), a standard test may be given. On occasion too, a test will be given because the clinician is devoid of ideas. This is a rare occurrence, it being more common for tests to be given to check on hypotheses arrived at on the basis of observation and interview, even though some clinicians may not appreciate that this is what they are doing!

In our view then, testing is one of several elements in the clinical process. The skill of the clinician in relation to test use consists of the ability to select appropriate tests, to interpret the resulting scores and to incorporate the information in a way that is relevant to assessment and treatment.

Although this chapter is not intended as a detailed guide to test use and interpretation there are several aspects of tests and testing that merit attention.

ADEQUACY OF TEST DATA

Being tested on psychological tests is not a neutral event. Individuals vary in their reactions and these reactions can influence test performance. For some, being tested is a noxious experience that can lead to scores that under-represent what the individual is capable of doing; for others the challenge of testing motivates performance to a degree that the individual does not normally manifest. Further, there are transient influences, such as illness, that can distort performance and hence the interpretations based on scores obtained during such times. Because of these or other intrusive influences, the tester has in the first instance to make a conscious decision about the adequacy of the test data: if for any reason it is felt that these unduly misrepresent what the testee might otherwise do, it is probably best to discard the data and start again.

TEST SPECIFICITY

A given psychological attribute or skill can be indexed in a variety of ways. For instance, reading accuracy, correctly deciphering the phonetic pattern of a word, can be tested using a disconnected set of words, prose passages, matching words to pictures and so on. Or, information about development can be obtained from a test, from interviewing someone who knows the child or from observing the child in a number of naturalistic settings. When two or more indices of the same attribute or skill are obtained, it is commonly found that the extent of agreement between them is limited. Thus, someone whose scores on a physical activity questionnaire indicate that they are very active may only be found to be moderately active on indices based on direct observations. This tendency of psychological test indices to show limited agreement is referred to as test specificity.

The implications of test specificity for clinical practice are quite important, the major consequence being that conclusions about things psychological should be based on at least two independent sources of information that are mutually supportive. It is good practice for test scores to be discussed with parents or others who are familiar with the individual to make sure that the conclusions make sense. The reasons for any disagreements should be investigated and no difference likely to be of importance should be left unremarked or if possible unresolved.

Another way of emphasising the importance of specificity is to point out that no single index is by itself sufficient, despite the tendency to argue for the greater objectivity of standardised tests or the acumen of the clinician or the special knowledge of parents or other caretakers. Each contributes something special, but none is so special as to be able to stand alone. For instance, although parents have good opportunities to observe their child, their skills as specialist observers are likely to be limited. They may therefore not see and hence not report on aspects of behaviour that the clinician regards as crucial. Similarly, tests can only sample a limited range of behaviours and tend to do so in specific ways. A person with a partial hearing loss may perform badly on a test that requires responses to spoken questions but not on a test with written instructions.

SIMILARITIES AND DIFFERENCES

Test score interpretation is based essentially on the identification of similarities and differences between the score of the individual and score patterns found in particular groups. Low ability for instance means that the score of the testee was *different*, i.e. below that of the average score of comparable individuals in the normative group.

We have already indicated that because of errors in measurement, score differences of a few points in the IQs of two people are likely to be psychologically irrelevant. For similar reasons, the score of an individual should not be invested with precision despite the seeming precision with which it is expressed: someone with a score of 87 when first tested could when retested get a score quite a few points above or below the original. This range is sometimes presented in test reports in the following way: 87 ± 9 where the '9' is the standard error of measurement and the '$\pm$' indicates that the direction of the error could be above or below the original score. It is not uncommon for the standard error to be misunderstood and misinterpreted (see Dudek 1979 for details). For present purposes it is sufficient to note the presence of error in all scores. This poses a further problem when comparing two scores because any difference between them could be a consequence of the errors in each and not because there is a real difference in the skills that gave rise to the score difference. This means that one has to be cautious in interpreting differences between two scores obtained by the same child. Let us take a common example. The WISC-R yields estimates of Verbal IQ and Performance IQ. We have noted that all test scores have an error component and that the shorter the test, the greater the error associated with a score. It should therefore come as no surprise that whereas the Standard Error for Full Scale at IQ at age ten and a half is 3.21, the standard errors for Verbal and Performance scales are respectively higher at 3.65 and 4.65.

By now, the reader will accept that it would not be appropriate to say that a Verbal IQ of 63 was really lower than a Performance IQ of 65. So how large must a (V-P) difference be before it is regarded as reflecting a real difference in cognitive function? Put another way, how large must the differences be to be regarded as *reliable?* As Sattler (1982) shows, a difference of 12 points is needed before it can be confidently accepted as not being due to random fluctuations, i.e. with less than a one in twenty chance, or $P < 0.05$.

However, differences of 12 points are very common. They are found in between 25 and 50 per cent of ten year olds. A difference of 29 points in the direction V lower than P is found in less than 3 per cent of the standardisation sample of ten year olds. Such a large difference could fairly be described as *statistically abnormal*.

Thus, a difference of one or 2 IQ points between Verbal and Performance IQs is so trivial as to be ignored; a difference of at least 12 points would indicate that the child was characteristically better at one type of activity than the other, but this would be a fairly common pattern, a difference of 29 points is found in less than 5 per cent of the population so it may indicate something unusual.

But what does it mean in psychological terms? It is often claimed that if a child has a Performance IQ significantly lower than his Verbal IQ that this indicates 'brain damage'. Putting aside the very real objection to using tests to diagnose 'brain damage' as if it were a global entity (Herbert 1964), let us examine evidence from the Isle of Wight population study that is relevant to this question (Rutter, Graham and Yule 1970). Out of 84 children with identifiable brain disorder, 13 children (15 per cent) were found to have their Verbal IQs significantly higher than their Performance IQs, by at least 25 points. This happened in only 7.5 per cent of a control group and this difference between the groups was itself statistically significant, thereby lending some credibility to the hypothesised link between

Table 2.1: Relation between abnormal (V-P) discrepancy and brain disorder

	Normal	Brain disorder	
No discrepancy	10,981	71	11,052
Abnormal (V-P) discrepancy	800 (7.5%)	13 (15%)	813
	11,781	84	11,865

Source: Rutter, Graham and Yule (1970).

Verbal-Performance discrepancies and brain disorder. There is, however, a flaw. *All* the children with brain disorder were tested, but only a sample of the remainder of the population was tested to act as a control group. Brain disorder is very rare; the total population amounted to 11,865 children. Thus, the true relation between abnormal V-P discrepancies and brain disorder can be seen in Table 2.1.

From this it can be seen that whereas *proportionally* twice as many children with identifiable brain disorder as controls have an abnormal (V-P) discrepancy, nonetheless for every one child with brain disorder who has such a discrepancy, there are about 61 with an equally large discrepancy who are perfectly normal. In passing, it should also be noted that only a minority of children with brain disorder share this famous V-P discrepancy, showing how useless it is, on its own, as a diagnostic index.

'DETERIORATION'

A commonly posed clinical problem with people who are mentally handicapped is whether their cognitive functioning has deteriorated. This question usually arises when a retest score turns out to be below an initial score, and is another form of difference score. Like many apparently simple questions, answering requires sophisticated knowledge of test construction and psychometrics.

Let us say that a boy obtained a Full Scale WISC-R IQ of 65 at age nine and a Full Scale IQ of 53 two years later. His 'IQ' has dropped by 12 points over this short period. Does this indicate some deterioration in his cognitive ability? Does it indicate some degenerative neurological condition? Before jumping to conclusions, frightening the parents or demanding expensive EEGs or CT scans, consider what questions need to be asked.

IQs can fluctuate dramatically so the first question is: Is this a *real* change in score? Put more formally, how often is such a change of scores observed in the normal population? The assumption is that if the change is seen in at least 5 to 10 per cent of the sample, it is unlikely that anything other than random variation is at work. Note that this is a probabilistic statement and it is possible for a loss of function both to be within normal limits and to be 'caused' by a neurological disorder. Such are the uncertainties operating in the real world.

Other factors have been taken into account. Scores which start below (or above) average will normally regress towards the mean on retesting. The same random errors are unlikely to operate the second time and the score appears to rise, although in practice this happens less often than the theory predicts (Silverstein 1982). Moreover, on retesting on the same test, practice effects occur and increases of 4 Verbal and 9 Performance points can be expected on the WISC-R (Kaufman 1979). Thus, on the grounds of regression and practice, very low scores should increase, making a *12*-point drop even more notable.

One has to know what goes on in making the IQ scores before one can really see what is happening. With these low IQ scores, a nine-year-old child is being tested on very few items. On some sub-tests, even when the child makes no score at all, the raw score of zero is transformed into a scaled score, i.e. age-corrected score, of 1 or 2. The resulting 'IQ' scarcely reflects the child's performance alone, but also the test's normative inadequacies. It is possible, as we have demonstrated elsewhere (Berger and Yule 1985) for a child to pass more items on a sub-test but because other children of the same age make even more gains, the tested child will appear to perform even worse as reflected in standardised scores. An examination of the raw scores is needed to investigate the question of deteriorating performances. In the example cited, on most sub-tests, the boy's raw scores remained static or increased. In no case did he lose any raw scores. Thus his previous skills remained intact — he just had not increased them at as fast a rate as normal. The IQ score was lower, but this did not reflect deterioration in the sense of loss of skills.

A similar effect can be seen in longitudinal studies of the cognitive development of individuals who are mentally handicapped. For example, in both Carr's (1975) and Cunningham and Mittler's (1981) longitudinal studies of infants with Down's Syndrome, radically different conclusions can be reached depending on whether

IQ or MA is used as the dependent variable. Where IQ is plotted, it appears that children with Down's Syndrome 'deteriorate' on this test performance. When MA is plotted, it is immediately apparent that the children are continuing to develop, but at a much slower rate than their normal peers. However, the psychological impact of the scores on parents and teachers is quite different.

'PROFILE ANALYSIS'

A particularly problematical approach to the differences between scores is 'profile analysis' in which the *pattern* of scores on a battery of tests is interpreted. Profile analysis is another manifestation of difference scores and takes various forms. One example is when a sub-test score such as Block Design on the WISC-R is below the other scores obtained by the individual. Such a low score might be interpreted as reflecting a spatial deficit in the person. Another example is where the pattern of sub-test scores is said to be similar to that of a particular clinical diagnostic group. Profile analysis is closely associated in practice with *diagnostic-prescriptive* remediation. In theory, the pattern of cognitive strengths and weaknesses should be reflected in the pattern of scores; and, in turn, knowledge of the cognitive pattern should guide the therapist to the appropriate intervention strategy.

As noted elsewhere (Berger and Yule 1972; Kaufman 1979; Sattler 1982), most sub-tests in a battery contain only a few items and are thus less reliable than tests with more than one item. Caution is necessary in interpreting scores on sub-tests and differences between sub-test scores have to be correspondingly large before any 'real' differences can be inferred. Further, without information on the temporal stability of a difference, the clinical significance of the findings may be highly questionable.

To date, the diagnostic-prescriptive approach has not proven of much practical value even in such an extensively researched area as that of reading difficulties (Bateman 1969; Hammill and Wiederholt 1973). This approach must be carefully distinguished from one which adapts a criterion-referenced approach to assessment. For example the use of the Portage materials (Shearer and Loftin 1984) pinpoints the skills and skill-deficits of individual children. Specific programmes are geared to improving each skill, working within a developmental-learning framework.

SOME COMMONLY USED IQ TESTS

Having mentioned the Gessel and Griffiths scales earlier, this section provides brief descriptions of some of the commonly used individual tests with children who are handicapped. More detailed descriptions and evaluative comments are contained elsewhere (Buros 1978; Anastasi 1982; Levy and Goldstein 1984).

The Wechsler Pre-school and Primary Scale of Intelligence (WPPSI)

The WPPSI (Wechsler 1967) follows a similar format to the other Wechsler scales for older children (WISC-R) and adults (WAIS-R) in that it consists of five short sub-scales which predominantly measure language development and functioning, and five sub-scales which provide an estimate of visual-spatial or performance skills. The scale yields estimates of Verbal IQ, Performance IQ and Full Scale IQ, expressed in terms of a mean of 100 and a standard deviation of 15.

The WPPSI covers the age range 4 to 6½ years. The sub-scales are:

VERBAL SCALE
1. Information — questions testing general knowledge.
3. Vocabulary — word definitions.
5. Arithmetic — simple counting and mental arithmetic items.
7. Similarities — children have to say in which way two words are alike.
9. Comprehension — questions on daily living.

PERFORMANCE SCALE
2. Animal House — place the correct coloured peg next to each animal picture.
4. Picture Completion — spot the missing part of the picture.
6. Mazes — draw a line through a maze without getting stuck.
8. Geometric Design — copy simple line drawing.
10. Block Design — copy patterns made from blocks.

All ten scales should be given and this takes 50 to 75 minutes to complete. When fewer scales are given, the score can be multiplied up, i.e. prorated, to give a rough idea of how the child is performing, but short form tests are less reliable and not to be recommended when important diagnostic or placement decisions are being made.

Each sub-test follows a similar path. That is, the child is given very easy items to start with. The items get progressively harder until a pre-determined number in a row are failed. The tester then moves on to the next sub-test in the WPPSI, verbal and performance items are alternated to keep up the child's interest.

The WPPSI was standardised on 1,200 American children. Some of the items have been reworded for use in Britain and studies in Britain find that it is generally a good test, with British children scoring marginally higher than their American counterparts (Yule, Berger, Butler, Tizard and Newnham 1969).

Overall, the test is quite 'reliable'. The test correlates well with other IQ tests and predicts later IQ and educational attainment quite well (Yule, Gold and Busch 1982).

The Wechsler Intelligence Scale for Children (revised) (WISC-R)

The WISC-R (Wechsler 1974) covers the age range 6 years 0 months to 16 years 11 months. The ten sub-scales are:

VERBAL SCALE
1. Information
3. Similarities
5. Arithmetic
7. Vocabulary
9. Comprehension

PERFORMANCE SCALE
2. Picture Completion
4. Picture Arrangement — set of pictures have to be rearranged to tell a story.
6. Block Design
8. Object Assembly — jigsaws have to be put together.
10. Coding — symbols have to be written against the correct shape or number.

Again, all the sub-scales should be administered in about 45 to 75 minutes. Points are scored in the performance items both for getting things right and for doing them within time limits. Children who are careful but very slow are thereby penalised.

The WISC-R was standardised on 2,200 American children. A British version is available and it is probably the most widely used of all IQ tests at present. It predicts academic success very well.

However, at the youngest ages it is quite difficult so that when assessing children of 6 to 16 years who may be mentally handicapped, it is better to use the WPPSI than the WISC-R.

The Wechsler Adult Intelligence Scale (Revised) (WAIS-R)

The WAIS-R (Wechsler 1981) covers the age range 16 to 74 years. It was standardised on 1,880 individuals. It has six Verbal sub-tests (the same five as in WISC-R) plus Digit Span which tests ability to recite strings of numbers forwards and backwards and five Performance scales.

In general, the Wechsler scales are very useful with people of normal range abilities. They can identify those who are moderately or severely mentally handicapped, but they do not discriminate within the group of individuals who are severely mentally handicapped. The Performance scales all require the testee to manipulate material so that people with physical handicaps may be at a disadvantage.

The Stanford-Binet Intelligence Scale

This grew out of the original Binet-Simon sub-scales. Different versions were developed and standardised on American samples in 1916 and 1937. Unfortunately the 1960 and 1972 versions were not properly standardised and are not recommended (Kaufman and Reynolds 1983).

The Stanford-Binet covers the age range two years to adulthood. Individuals are tested on a range of items according to how well they do. The test takes 30 to 40 minutes with young children and up to 90 minutes with adults. Although there are some performances items on the test, studies have found that it is very largely a measure of verbal intelligence. This makes it very difficult to interpret when testing children with mental handicap. Children with specific language delays and disorders will score poorly on the test, but may have normal nonverbal intelligence which is not reflected in their scores. Such misdiagnosis can have serious effects.

McCarthy Scales of children's abilities

The McCarthy (1972) Scales cover the age range $2\frac{1}{2}$ to $8\frac{1}{2}$ years. There are 18 tests which supposedly contribute to six sub-scales — Verbal, Perceptual Performance, Quantitative, General Cognitive, Memory and Motor. The General Cognitive Index is presented as a measure of general abilities. The test was standardised on 1,032 children in America but there are few studies of its validities. Indeed, recent studies in Britain (Lynch, Mitchell, Vincent, Truman and Macdonald 1982; Tierney, Smith, Axworthy and Ratcliffe 1984; Truman, Lynch and Braithwaite 1984) found that the sub-scale did not work in the way expected and that only the General Cognitive Index could be interpreted.

British Picture Vocabulary Test (BPVT)

This is a recently standardised version (Dunn, Dunn and Whetton 1982) of the older Peabody Picture Vocabulary Test. The child is shown a card with four line drawings on it and is asked to point to one specified picture. Children can point or indicate by eye movements if physically disabled. The test covers the age range 3 to 18 years 11 months, and the British version was standardised on 3,334 children. The scores can be presented as language ages or as standard (IQ) scores.

The BVPT is essentially a test of language comprehension. It is useful as a quick screening test or as a rough measure when children refuse to co-operate with more complex testing. However, it has been argued (Mittler 1972; Wheldall and Jeffree 1974) that it can *over*estimate the ability of some children with mental handicap who have been coached in pointing to objects in story books.

The British Ability Scales

The British Ability Scales (Elliot, Murray and Pearson 1983) appeared after many years of development only to be substantially revised almost immediately. The scales are intended to provide measures of separate psychological processes and academic attainment and there are 23 different scales in all. Various combinations of scales are recommended for different age levels and different assessment purposes, and it is possible to obtain an overall index of

IQ. The scales cover the age range 2 years 6 months to 17 years 6 months.

The tests are broadly grouped into measures of Speed, Reasoning, Spatial Imagery, Perceptual Matching, Short-Term Memory and Retrieval and Application of Knowledge. In addition to familiar test items such as vocabulary, block design and digit span, other scales are included to reflect Piagetian views of development.

Three thousand four hundred and thirty-five children were used to standardise the scales. Scores on individual scales are given as T-scores (Mean of 50, Standard Deviation of 10) and T-scores can be converted into conventional IQ scores. Most sub-scales are reported to have satisfactory reliability. The scale, overall, seems to measure one general factor and two sub-factors — visual and verbal IQ.

The development of the scales was an ambitious project. The need to revise many of them even before the original manuals were fully available does not inspire confidence in their construction. Reviewers have been cautious in their welcome (Blinkhorn 1984). Very few studies have so far been published using them, and these few have found the norms to be inappropriate for the samples investigated (Cockburn and Oundstead 1983). There are no published studies of their use with children who are mentally handicapped.

The Merrill-Palmer Scale

This is a very old, predominantly nonverbal scale (Stutsman 1931) which is still found of value in testing young children who are handicapped. It is suitable for testing in the one to six year range and as items are scored at a variety of age levels, performance on three to four tests can yield a rough guide to mental age level. For example, the Seguin Form Board is given three times to the child. Scores span the age range from 30 to 71 months giving an indication of MA.

Although at earlier ages there are a few verbal items, the bulk of the items are nonverbal. The test can be scored to take account of the child's refusal to do some items or the lack of time to administer them. This is a feature vital in testing children who are mentally handicapped and a feature sadly missing from most later standardised instruments.

The test is useful in *ruling out* overall low functioning, although one has to be careful not to be overoptimistic in prognostications based on a nonverbal IQ.

TESTS OF LANGUAGE DEVELOPMENT

One of the main problems posed by people who are severely mentally handicapped is their slow language development. While there is controversy as to whether the language is delayed or deviant (Rondal 1985), advances in recent years in the field of developmental psycholinguistics have brought greater precision to describing and measuring language development. It is now considered necessary not only to distinguish speech from language, comprehension of language from expression of language, but also to differentiate syntax, semantics and pragmatics (Bishop and Rosenbloom 1985). Unfortunately, test development has not kept pace with these advances. The following instruments and tests can each help index different aspects of the total processes we call language:

The Reynell Scales of language development

Probably the most useful tests for indexing the level of children's language development are those developed by Reynell (1977). The scales are in two forms for children who are nonhandicapped and those who are severely physically handicapped. They cover the age range one month to six years, and provide separate measures of Comprehension of Lanaguage and Expressive Language.

The tester uses small toys and dolls to elicit responses from the child. In testing comprehension, the child need only point to objects if they are nonhandicapped; children who are physically handicapped are tested in such a way that they can indicate responses with eye movements. Verbal expression is recorded verbatim and scored according to detailed protocols.

The Illinois Test of Psycholinguistic Abilities (ITPA)

The ITPA (Kirk, McCarthy and Kirk 1968) was developed to reflect Osgood's theoretical model of language processes — a model that now seems sadly dated in the light of recent developments. The test still finds favour in some quarters and so it is important to know that studies of its use will find little empirical support for the view that the sub-scales are measuring separate language functions (e.g. Mittler and Ward 1970). At best, one can place some reliance on the overall index of language ability but it is a cumbersome way to arrive at a simple measure of language level.

Language Assessment, Remediation and Screening Procedure (LARSP)

LARSP was developed by Crystal, Fletcher and Garman (1976) to describe the linguistic competencies of language-delayed children. Transcripts of samples of the child's speech are subjected to detailed analysis of their structure and so this is more properly a criterion-referenced procedure, although approximate levels of language development are produced. It is mentioned here as it is currently gaining favour with speech therapists and linguists in Britain. It is one of a number of such procedures which, unfortunately, tend to produce different estimates of children's level of difficulty (Klee and Paul 1981).

TESTS OF ACADEMIC ATTAINMENT

A number of Graded Word Reading Tests such as the Burt and Schonell tests are still widely used in Britain. Printed words are presented in increasing order of difficulty and the child or adult has to pronounce them aloud. The major problem with these tests is that they measure only one aspect of reading — the ability to sound out words, or Accuracy of Reading. The results tell nothing about Comprehension of Reading — whether the child *understands* what has been read. While Accuracy and Comprehension relate highly in normal groups, it is not uncommon to find children who are handicapped, especially those who are autistic, who have good accuracy but very poor comprehension. They truly are just 'barking at print'. For these reasons, it is best to test both aspects of reading.

The *Neale Analysis of Reading Ability* (Neale 1958) consists of three parallel forms, each containing six short passages. The child is asked to look at a picture, then to read a story out aloud and finally to answer factual questions about each story. Three measures of reading are obtained — Rate (speed) of reading, Accuracy and Comprehension. The latter two are stable indices. The test is suitable for reading ages 6 years 0 months to 11 years 0 months.

There are other experimental and criterion-referenced tests of reading skills which are too numerous to mention here.

Of the other test of scholastic attainment, it is worth mentioning the Vernon Graded Word Spelling Test (Vernon 1977) and the Vernon Graded Arithmetic Mathematics Test (Vernon and Miller 1976) as both have been recently standardised. It should be emphasised that one cannot assume in a handicapped group that reading and spelling go hand in hand. It is always worth testing both separately. In this age of augmented communications systems using microprocessors, it is increasingly important to consider the spelling ability of people who are mute and handicapped.

Similarly, where one is interested in a person's computational skills, it is not sufficient to rely on brief testing as undertaken on a sub-test of the Wechsler scales. More reliable and detailed measurement is usually necessary.

THE VALUE OF NORM-REFERENCED TESTS

Norm-referenced tests were originally developed to identify children who are mentally handicapped who are not benefiting from ordinary schooling *so that they would receive appropriate special help.* IQ tests still have an important part to play in contributing to the diagnosis of mental handicap in particular, the distribution between mild (50 to 70) and severe (below 50) mental handicap has important diagnostic and prognostic implications (Madge and Tizard 1980; Clarke, Clarke and Berg 1985). However, a diagnosis of mental handicap should never be made on the basis of an IQ score alone. Other information on social adjustment and developmental history must also be gathered and given due consideration.

Even so, the need for standardised, normative assessment remains. It is still common, in one's clinical experience to find socially outgoing children being overestimated with respect to their general abilities. This was recently shown with respect to children with infantile hypercalcaemia who are socially disinhibited, have good expressive language but poor understanding of language (Arnold, Yule and Martin 1985). In the opposite direction, it is not uncommon to find children with specific language disorders being labelled as globally mentally handicapped when they have been assessed on an inappropriate test like the Stanford-Binet.

However, as noted earlier, IQ and many other norm-referenced tests are of less value in differentiating within a group of mentally handicapped children or making predictions about their progress. In part, this is because the tests were not designed to do this and so were not standardised on many such individuals; in part, they are poor predictors because of the restricted range of scores necessarily obtained (see Berger and Yule 1985 for a fuller discussion).

There is no doubt that IQ tests have been misused, misinterpreted and abused and that they will continue to be used in the hands of some in the future. But this should not divert us from employing them if such use can be justified with regard to the clinical and other needs of people who are handicapped and on the basis of adequate empirical evidence:

> ... the intelligence test is one of major achievements of psychology. It is objective, reliable and valid. Although it is not perfect, can be misused, and does not provide a real definition of intelligence, it is the best working definition that we have of intelligence regarded as a trait.
>
> Betty House (1977, p. 537)

REFERENCES

Anastasi, A. (1982) *Psychological Testing,* 5th edn, Macmillan, New York

Arnold, R., Yule W. and Martin, N. (1985) 'The Psychological Characteristics of Infantile Hypercalcaemia: A Preliminary Study', *Developmental Medicine and Child Neurology, 27,* 49–59

Bateman, B. (1969) 'Reading, A Controversial View: Research and Rationale' in L. Tarnopol (ed.), *Learning Disabilities: Introduction to Educational and Medical Management,* C.C. Thomas, Springfield, Ill.

Bayley, N. (1969) *Bayley Scales of Infant Development: Birth to Two Years,* Psychological Corporation, New York

Berger, M. (1985) 'Psychological Assessment and Testing' in M. Rutter and L. Hersov (eds.), *Child and Adolescent Psychiatry: Modern Approaches,* 2nd edn, Blackwell, Oxford

Berger, M. and Yule, W. (1972) 'Cognitive Assessment in Young Children with Language Delay' in M. Rutter and J.A.M. Martin (eds.), *The Child with Delayed Speech,* Heinemann Medical, London

Berger, M. and Yule, W. (1985) 'IQ Tests and the Assessment of Mental Handicap' in A.D.B. Clarke, A.M. Clarke and J.M. Berg (eds.), *Mental Deficiency: The Changing Outlook,* 4th edn, Methuen, London and New York

Bishop, D.V.M. and Rosenbloom, L. (1985) 'Childhood Language Disorders: Classification and Overview' in W. Yule, M. Rutter and M. Bax (eds.), *Language Development and Disorder,* Spastics International Publications, London

Blinkhorn, S. (1984) 'Review of British Ability Scales' in P. Levy and H. Goldstein (eds.), *Tests in Education: A Book of Critical Reviews,* Academic Press, London and New York

Buros, D. (1978) *The Eighth Mental Measurement Yearbook,* Gryphon

Press, New York
Carr, J. (1975) *Young Children with Down's Syndrome*, Butterworths, London
Clarke, A.D.B. and Clarke, A.M. (1974) 'The Changing Concept of Intelligence: A Selective Historical Review' in A.D.B. Clarke and A.M. Clarke (eds.), *Mental Deficiency: The Changing Outlook* 3rd edn, Methuen, London and New York
Clarke, A.D.B. and Clarke, A.M. (1984) 'Consistency and Change in the Growth of Human Characteristics', *Journal of Child Psychology and Psychiatry, 25*, 191–210
Clarke, A.D.B., Clarke, A.M. and Berg, J.M. (eds.) (1985) *Mental Deficiency: The changing outlook*, 4th edn, Methuen, London and New York
Cockburn, J. and Ounstead, M. (1983) 'The British Ability Scales: Some Differences Between Scores for Oxfordshire Children and the Standardisation Sample', *Bulletin of the British Psychological Society, 36*, 83–4
Crystal, D., Fletcher, P. and Garman, M. (1976) *The Grammatical Analysis of Language Disability: A Procedure for Assessment and Remediation*, Edward Arnold, London and Baltimore
Cunningham, C.C. and Mittler, P. (1981) 'Maturation, Development and Mental Handicap', in K. Connolly and H.V. Prechtl (eds.), *Maturation and Development: Biological and Psychological Properties*, Heinemann Medical, London
Dudek, F.J. (1979) 'The Continuing Misinterpretation of the Standard Error of Measurement', *Psychological Bulletin, 86*, 335–7
Dunn, L.M., Dunn, L.M. and Whetton, C. (1982) *British Picture Vocabulary Scales*, NFER-Nelson, Windsor
Elliot, C., Murray, D.J. and Pearson, L.S. (1983) *The British Ability Scales (New Edition)*, NFER-Nelson, Windsor
Goodman, J.F. and Cameron, J. (1978) 'The Measuring of IQ Constancy in Young Retarded Children', *Journal of Genetic Psychology, 132*, 109–19
Griffiths, R. (1954) *The Abilities of Babies*, University of London Press, London
Hammill, D.A. and Wiederholt, J.L. (1973) 'Reviews of the Frostig Visual Perception Test and the Related Training Program' in L. Mann and D. Sabrotino (eds.), *The First Review of Special Education*, Buttonwood Farms, Philadelphia
Herbert, M. (1964) 'The Concept and Testing of Brain Damage in Children: A Review', *Journal of Child Psychology and Psychiatry, 5*, 197–216
Hindley, C.B. and Owen, C.F. (1978) 'The Extent of Individual Changes in IQ for Ages Between 6 Months and 17 Years, in a British Longitudinal Sample', *Journal of Child Psychology and Psychiatry, 19*, 329–50
Hogg, J. and Mittler, P.J. (1980) 'Recent Research in Mental Handicap: Issues and Perspectives' in J. Hogg and P.J. Mittler (eds.), *Advances in Mental Handicap Research (Vol. 1)*, Wiley, New York and Chichester
House, B.J. (1977) 'Scientific Explanation and Ecological Validity: A Reply to Brooks and Baumeister', *American Journal of Mental Deficiency, 81*, 534–42
Illingworth, R.S. (1971) 'The Predictive Value of Developmental Assessment in Infancy', *Developmental Medicine and Child Neurology, 13*, 721–5

Kaufman, A.S. (1979) *Intelligent Testing with the WISC-R,* Wiley, New York

Kaufman, A.S. and Reynolds, C.R. (1983) 'Clinical Evaluation of Intellectual Functioning' in I.B. Weiner (ed.), *Clinical Methods in Psychology,* Wiley, New York

Kirk, S.A., McCarthy, J.J. and Kirk, W. (1968) *The Illinois Test of Psycholinguistic Abilities,* revised edn, University of Illinois, Urbana, Ill.

Klee, T.M. and Paul, R. (1981) 'A Comparison of Six Structural Analysis Procedures' in J.F. Miller (ed.), *Assessing Language Production in Children,* University Park Press, Baltimore, Md.

Knobloch, H. and Pasamanick, B. (1974) *Gesell and Amatruda's Developmental Diagnosis: The Evaluation and Management of Normal and Abnormal Neuropsychologic Development in Infancy and Early Childhood,* 3rd edn, Harper & Row, Hagerstown, Md.

Levy, P. and Goldstein, H. (1984) *Tests in Education: A Book of Critical Reviews,* Academic Press, London and New York

Lynch, A., Mitchell, L.B., Vincent, E.M., Truman, M. and Macdonald, L. (1982) 'The McCarthy Scales of Children's Abilities: A Normative Study on English Four-year-olds', *British Journal of Educational Psychology, 52,* 133–43

McCarthy, D.A. (1972) *Manual for the McCarthy Scales of Children's Abilities,* Psychological Corporation, New York

Madge, N. and Tizard, J. (1980) 'Intelligence' in M. Rutter (ed.), *Scientific Foundations of Developmental Psychiatry,* Heinnemann Medical, London

Mittler, P. (1972) 'Psychological Assessment of Language Abilities' in M. Rutter and J.A.M. Martin (eds.), *The Child with Delayed Speech,* SIMP/Heinemann Medical, London

Mittler, P. and Ward, J. (1970) 'The Use of the Illinois Test of Psycholinguistic Abilities with English Four-year-old Children: A Normative and Factorial Study', *British Journal of Educational Psychology, 40,* 43–54

Neale, M.D. (1958) *The Neale Analysis of Reading Ability,* Macmillan, London

Reynell, J. (1977) *Reynell Developmental Language Scales (Revised),* NFER, Windsor

Rondal, J.A. (1985) 'Language Development and Mental Retardation' in W. Yule, M. Rutter and M. Bax (eds.), *Language Development and Disorders,* Spastics International Publications, London

Rutter, M., Graham, P. and Yule, W. (1970) *A Neuropsychiatric Study in Childhood,* Heinemann Medical, London

Rutter, M., Tizard, J. and Whitmore, K. (eds.) (1970) *Education, Health and Behaviour,* Longmans, London

Sattler, J.M. (1982) *Assessment of Children's Intelligence and Special Abilities,* 2nd edn, Allyn and Bacon, Boston

Shearer, D.E. and Loftin, C.R. (1984) 'The Portage Project: Teaching Parents to Teach their Pre-school Children in the Home' in R.F. Dangel and R.A. Polster (eds.), *Parent Training: Foundations of Research and Practice,* Guilford Press, New York

Silverstein, A.B. (1982) 'Note on the Constancy of the IQ', *American Journal of Mental Deficiency, 87,* 227–8

Stutsman, R. (1931) *Guide for Administering the Merrill-Palmer Scales of Mental Tests,* Stoelting Co., Chicago, Ill.

Tew, B.J. and Laurence, K.M. (1983) 'The Relationship between Spina Bifida Children's Intelligence Testscores on School Entry and at School Leaving: A Preliminary Report', *Child: Care, Health and Development, 9,* 13–17

Tierney, I., Smith, L., Axworthy, D. and Ratcliffe, S.G. (1984) 'The McCarthy Scales of Children's Abilities — Sex and Handedness Effects in 128 Scottish Five-year-olds', *British Journal of Educational Psychology, 54,* 101–5

Truman, M., Lynch, A. and Branthwaite, A. (1984) 'A Factor Analytic Study of the McCarthy Scales of Children's Abilities', *British Journal of Educational Psychology, 54,* 331–5

Vernon, P.E. (1977) *Vernon Graded Word Spelling Test,* Hodder and Stoughton, London

Vernon, P.E. (1979) *Intelligence, Heredity and Environment,* W.H. Freeman, San Francisco

Vernon, P.E. and Miller, K.M. (1976) *Vernon Graded Arithmetic Mathematics Test,* Hodder and Stoughton, London

Wechsler, D. (1967) *The Wechsler Pre-School Primary Scales of Intelligence,* Psychological Corporation, New York

Wechsler, D. (1974) *The Wechsler Intelligence Scale for Children — Revised.* Psychological Corporation, New York

Weschler, D. (1981) *The Wechsler Adult Intelligence Scale — Revised,* Psychological Corporation, New York

Wheldall, K. and Jeffree, D. (1974) 'Criticisms Regarding the Use of the EPVT in Subnormality Research', *British Journal of Disorders of Communication, 9,* 140–3

Wilson, R.S. (1983) 'The Louisville Twin Study: Developmental Synchronies in Behavior', *Child Development, 54,* 298–316

Yule, W., Berger, M., Butler, S., Tizard, J. and Newnham, V. (1969) 'The WPPSI: An Empirical Evaluation with a British Sample', *British Journal of Educational Psychology, 39,* 1

Yule, W., Gold, R.D. and Busch, C. (1982) 'Long-term Prediction Validity of the WPPSI: An 11 Year Follow-up Study', *Personality and Individual Differences, 3,* 65–71

3

Early Development and Piagetian Tests

J. Hogg

GENERAL CHARACTERISTICS OF APPROACH

Historical and theoretical background

The past 15 years has seen a marked growth in the application of tests of early cognitive development to children who are moderately, severely and profoundly mentally handicapped, and to adults who are profoundly mentally handicapped. A number of related influences account for this trend and for the growing enthusiasm among professionals for this form of assessment. While radical behaviourism has continued to determine much of the mainstream of intervention approaches in the UK and the USA, there has been a persistent unwillingness to accept the theoretical assumption of behaviourism that we should not interest ourselves in unobservable cognitive processes. This was first clearly stated in the literature on mental handicap by Bricker (1970) who argued coherently that the use of behavioural techniques should be informed by our growing knowledge of developmental psycholinguistics and of cognitive development. In the wider field of developmental psychology, a number of workers were evolving assessment procedures to assess cognitive change as an aid to research into the processes underlying such development. The availability of these assessment instruments provided the natural vehicle for realising Bricker's proposed link between theory and technique and has led to a considerable body of work on both the development of people with mental handicap and their cognitive assessment with a view to devising appropriate intervention procedures.

Most of these instruments derive ultimately from the writings of the Swiss genetic epistemologist, Jean Piaget. With respect to the field of mental handicap, this origin is quite appropriate as there has been a tradition of work that has tried to understand the nature of cognitive delays and deficits in this population within a Piagetian framework. Though a controversial theory, there is agreement among widely differing groups of professionals on the heuristic value of Piaget's theory and at the very least it is in this spirit that we can employ assessment devices derived from this position.

A detailed account of Piagetian theory and its relation to the development of children with mental handicap is beyond the scope of this chapter. The interested reader should refer to Woodward's (1979) chapter 'Piaget's Theory and the Study of Mental Retardation' in conjunction with one of the many available primers of which I have found Philips's (1981) brief account excellent. Ideally reading of commentaries of this sort should be complemented by some study of Piaget's original writings. With respect to the periods of early development covered here, *The Origin of Intelligence in the Child* (Piaget 1953) and *The Child's Construction of Reality* (Piaget 1955) are particularly relevant. These writings are rich in examples of behaviour observed in children and enhance understanding of the often abstract concepts with which commentaries necessarily concern themselves.

With respect to the assessment instruments described in this chapter, the reader should, through the above sources, be familiar with the following concepts: (1) That Piaget's theory attempts to account for how the child comes to understand the world by interacting with it, initially through motor actions in the first two years of life which are referred to as the Sensorimotor period. (2) That this period gives way to the Preoperational period. Here mental representation of the world has developed, but the child works with representations of objects and events as already experienced. True operational thought in which these representations can be manipulated mentally does not emerge until round seven years of age — hence the difficult term '*pre*operational'. (3) That these general periods are divided into stages, the sensorimotor stage in more detail than the preoperational stage. The sensorimotor stage is divided into six stages conventionally numbered I–VI. Several different domains of development are considered in relation to these stages, e.g. development of understanding about objects and of space both pass through Stages I–VI. The belief that development in each domain is parallel, e.g. that Stage IV in understanding about objects and space will be reached at the same time, is referred to as the 'stage congruence hypothesis'. A full understanding of sensorimotor stages and domains will be gained from reading the actual description of the instruments noted. The preoperational period is divided into the Preconceptual Sub-stage (2–4 years) and the Intuitive Sub-stage (4–7 years). Here we are concerned essentially with the first of these stages and again it is hoped that the detailed description of some of the assessment devices will clarify the nature of development change in this sub-period. (4) That the development of mental representation is closely bound up with the emergence of symbolic play and language. In this chapter, therefore, we see assessment of the former as an essential aspect of early cognitive assessment. There is a variety of other concepts necessary to fully understand Piagetian theory, notably those concerned with the actual mechanisms of developmental change. These are not directly dealt with in the assessment instruments, though observations of behaviour in the assessment can well be interpreted in Piagetian terms over and above the immediate achievements demonstrated. I do not deal with this aspect in the present chapter either at a theoretical or at a practical level. However, reference back to many of the original sources will provide illustrative material on this more advanced stage of assessment.

Piagetian assessment instruments and intelligence testing

Though Piaget's theory has been criticised for being too abstract and having too little to do with the real world, the crucial developments in the child's understanding of the world have made it a rich source of ideas for those working with individuals who are mentally handicapped. As in nursery education generally, curricula have been developed not only out of the specific kinds of material and situations employed by Piaget himself, but also from situations considered useful in increasing understanding in real-life skills. This interest has in turn led to the need to employ assessment instruments that reflect the content of Piaget's account, and which also place the child within the period-stage framework just described. As we shall see, this has led to the use of existing, though only recently developed, instruments, and to the development by practitioners themselves of suitable devices.

The development of tests of specific aspects of cognitive functioning shows a marked departure from traditional ways of measuring intelligence in which an attempt is made to establish an overall measure, usually expressed as an Intelligence Quotient (IQ) or a Developmental Quotient (DQ) and often some Mental Age (MA) equivalent based on the relation between rate of development as measured by IQ or DQ and the child's actual or Chronological Age (CA) (see Chapter 2 of this volume). The need to go beyond such assessments in developmental psychology in general and in mental retardation in particular was expressed many years ago by Inhelder in a book published in 1943 and titled *The Diagnosis of Reasoning in the Mentally Retarded* (English translation, Inhelder 1968). In this she commented on the usefulness of intelligence testing for the rapid detection of 'mental anomalies', but the limitation of such an approach when it came to saying something about the nature of thought processes and any inadequacies that might exist. Her reason for this statement still holds today, and have been reiterated in various forms by many subsequent writers. Her criticisms are:

(1) IQ Tests, and their downward extension into infant development tests such as the Bayley Scales of Infant Development (Bayley 1969) or the Griffiths Mental Development Scales (Griffiths 1970), are essentially concerned with outcomes or products. Can the child achieve such and such a behaviour which we would typically expect for that particular CA? Indeed, the very items of such tests are in large measure chosen because they reliably distinguish between children at different age levels. Such testing is not concerned with the cause of behaviour, nor with the overall structure of the child's beahviour at a given time (see Chapter 7 for a further discussion).
(2) Psychometric tests tell us nothing about the stages of development. All we have is a simple series of increments that add to a continuously increasing score. Even if the idea of stages of development is not accepted, we must agree with Inhelder's related criticism that this total global score can be achieved in several ways. Hogg and Moss (1983), for example, have shown how young Down's Syndrome children can achieve the same MA as nonhandicapped children despite performing more poorly on fine motor items, by achieving a relatively higher score on certain aspects of language development.
(3) Psychometric testing tells us nothing about the way in which behaviour is transformed at successive levels of mental development.

With respect to people with mental handicap, the value of

psychometric testing is reduced further by the fact that the tests have not been developed on, or standardised with, this particular group. Where additional impairments exist, this state of affairs is exacerbated. Testing such a child on an IQ test and finding an MA of twelve months will not have involved the same procedure, or mean the same thing, as for a nonhandicapped 12 month old. At the very best, all we have is an imperfect shorthand expresion of the extent to which a child lags behind CA expectations. Employed in this way, however, IQs and MAs do have a useful function in description of people who are mentally handicapped and in their preliminary screening.

What Inhelder sought was a technique of assessment that would enable the operations of mental activity to be assessed by placing children in a situation in which it can be established whether children who are mentally handicapped are fixated at a lower operational stage than would be expected for their age. This entailed presenting a child with a variety of problems in which evidence of operational thought could be assessed. Questions and answers dependent upon the child's observation of a situation were used and the approach was essentially clinical or experimental, rather than standardised as in the case of psychometric tests. The tasks actually used by Inhelder are generally more advanced than those with which we are concerned here, and indeed, she excludes from her study children who were severely or profoundly mentally handicapped. Thus her concern in Piagetian terms was with the later stages of intuitive thinking and with concrete operations.

The extent of Inhelder's approach to the functioning of less able retarded children in the sensorimotor period, came some years later with Woodward's (1959) important paper on this topic. Here, for the first time, an attempt was made to present a consistent procedure for undertaking a developmental assessment in a Piagetian framework with children who were profoundly mentally handicapped. Further studies by other authors have on occasions also employed scales and test items devised by the author for the specific purpose of the study. Increasingly, however, Piagetian-based tests developed with nonhandicapped children have been extended to people with mental handicap, a similar extension to that which has occurred with many psychometric infant development tests.

Further differences between Piagetian-based tests of development and traditional psychometric tests are noted by Dunst (1980). In the latter, composition of the global score, MA, usually takes into account the highest item passed (the ceiling item) and the item before the first failure, i.e. the basal item. This is necessary because it is rare to find a distinct break in the child's performance where passes stop and failures begin, there usually being a grey area where failures occur but higher level items are passed. In contrast, the Piagetian tests take the highest pass as representing the child's ceiling and actual level of development, the assumption being that the items form a rank order or ordinal scale in which a pass on an item assumes passes on all previous items. Secondly, Dunst points out that the general administrative procedures for psychometric tests are much more rigid than for Piagetian testing. Taking their cue from Inhelder's flexible approach to Piagetian assessment, the authors of these tests vary material and context and utilise informal observations. Thirdly, while psychometric tests yield Intelligence or Developmental Quotients, Piagetian tests do not, though Dunst points out, for any particular activity it is possible to establish a Mental Age equivalent.

A more positive note with respect to IQ testing is sounded by Lunzer (1970) who considers the standardisation of the test situation may more adequately cue the child:

> In other words, such tests may be purer measures of intellectual power than Piaget tests themselves. Even granted this were so, (and it has not been proven), it is still possible that the very fact that the Piagetian situations tap the spontaneous behaviour of the child renders them a better instrument for educational diagnosis and prediction, for a measure of effective intelligence may be more informative than one of (relatively) 'pure' mental power. (pp. 54–5).

Piagetian scales that have been used with retarded people fall broadly into two categories: (1) those that have been published as scales with something approaching standardisation; and (2) those appearing in experimental studies that have been developed for specific purposes. In reality, the distinction is often blurred. Assessments falling in group (1) are reviewed first.

THE INSTRUMENTS AND THEIR APPLICATION

Sensorimotor assessment

Uzgiris and Hunt's 'Ordinal Scales of Psychological Development'

These scales, which cover key Piagetian areas of sensorimotor development, were devised (1) in response to shortcomings perceived by the authors in traditional psychometric tests, and (2) to provide an instrument that would enable studies to be made of theoretical issues in child development. With respect to the former, Uzgiris and Hunt (1975) draw attention to the limitations of DQ or IQ testing that were noted above, particularly with respect to global measures that assume some general factor of intelligence or developmental status, and also with respect to measuring this status with reference to a performance of a standardisation group at a given age.

While disregarding Piaget's stage placements and any link between their test items and CA, Uzgiris and Hunt draw heavily on Piaget's observations for the ordinal scales they propose. It is, however, the sequential nature of development in various sensorimotor domains that is their main concern, not the six stages that were described earlier. One important reason for this, they argue, is that the Piagetian position is as yet unproven. That is, achievement of the same stage in different sensorimotor domains at the same time has not been demonstrated and, indeed, it would only be through the development of scales such as their own that a test of this hypothesis could be achieved. The Uzigiris-Hunt Scales, therefore, are independent of both CA and Piagetian Stage placements, though in Phase I of the instrument's development described below, Stage placements were still attempted. Uzigiris and Hunt describe four phases in the development of the scales:

Phase I: Selecting the eliciting situations and the critical actions. On the basis of Piaget's writings on infancy, situations that could realistically be established in the home were selected in which critical actions indicative of cognitive development were chosen. An emphasis was placed on a form of standardisation quite different from that obtaining in psychometric procedures:

> ... another form of standardisation was to be achieved by aiming always for a state of optimal cooperation from the infant and by assuring always that his interest in the test materials extended to manipulating the materials provided in a manner which produced relevant information for the examiner. This meant that the infant

was presented with the eliciting situations in his own home, usually on the floor of his living room, rather than in a standardized testing room and in a standardized baby seat.

Furthermore, the toys and materials used to structure the various situations were to be varied in accordance with the experience and interests of each infant examined, instead of being fixed and unchanged from infant to infant. The order of presenting the eliciting situations was also to be varied in accordance with the interests of each infant. (p. 53).

Thus, flexibility and optimisation of performance were to be the keynotes of assessment sessions.

Phase II: Reliability of assessment by sensorimotor stage with the second version of the instrument. The reliability of independent assesssments was considered and further revision of the administration procedure undertaken. It was then that Stage placement was abandoned because it became clear that Piaget's six sensorimotor stages did not fully reflect the variety of actions that children displayed in the eliciting situations. However, the various domains of development were retained. Five sets of eliciting situations were established in which the 63 situations were grouped in order to facilitate administration.

Phase III: Inter-examiner reliability and inter-session stability of infant actions in the eliciting situations. Good inter-observer agreement was established and stability (test-retest reliability) was generally acceptable especially for well-established actions.

Phase IV: Revision of the instrument: the six series with evidence of their reliability and stability. A further revision was undertaken in the light of Phase III. Lack of reliability was partly attributable to failure to anticipate some of the infant's actions and these were, therefore, further enumerated. Some situations leading to infant behaviour that was difficult to interpret or otherwise problematical, were dropped.

Ordinal scales for different domains of development were produced concerned with development in:

I   Progress in visual pursuit and the permanence of objects.
II   Means for obtaining desired environmental events.
III   Imitation: I Vocal; II Gestural.
IV   Operational causality.

V   Construction of object relations in space.
VI Schemes for relating to objects.

Highly satisfactory reliabilities, both inter-observer and test-retest, were established for most of the items on each of these scales. The scalability of the items within a scale was also considered. The term 'ordinal' in fact refers to the order in which a child passes various items. For example, with respect to the visual pursuit, consider the following items:

(1) Does not visually follow an object.
(2) Follows object, but jerkily.
(3) Follows object through part of arc smoothly.
(4) Follows object through complete trajectory smoothly.

We would expect the child's visual tracking to follow this order, i.e. passing (1), then (2), (3), and (4). In an unimpaired child, we would not expect (2) to be passed, then (4), then (3). Statistical measures of the consistency with which items form an ordinal scale can be established and application to the Uzgiris-Hunt scales were highly satisfactory.

The authors conclude that their instrument does permit description of an infant's psychological development without having to refer to a standardised group of infants or to CA as in the case of DQ or IQ testing. In order to give a clear indication of the instrument, the Development of Visual Pursuit and the Permanence of Objects in one child will now be illustrated.

Figure 3.1 reproduces Scale I from Uzgiris and Hunt (1975, pp. 206–9) completed for a child who is profoundly retarded and multiply handicapped (LP). As may be seen, there are 15 situations, starting with 'Following a Slowly Moving Object through a 180° Arc' (No. 1) to 'Finding Object Following a Series of Invisible Displacements by Searching in Reverse of the Order of Hiding' (No. 15). In each situation a range of possible behaviours is listed, with those asterisked indicating that the child has accomplished the skill. Again, taking Situation 1 a–c, behaviours do not give evidence of the accomplishment of smooth tracking while 'd' does. The recording form permits repeated presentations, though the recommended number appears in parentheses after each situation description. As may be seen, from the summary form in Figure 3.2, this child passed all situations up to and including Scale step 9, with the exception of Scale step 4. Her pass on No. 9, Finding an Object Following One Invisible Displacement, is then the highest item and this places

EARLY DEVELOPMENT AND PIAGETIAN TESTS

Figure 3.1: Samples record for child with profound retardation and multiple impairments of scale I (the Development of Visual Pursuit and the Permanence of Objects) from the Uzgiris and Hunt Scales of Ordinal Development

SAMPLE EXAMINATION RECORD FORMS

SCALE I: THE DEVELOPMENT OF VISUAL PURSUIT AND THE PERMANENCE OF OBJECTS

Name: LP
Birthdate: 1 : 5 : 69
Date of Examination: 14/15 : 3 : 83

PRESENTATION
(Suggested number of presentations for each situation is indicated in parentheses)

SITUATION	1	2	3	4	5	6	7
1. *Following a Slowly Moving Object through a 180° Arc* (3–4)							
a. Does not follow object							
b. Follows jerkily through part of arc							
c. Follows smoothly through part of arc							
*d. Follows object smoothly through complete arc	✓	✓	✓				
Other:							
2. *Noticing the Disappearance of a Slowly Moving Object* (3–4)							
a. Does not follow to point of disappearance							
b. Loses interest as soon as object disappears							
*c. Lingers with glance on point of disappearance	✓	✓	✓				
*d. Returns glance to starting point after several presentations							
e. Searches around point of disappearance							
Other:							
3. *Finding an Object Which Is Partially Covered* (3)							
a. Loses interest	✓						
b. Reacts to the loss, but does not obtain object							
*c. Obtains the object		✓	✓				
Other:							
4. *Finding an Object Which Is Completely Covered* (3)							
a. Loses interest	✓						

SCALE I (*continued*)

	PRESENTATION
SITUATION	(Suggested number of presentations for each situation is indicated in parentheses)
	1 2 3 4 5 6 7

    b. Reacts to loss, but does not obtain object   ___ ___ ___ ___ ___ ___ ___
    c. Pulls screen, but not enough to obtain object   ___ ___ ___ ___ ___ ___ ___
   *d. Pulls screen off and obtains object   ___ ✓ ✓ ___ ___ ___ ___
    Other: ___ ___ ___ ___ ___ ___ ___

5. *Finding an Object Completely Covered in Two Places* (2)
    a. Loses interest ___ ___ ___ ___ ___ ___ ___
    b. Searches for object where it was previously found ___ ___ ___ ___ ___ ___ ___
    c. Searches for object where it is last hidden ✓ ✓ ___ ___ ___ ___ ___
    Other: ___ ___ ___ ___ ___ ___ ___

6. *Finding an Object Completely Covered in Two Places Alternately* (3–5)
    a. Becomes perplexed and loses interest ___ ___ ___ ___ ___ ___ ___
    b. Searches haphazardly under one or both screens ___ ___ ___ ___ ___ ___ ___
   *c. Searches correctly under each of the screens ✓ ✓ ✓ ___ ___ ___ ___
    Other: ___ ___ ___ ___ ___ ___ ___

7. *Finding an Object Completely Covered in Three Places* (5–7)
    a. Loses interest ___ ___ ___ ___ ___ ___ ___
    b. Searches haphazardly under some or all screens ___ ___ ___ ___ ___ ___ ___
   *c. Searches directly under correct screen ✓ ✓ ✓ ✓ ✓ ___ ___
    Other: ___ ___ ___ ___ ___ ___ ___

8. *Finding an Object after Successive Visible Displacements* (3–5)
    a. Does not follow successive hidings ✓ ✓ ✓ ___ ___ ___ ___
    b. Searches only under the first screen ___ ___ ___ ___ ___ ___ ___
    c. Searches under screen where object was previously found ___ ___ ___ ___ ___ ___ ___
    d. Searches haphazardly under all screens ___ ___ ___ ___ ___ ___ ___
    e. Searches in order of hiding ___ ___ ___ ___ ___ ___ ___

SCALE I (*continued*)

Situation	Presentation (Suggested number of presentations for each situation is indicated in parentheses)						
	1	2	3	4	5	6	7
f. Searches directly under the last screen in path	—	—	—	—	—	—	—
Other:	—	—	—	—	—	—	—
9. *Finding an Object under Three Superimposed Screens* (2–3)							
a. Loses interest	✓	—	—	—	—	—	—
b. Lifts one or two screens, but fails to find object	—	—	—	—	—	—	—
*c. Removes all screens and obtains object	—	✓	✓	—	—	—	—
Other:	—	—	—	—	—	—	—
10. *Finding an Object Following One Invisible Displacement* (3)							
a. Loses interest	—	—	—	—	—	—	—
b. Reacts to loss, does not search	—	—	—	—	—	—	—
c. Searches only in the box	—	—	—	—	—	—	—
*d. Checks the box and searches under the screen	✓	—	—	—	—	—	—
*e. Searches under screen directly	—	✓	✓	—	—	—	—
Other:	—	—	—	—	—	—	—
11. *Finding an Object Following One Invisible Displacement with Two Screens* (2)							
a. Searches only in box	—	—	—	—	—	—	—
b. Searches under screen where object was previously found	—	—	—	—	—	—	—
*c. Searches directly under correct screen	—	—	—	—	—	—	—
Other:	Loses interest	—	—	—	—	—	—
12. *Finding an Object Following One Invisible Displacement with Two Screens Alternated* (3)							
a. Loses interest	✓	—	—	—	—	—	—
b. Searches haphazardly under screens	—	—	—	—	—	—	—
*c. Searches directly under correct screen	—	—	—	—	—	—	—
Other:	—	—	—	—	—	—	—
13. *Finding an Object Following One Invisible Displacement with Three Screens* (5–7)							
a. Loses interest	✓	—	—	—	—	—	—
b. Searches haphazardly under all screens	—	—	—	—	—	—	—

SCALE I (continued)

SITUATION	PRESENTATION (Suggested number of presentations for each situation is indicated in parentheses)						
	1	2	3	4	5	6	7
*c. Searches directly under correct screen	—	—	—	—	—	—	—
Other:	—	—	—	—	—	—	—
14. Finding an Object Following a Series of Invisible Displacements (4-6)							
a. Searches only in E's hand	_loses interest_			—	—	—	—
b. Searches only under first one or two screens in the path	—	—	—	—	—	—	—
*c. Searches under all screens in the path in the order of hiding	—	—	—	—	—	—	—
*d. Searches directly under the last screen in the path	—	—	—	—	—	—	—
15. Finding Object Following a Series of Invisible Displacements by Searching in Reverse of the Order of Hiding (2)							
a. Searches only under last screen	_loses interest_			—	—	—	—
b. Searches haphazardly under all screens	—	—	—	—	—	—	—
*c. Searches systematically from the last screen back to the first	—	—	—	—	—	—	—
Other:	—	—	—	—	—	—	—

Source: Uzgiris and Hunt (1975).

Figure 3.2: Sample summary assessment of Figure 3.1.

SCALE I: THE DEVELOPMENT OF VISUAL PURSUIT AND THE PERMANENCE OF OBJECTS

Infant Code Number: LP

Age: 13 yrs 10

Scale Step	Relevant Situation Number	Critical Infant Action	Infant Actions Observed (List situation by no. and response by letter)
1	1	d	1d
2	2	c	2c
3	3	c	3c
4	2	d	—
5	4	d	4d
6	6 (and 5)	6c (and 5c)[a]	5c & 6c
7	7	c	7c
8	9	c	9c
9	10	d or e	10d & e
10	11	c	
11	12	c	
12	13	c	
13	14	c	
14	14 and 15	14d plus 15c	

[a] Infant actions in situations 5 and 8 were not included in the scaling analysis. The scale step for which actions in situation 5 may be relevant is indicated in parentheses.

Source: Uzgiris and Hunt (1975).

her developmentally in this scale. A full description of the location of testing, choice of objects and administrative directions are also given for each situation.

In their original form, the Uzgiris-Hunt Scales retain all the central distinctions between psychometric developmental testing and cognitive ordinal assessment that we have noted. Most importantly, they represent an attempt to assess a child's sensorimotor development within a Piagetian framework eschewing not only derived measures of Mental Age but even Stage placements. As we have seen, the authors did not envisage that their scales would be evolved or used in a direction that moved them towards more traditional approaches to assessment. Nevertheless, there has been a real interest in applying these scales to the cognitive assessment of children with mental handicap, and in the use of the information for development of intervention programmes.

Kahn (1985) has provided a detailed review on the applicability of the Uzgiris-Hunt Scales to people who are severely and profoundly retarded, many of his conclusions being based on unpublished work from the USA. Rather than reconsider his sources in detail, I will here note his general conclusions and refer the interested reader to his original paper. The reliability of the scales with this population is generally high, i.e. different assessors will arrive at highly comparable assessments of the same person as will the same assessor on different occasions. The validity of these scales also receives some confirmation with comparable developmental behaviour assessed in other ways matching those assessed by the Uzgiris-Hunt Scales. Kahn suggests, however, that considerably more work on the validity of the scales is called for. The issue of ordinality must also be considered. As noted earlier, the items on each of the scales are intended to indicate a progression in which a pass on any given item assumes that all lower items will also have been passed. Kahn reports that this has only been fully demonstrated for Scale I, The Development of Visual Pursuit and the Permanence of Objects. Specially problematical is Scale V, The Construction of Object Relations in Space, where doubt has been cast on the applicability of this scale with this population. From the practical point of view, Kahn suggests caution in assuming that when an individual fails an item then he or she will not pass higher items. Testing should be continued to establish whether, for that person, ordinality has for some reason broken down.

An order form is available with Uzgiris and Hunt (1975) for both 16 mm films and video cassettes for demonstrating each of the scales. At the time of going to press (1975) prices ranged from $235 to $400.

Dunst's 'Clinical and Education Manual for Use with the Uzgiris and Hunt Scales of Infant Psychological Development'

Dunst (1980) has responded to the need for more standardisation by formalising the Uzgiris-Hunt Scales in a way that makes them usable for assessment and intervention. Here I will summarise the procedure he advocates with respect to the former, i.e. assessment, and illustrate the outcome from some of our own assessments.

The 73 items in Uzgiris and Hunt's seven scales are spread unevenly among these domains, and to them Dunst adds a further 53 experimental items which are designated with a prefix 'E' in the various recording sheets. Thus, for Stage V, 'Object Permanence', the items in ascending order are 6, 7, E_6, 8 and 9. E_6 is here a Dunst addition, while the remainder are from the original Uzgiris-Hunt Scales. These items are administered in a semi-standardised fashion, but allowing for greater flexibility than would be acceptable in a standardised developmental test. Thus, the position of the child, suitable objects, directions for administration and critical responses are all described (Dunst 1980, Appendix B).

The information that these assessments yield can best be described by reference to the recording forms. Figure 3.3 shows the recording form for Visual Pursuit and the Permanence of Objects and has 21 items, the original Uzgiris-Hunt items and additional 'E' items provided by Dunst to create a finer progression through the series. In the second column, Estimated Age Placements (EDAs) are given, based on a variety of psychometric tests and experimental studies and marking a clear departure from Uzgiris and Hunt's conception of the assessment procedure, though the possibility of such a procedure is considered by them (Uzgiris and Hunt 1975, pp. 18–19). The validity of these EDAs has been established by Dunst correlating them with a psychometric assessment of developmental level. Dunst cautions that the EDAs are not predictive and have no normative value. While the former claim is certainly the case, it is difficult not to see the introduction of EDAs in the assessment as anything other than a legitimate attempt to place the outcome of sensorimotor assessment within a normative framework.

In column 3 the appropriate Stage placement is given, again an extension to Uzgiris and Hunt's procedure. In practical terms, Dunst's decision to include Stage placements is based on the need to establish a Stage profile in which strengths and weaknesses in different areas can be indicated. The value of such an approach is that it permits identification of recurrent deficits in specific sensorimotor domains and points to areas requiring special remediation. From a

Figure 3.3: Assessment of a Child with Profound Retardation and Multiple Impairment on Scale I of the Uzgiris and Hunt Scales of Ordinal Development in the Framework of Dunst's Revision. Source: Dunst (1980)

Child's Name: **LP** Date of Birth: 1:5:69 Date of Test: 14/5:3:83

I: VISUAL PURSUIT AND THE PERMANENCE OF OBJECTS

SCALE STEP	AGE PLACEMENT (Months)	DEVELOP MENTAL STAGE	ELICITING CONTEXT	CRITICAL ACTION CODE	CRITICAL BEHAVIORS	SCORING 1	2	3	4	5	OBSERVATIONS
E₁	1	I	Visual Fixation	1a	Fixates on object held 8 to 10 inches above the eyes	+	+	+	+		
1	2	II	Visual Tracking	1d	Tracks object through a 180° arc	+	+	+	+		
2	3	II	Visual Tracking	2c	Lingers at point of object's disappearance — child in supine position or on an infant seat	+	+	+	+		
E₂	4	III	Visual Tracking	—	Searches for object at point of disappearance — child seated on parent's lap	—	—	—	—		
3	5	III	Visible Displacement	3c	Secures partially hidden object	—	+	+	+		
4	6	III	Visual Tracking	2d	Returns glance to position above the head after object moves out of visual field	—	—	—	—		
E₃	7	IV	Visual Tracking	—	Reverses searching for object in anticipation of reappearance — child seated on parent's lap						NOT APPLICABLE
E₄	7	IV	Visible Displacement	—	Withdraws object held in hand following covering of hand and object with cloth						
5	8	IV	Visible Displacement	4d	Secures object hidden under a single screen		+	+			
E₅	9	IV	Visible Displacement	5b	Secures object hidden with two screens (A & B) — hidden under A twice then B — searches under A only	—	—				
6	9	V	Visible Displacement	6c	Secures object hidden under one of two screens — hidden alternately	+	+	+	.		
7	9	V	Visible Displacement	7c	Secures object hidden under one of three screens — hidden alternately	+	+	+	+	+	
E₆	10	V	Successive Visible Displacement	8e	Secures object hidden through a series of successive visible displacements with three screens	—	—	—			
8	10	V	Superimposed Screens	9c	Secures object under three superimposed screens	—	+	+			
9	13	V	Invisible Displacement	10d 10e	Secures object hidden with a single screen	+	+	+			
10	14	VI	Invisible Displacement	11c	Secures object hidden with two screens (A & B) — hidden under A twice then B	—					
11	14	VI	Invisible Displacement	12c	Secures object hidden under one of two screens — hidden alternately	—					
12	15	VI	Invisible Displacement	13c	Secures object hidden under one of three screens — hidden alternately	—					
13	18	VI	Successive Invisible Displacement	14c	Secures object hidden with three screens - object left under last screen — child searches along pathway	—					
E₇	22	VI	Successive Invisible Displacement	14d	Secures object hidden with three screens — object left screen — child searches directly under last screen	—					
14	23	VI	Successive Invisible Displacement	15c	Secures object hidden with three screens — object left under first screen — child searches in reverse order	—					

theoretical point of view, Dunst hopes that this procedure will tell us what cognitive operations the child can perform in the various domains since equivalent Stage placements are assumed to reflect equivalent cognitive operations.

Column 4 indicates the eliciting context, essentially a cue to the assessor as to the situation or behaviour of interest. In column 5 the behaviour required of the child to indicate that a given level of functioning has been achieved is noted. The number indicates the eliciting situation in which the behaviour is assessed and the letter, the critical behaviour which is described in the 'Critical Behaviour' column. These codes relates in general to the original Uzgiris-Hunt codes.

Critical behaviours are listed in column 6 and Dunst suggests that taken with the eliciting context information, a reasonable description of what is required in administration and scoring can be inferred, always assuming that the assessor is familiar with the background provided in the original Uzgiris-Hunt procedure. Provision is then made (column 7) for up to five assessments and a code for 'pass' on the critical item, 'pass following demonstration', 'critical behaviour in the course of emerging' and 'not manifest' is given. Subsidiary codes for the item — omission, other reports of behaviour and mistrials — are given. These codes are not shown on the figure. In the final column space is provided for observations on the child's behaviour that are deemed of interest.

Dunst provides a detailed account of how the items should be administered and emphasises the need to be familiar with Uzgiris and Hunt's general and specific procedures. General indications on establishing rapport between infant and assessor, environmental considerations, order of presentation of scales and initial approach are given. More detailed suggestions on administering the seven individual scales are then offered. A summary form is also provided on which information from the seven individual scale administrations can be collated.

The form for producing a profile of a child's sensorimotor abilities is given here in Figure 3.4. The six sensorimotor stages are indicated on the left of the profile in Roman numerals I–VI. The profile is generated by simply ringing the Scale step passes in each domain and joining these. As noted earlier, this allows a clear visual representation of the extent to which the child is performing consistently with respect to cognitive operations and the pattern of strengths and weaknesses exhibited.

The applicability of this assessment to both children who are

Figure 3.4: Dunst's Profile of Ability Form for a Child with Profound Retardation and Multiple Impairment Across All Sensorimotor Domains

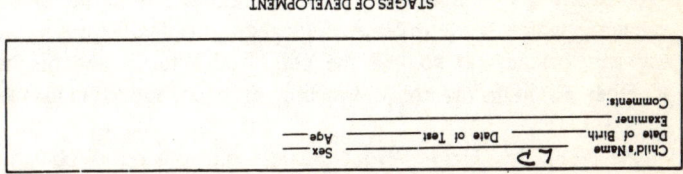

Source: Dunst (1980).

nonhandicapped as well as those who are mentally handicapped is clearly demonstrated by Dunst with illustrative profile data on children from both groups. Work by this author has also shown the utility of the scales with children who are multiply impaired and profoundly retarded. Here, the passes for LP indicated in Figures 3.1 and 3.2 have been transcribed on Dunst's form in Figures 3.3 and 3.4.

Woodward's Assessment of Sensorimotor Development

Woodward's (1959) approach to Piagetian assessment is of particular interest on at least two counts. First, this represented the first published attempt to extend Inhelder's work with more able retarded children with mental handicap downwards to those who are profoundly retarded. Second, the emphasis is essentially on a semistructured play context from which inferences about the child's sensorimotor development could be made. In the tests, six problems were presented, two each derived from Stages IV, V and VI. In Stage IV two object-behind-screen tasks were presented, one with a transparent and the other with an opaque screen. In Stage V retrieval of an object by pulling a support or pulling a piece of string attached to it were presented. In Stage VI retrieval of an object with a rake and reorienting object to draw it through the bars was required. It is, of course, possible to observe Stages I–III behaviour within this context, for example, sucking one of the presented objects indicating Stage I. Though a flexible procedure for administration is described, Woodward gives details of presentation, and also an eliciting sequence which is the reverse of Piaget's grasping sequence: 'The toy was placed, (a) so that the child could see it and his hand together, (b) in his mouth, (c) touching his hand, and (d) in his palm' (p. 63).

As with the Uzgiris-Hunt Scales and others, Woodward's development of an assessment procedure was dictated by experimental considerations. Like Uzgiris and Hunt, she has been insistent on the fact that her approach is exploratory and she has made no attempt to evolve it into a standardised technique. In making her approach more widely available later (Woodward 1967) she emphasised the nonstandardised nature of her approach and her intention not to formalise the procedure. Her reservations about such formalisation of her own and other scales have recently been reiterated (Woodward 1984), not only with respect to the nature of Piagetian assessment itself, but also in relation to the special problems of assessing severely and profoundly retarded children.

Gouin Décarie's Scale of Object Permanence

This scale was employed in her study of thalidomide-damaged children (Gouin Décarie 1969), and reported fully in Gouin Décarie (1962). It consists mainly of visual-manual items and allows the assessor to locate the child in one of six sequential stages of the sensorimotor period. It also permits location at the start and end of each scale, e.g. Ia or Ib. In line with the application of ordinal scale tests of this sort, flexibility of administration permits assessment of children with additional impairments. Thus, in assessing thalidomide children, Gouin Décarie permitted children to move screens with mouth or toes.

The Corman-Escalona Scales of Sensorimotor Development

As with all other scales of sensorimotor development, those developed by Corman and Escalona (1969) began life with a specific experimental aim in view. The authors were beginning a longitudinal study of personality development and on the basis of Piaget's observations set about constructing three separate scales:

Prehension. This assesses developmental changes in hand use, from Stage II — primary circular reactions — through to Stage III — secondary coordinations involving hand, eye and other modalities.
Object Permanence. This reflects development of the object concept in itself and the relation between action and object. It covers behaviour from Stage III (failure to search for a hidden object) through to Stage VI where the object is found after complex displacements.
Spatial Relations. Again, this covers from Stage III to Stage VI, i.e. from movement in space that is limited by the child's own range of movement to a fuller construction of the understanding of space in which the child can invent new routes and employ complex detours. (The authors comment on future development of a causality scale.)

Data are reported showing a high degree of reliability in administering the scales, and general confirmation of the sequences described by Piaget. A longitudinal study shows almost perfect sequencing of the hypothesised stages by all children. For example, Child 1 on the Object Concept Scale achieves the various stages at the following months: III — 4 months, IV — 6.3 months, V — 8.7 months, VI — 19.7 months, completing all Stages VI items at 20.0 months.

In this publication, the authors indicate that a manual is available and two films dealing with the object concept and spatial relation scales are also stated to be available (Escalona and Corman 1971a and 1971b) though it has not proved possible to get further information on access to the films.

Chatelanat and Schoggen's observation system to assess spontaneous infant environment interactions

The instruments described so far typically take place in a flexible one-to-one test situation. Clearly, however, it is possible to observe many aspects of sensorimotor behaviour by watching a child interact spontaneously with his or her environment. Chatelanat and Schoggen (1980) devised an observation scheme in order to assess sensorimotor development in just this way. Their on-the-spot coding scheme covers 44 categories ranging from Stage I exercising reflexes to Stage VI behaviours concerned with tool use and means-end behaviour. A coding scheme is presented and highly acceptable inter-observer reliabilities found. The authors point out that the descriptions of the at-risk children they studied:

> . . . cannot be equated with tests or assessment procedures which are an attempt to describe what the children *can* do. However, the fact that behaviour-on-demand was not required and that the child was observed in situations with which he was familiar resulted in a description of specific behaviour patterns the child was actually practising in the particular situation. (p. 77)

It is worthwhile to emphasise the implications of this comment. Formal cognitive tests will typically overestimate the person's performance in nontest situations. In a sense, it is limits that are being established. Since it is now widely agreed that intervention should be shown to have an impact in the person's actual world, Chatelanat and Schoggen's instrument points the way to evaluating cognitive functioning in everyday situations to which it is always our hope that teaching will generalise. Far more emphasis on assessment through observation is called for in all areas and it is discussed in detail in Chapter 8 of this volume.

Other Piagetian Assessments of Sensorimotor Development

The major authors noted above are all insistent on the need for those undertaking Piagetian assessments to be well grounded in the theory underlying specific observations. Such a requirement is in marked contrast to standardised psychometric or developmental testing. Such is the relevance of the approach to assessment of children with mental handicap, particularly those who are profoundly so, that practitioners have increasingly developed and modified existing Piagetian instruments in order to make them more directly applicable in their own clinical or educational practice. One aspect of such relevance is the consideration of time, where abbreviated scales are more viable. Foxen (1977), for example, employed the Object Schemes Scale of the Uzgiris and Hunt Assessment as an observational procedure for training professionals in the assessment of children who are severely and profoundly retarded. Working in a teaching context, Coupe and Levy (1985) have developed the Object Schemes Scale specifically in relation to children who are severely and profoundly retarded: 'The Object Related Scheme Assessment Procedure: A cognitive assessment for developmentally young children who may have additional physical or sensory handicaps.' The approach differs in that details are given of presentation to children who are multiply impaired and suggestions are made for remedial activity. As yet no formal standardisation or evaluation of the approach has been attempted.

Preoperational assessment

A general lack of research into the preoperational period is reflected in the dearth of assessment instruments compared with those generated by sensorimotor studies. The increasing differentiation of function towards the end of the sensorimotor period that we have noted becomes even more apparent during the preoperational period and there is no comparable instrument to, say, the Uzgiris-Hunt Scales. Instead, various attempts to assess manipulative, symbolic or linguistic function can be noted. Clearly, many specialised instruments, including language assessment devices, will be excluded from this review (but see relevant chapters elsewhere in this volume).

Cognition

Earlier I gave some account of changes in cognitive functioning. For Woodward (Woodward 1972; Woodward 1983; Woodward and Hunt 1972), the interest in assessment is not in the simple achievement of nesting beakers or matching shapes but in the general elimination of inappropriate strategies as the child acquires mastery through increasingly complex mental operations.

One particular attraction of her approach is the familiarity and availability of the material employed:

Fitting tasks

(1) Round hole pegboard with ten holes arranged in pairs.
(2) Round hole pegboard with nine holes grouped irregularly and one displaced from group.
(3) Twelve rings of different size and colour for placement on a stick.
(4) Four-item formboard with circle, cross, square and triangle.
(5) Five 'trees' with five sticks each onto which beads could be fitted.

Material for spontaneous handling This consists of four sets of items varying in their characteristics:

(1) Thirty one-inch cubes in six colours.
(2) Twenty-four triangular pieces in six colours.
(3) Twenty-seven items varying in colour, shape and size (cubes, triangles, rods, in three sizes and three colours).
(4) One hundred identical counters.

Induced matching tasks Matching linear and circular arrays of cubes or beads on basis of colour, e.g. nine cubes of different colours as standard, eight matches to be selected from an array of twenty-three cubes of twelve different colours.

Spatial order tasks Here matching requires location of beads on a rod, again involving the same standard and match numbers as in the induced matching task.

Positioning tasks Location of four cubes into a tray into which they fitted exactly if correctly positioned permitting observation of error correction and anticipation.

Any attempt to use Woodward's materials to assess cognition requires the same grounding in her conception of development as does use of sensorimotor tests in Piagetian theory. In addition, for most teachers, some co-ordination with available rating scales would be feasible. For example, many checklists in the cognitive or manipulative areas will embody some of Woodward's material and concepts, e.g. 'can place peg in hole'.

Smith (1982) drew on Lunzer (1970), Woodward (1972) and Woodward and Hunt (1972) to develop an instrument for assessing preconceptual and intuitive development in the preoperational period. Though at present available only in her Ph.D. thesis, 'A Study of Mental Growth in Young Severely Subnormal Children', this development does illustrate the way in which assessment procedures of this sort can be evolved into usable instruments. Detailed procedures for presenting tasks and standardised recording forms are presented in her Appendices B and C (pp. 294–306), with response coding in Appendix D (pp. 307–17).

Smith's developmental areas are comparable to those of Woodward's in a number of respects:

A1 Classification:	(a) Sorting by colour or shape
	(b) Sorting into piles where colour or shape can be used as an attribute
A2 Seriation:	(a) Stacking of cups
	(b) Seriation of wooden rods (scoring based on Lunzer 1970)
A3 Number:	(a) Copying models with given number of blocks
	(b) Number matching and conservation of numbers (again based on Lunzer)
A4 Spatial Relations:	(a) Spontaneous arrangements of blocks
	(b) Copy of models with varying horizontal and vertical arrangements
	(c) Matching linear spatial order

Of particular interest is the emphasis placed by Smith on the strategies employed to achieve the various outcomes rather than a simple pass-fail approach. In adopting this approach Smith again draws on Woodward (1972) and on Woodward and Hunt (1972). To illustrate more fully the procedure we will follow through one example, from A2 (Seriation) above, i.e. the use of stacking cups to assess the ability to seriate and the strategies employed:

CUPS: (2 trials). Materials 12 stacking cylindrical cups.
Present the cups already stacked.
Say *'Let's take them apart'* and encourage S. to help.
Place cups singly on the base with the largest in front of the child and the others to the right or left.
Say *'Put the cups back in there'* indicating the largest cup.
A coding system has been derived from Woodward which records each move the child makes in the sequence of stacking the cups.

If S. is not successful on the first trial demonstrate and give second trial.

Correct cup (largest from array) put in nest.

STRATEGIES WHEN OTHER THAN LARGEST IS PLACED:
1. The placed cup is consecutive in size but a larger one has been omitted earlier;
2. A cup of the wrong size (not the largest in the array) is held inside the top of the last cup nested, and then returned to the collection, without being dropped in;
3. A cup of the wrong size is dropped into the last one nested, and then removed and returned to the collection.

OBSTRUCTION SITUATION:

When this occurs, various strategies may be applied (4–9):

4. The obstructed cup is taken off the nest and the obstructing cup(s) removed, the obstructed cup is then placed in the nest. Strategy 4 may result in restoration of the sequence or may be abortive in that too few or too many cups are removed and the cup placed in the nest is not the next consecutive one. The different outcomes are recorded in brackets thus: 4 ( ) Result of strategy 4 was that the cup placed in the nest was not the next consecutive one. If S. removed the obstructing cup as he approached the nest, i.e., he anticipated the obstruction, record this in brackets as (ant) after the outcome, e.g. 4 ( ) or 4 (x) (ant);
5. The obstruction is taken off the nest and the obstructing cup removed; both are returned to the collection of unnested cups;
6. The obstructed cup is taken off and placed underneath the main nest, then returned to the collection, or nested, if it is bigger than the main nest;
7. The obstructed cup is taken off and placed successively on cups not nested until it goes on;
8. The obstructed cup is taken off and returned to the collection of unnested cups;
9. No action, the obstructed cup is left where it is. (Smith 1982, pp. 297–8)

An appropriate recording form is presented in p. 305 of Smith (1982) permitting recording on each of the two recommended trials. Both success and strategy are covered as well as whether several separate nests were made or other uses to which cups were put. Computer coding of these responses is also described (p. 314). Some other tasks are included in the preoperational assessment form in

Appendix B, namely pegboards, rings or stick and formboards though Smith (1984) recently considered that these would be better viewed as late sensorimotor items. Three- or four-point scales were developed for rating the relation between strategy sophistication and degree of success.

Smith describes three main levels of functioning, 'nonoperational', 'transitional' and 'operational', the latter implying the ability to use some degree of cognition prior to the response rather than just an action strategy. Strategy hierarchies were determined for most tasks. By considering achievement of strategy scores across qualitatively different tasks some statement of stage congruence can be made and what Smith calls a 'rough and ready' (p. 95) estimate of cognition made. On this basis, groups of items constituting preoperational sub-stages are derived.

Smith emphasises that in administering the assessment allowance must be made for attention, mood, fatigue and motor problems. Nevertheless, the items achieved good scalability and construct validity when considered in relation to the children's special education category and the extent to which the instrument predicts language and social skills. Reliability, however, proved difficult to assess in conventional psychometric terms.

Symbolic Functions

Much work in the field of early development has explored the proposed relation between play and the development of symbolic function and language. Among such studies is that of Lowe (1975), from which emerged her 'Symbolic Play Test'. Lowe and Costello (1976) describe the need for such a test: 'The presumed close, though probably complex, relationship between non-verbal semantic functions (particularly the ability to use symbols in any form) and the development of verbal language prompted the development of a diagnostic tool that would aim at evaluating the language potential of children who for some reason have failed to develop receptive or expressive language' (p. 5). Such a test, while being language-free and therefore a kind of performance test, '. . . should explore the child's ability to appreciate semantic rather than spatial relationships, his early concepts, and his ability to deal with symbols in their simplest form to express his own experience and phantasies' (p. 5).

The test is aimed at children who are developmentally in the 12–36 months range, and involves spontaneous play with miniature objects derived from Lowe's (1975) study. It is not intended to replace other existing tests for children in this period, but to complement them and provide a comparison with other areas of development. Thus, at its simplest, it is directed at finding whether language development and symbolic function are proceeding in the expected way, or whether discrepancies exist. For example, is there a discrepancy between language development and symbolic function with the latter lagging behind the former in such a way that we might be led to search for sensory or environmental factors that may have retarded language development?

Four situations are presented:

(1) (a) large doll, sitting; (b) add saucer, spoon, cup; (c) add brush, comb.
(2) bed, pillow, blanket, small girl doll.
(3) chair, table, table cloth, fork, small boy doll, knife, plate.
(4) trailer, tractor, man, logs in random positions.

These were selected in order that:

(1) the toys in a situation should lend themselves to meaningful inter-relationships;
(2) have spontaneous appeal to both sexes;
(3) should appeal to children of different backgrounds; and should permit:
(4) short administration time (10–15 minutes);
(5) simple administration;
(6) administration independent of verbal comprehension and expression;
(7) scoring based on direct observation.

The scalability of the types of play within the situations was found to be good, i.e. if the child showed a given level of play on one item, he or she would also have 'passes' on earlier items. Reliability was also acceptable, and validity was assessed in relation to the child's present and future performance in expressive language. While correlations between Play-Test score and present language tended to be low, much higher correlations were found between the score and language development at a later date. Lowe and Costello (1976) comment: 'Moreover there is a tendency for the correlations to rise as the time interval increases, which argues that there may be a time-lag before complexity of thought is manifest in speech (p. 14).

Detailed descriptions of administration are given (p. 20) with the emphasis on encouraging spontaneous play. A detailed scoring guide is included (pp. 30–3). This may be illustrated from Situation 1 activity of 'Feeds, combs or brushes self or other person'. Here the criteria for a positive (+) or negative (−) score are given thus:

+ 'drinks' from cup; 'eats from spoon'; feeds or offers food to person present.
+ also, if brush is clearly used as a cloth, or toothbrush e.g. dipped in the cup and moved to and fro in the mouth.
− indiscriminant mouthing, e.g. if cup and spoon are in wrong position; puts brush in mouth; puts brush in cup. (p. 30).

A scoring sheet permitting further observations is also provided (pp. 34–5). In addition to the score, an age equivalent can also be derived (cf. Dunst's Mental Age Equivalent).

The overall function of the test is to provide information in the form of a score and age equivalent to permit a critical evaluation of the child's play which can in turn be related to other types of assessment as described above. Whittaker (1980) has applied the Symbolic Play Test to the assessment of children with profound retardation. He emphasises that implements such as the knife, fork and spoon should be scaled up in size in order to make them manipulable and discriminable by children with impairments.

In the experimental literature on symbolic play a variety of other, often comparable approaches are employed. One of the most elaborate is that of Nicolich (1977) who selected her toys on the basis of a list used by Sinclair (1971). Here 30 toys are presented in a similar configuration on each occasion in a bucket. The child is observed playing with the toys and a transcription of play and transitions between play made. The judgement as to placement of the child at a given level is essentially a clinical one. The stages of play as defined by Piaget (1962) are used by Nicholich as a framework with levels, criteria and examples indicated.

Both Lowe's (1975) and Nicolich's (1977) procedures were employed in Riguet, Taylor, Benaroya and Klein's (1981) study of symbolic play in Down's Syndrome, autistic and nonhandicapped children. Again, these authors give detailed descriptions of material, some presented with modelled actions by the adult and some without.

Play was rated with respect to actual play, stereotyped activity and off-task behaviour. The highest level of play was recorded even if it only occurred once. Where play was observed it was rated as follows: (1) motor; (2) transitional; (3) symbolic; (4) animation or nonanimated sequence; (5) animated sequence.

Measures of 'symbolic fluency' and imitation were also taken. 'Symbolic fluency was assessed for each child by determining the number of different substitute symbolic uses of the objects, such as using the pill container as a cup to give the toy a drink . . .' (p. 444). Imitation was scored on a six-point scale.

Standardised observations have also been made by Wing, Gould, Yeates and Brierly (1977) of children with mental handicap employing Sheridan's (1969) observational procedure of play as a means of assessing symbolic representation.

ISSUES IN THE USE OF PIAGETIAN-DERIVED TESTS

Empirical relation to psychometric tests

Even among proponents of Piagetian-derived assessment there is agreement that psychometric tests have value in diagnosing marked deviations from normative development. To this should be added the reservation that such a diagnosis will only be convincing for people who are multiply impaired where sufficient care is taken to ensure that responses available to the child are permitted and indeed engineered by the tester where required. Similarly, the more selective assessment of particular areas of cognition linked at least in part to a wider theory of development has special advantages in both 'placing' the child developmentally and developing appropriate educational strategies. It should be noted, however, that relations *do* exist between the two types of assessment. Both Wachs (1975) and DeVries (1974) found significant correlations between standardised measures of IQ and Piagetian-based assessments. DeVries (1974) concluded that:

> This evidence indicates that intelligence as defined by Stanford-Binet mental age overlaps to a moderate degree with Piagetian intelligence, but that they are not identical. Therefore, the theoretical differences between Piagetian and Psychometric intelligence do seem to correspond to real differences in cognitive measurement. (p. 750)

Similarly, with Down's Syndrome children, McCune-Nicolich and Hill (1981) found significant correlations between symbolic development as assessed through play and psychometrically assessed mental age.

Studies of individuals with mental handicap

It is beyond the scope of this chapter to review all studies of cognitive development in mentally handicapped people which have employed the instruments described here. We have already pointed to Kahn's (1985) review of work with the Uzgiris-Hunt Ordinal Scales while Hogg and Sebba (1986a, Chapter 8) have considered work using a variety of instruments relevant to profoundly retarded multiply impaired people. Kahn's review is encouraging with respect to this population, though he urges the need for more research. Hogg and Sebba argue that the movement towards viewing even the most impaired children within the framework of development derived from nonimpaired children seems justified by the available information. Not only can such people be assessed within this framework, but in many respects their development is extraordinarily similar, though extremely prolonged, when compared with their nonhandicapped peers. Additional sensory and physical impairments in individuals who are profoundly retarded also appear to have similar effects on development as they do in children who are not mentally handicapped, though here the evidence is very restricted. It is also clear, however, that extensive brain damage, epilepsy, and failures of social development can disrupt sequences of development and may preclude advances in a given area. This state of affairs should not be seen as a limitation to the applicability of the developmental frame of reference, but as a pointer to psychological, social or medical mediation that places the person firmly within that context.

Smith (1982) also undertook a number of assessments of language, symbolic functioning, self-help, number work and motor abilities in addition to her cognitive assessment. The children assessed were between CA seven to thirteen years. Significant correlations between all these measures (including cognition) were found, with the exception of expressive language. Smith presents her results separately in five groups: (1) No specific pathology. (2) Down's Syndrome. (3) Specific medical diagnosis. (4) Trauma. (5) Arrested development. For average data there was no dramatic improvement across the years although steady progress was noted. Between eleven and twelve years significant improvements were found in cognition, representational drawing and ability to copy forms.

Relation to curriculum development

A major weakness in much curriculum planning for individuals with mental handicap has been the often arbitrary way in which teaching objectives are selected. While a developmental perspective in the development of such curricula is essential, a starting point in psychometric tests has often led to a choice of objectives that have little bearing on the wider competence of the person (see Chapter 7 of this volume). A similar danger exists with respect to the Piagetian-based tests. While it has been amply demonstrated that it is possible to teach the specific activities described in these tests, it is essential that a wider view be developed of the general applicability of the cognitive advances they reflect. Thus, snack-time offers a good opportunity to encourage preoperational thought with respect to number (e.g. of biscuits), volume (of juice) and spatial experience (equivalence of place settings when viewed from different sides of the table). For a full description of teaching content and methods in the sensorimotor and preoperational periods, see Hogg and Sebba (1986b).

In the sensorimotor period, much of this generality will be reflected in structured play situations, though many self-help activities will tap advances. Woodward and Stern (1963) were the first to explore this link and their results will merit a detail comment. Children were classified as being at Sensorimotor Stage III, IV or VI. This placement was then cross-tabulated with three aspects of self-feeding:

(1) *Does not drink from cup.* No Stage VI children were thus classified, while all Stage III, 70 per cent of Stage IV and 24 per cent of Stage V could not drink from a cup. *Drinks if cup held.* Again no Stage VI children came into this category, nor any at Stage III. All who did were either Stage IV or V. *Helps to hold cup.* The majority here were Stage V, with a small proportion of Stage VI requiring such assistance (6 per cent). No Stage III or IV children were able to use a cup even with help. *Hold cup without help.* Again no Stage III or IV children were able to drink independently, while 31 per cent of Stage V children were able to and 94 per cent of Stage VI children could drink from a cup independently.

(2) *Use of fingers for feeding.* All Stage VI children feed themselves with their fingers, and this was also noted for some children in Stage IV and a substantial number at Stage V. No Stage III children fed themselves with their fingers.

(3) *Spoon use*. The majority of Stage VI children could use a spoon without spilling the food, and most of those who could not do so did use a spoon though with some spillage. Only 24 per cent of Stage VI children could not use a spoon. In contrast, most Stage V children and all Stage III and Stage IV could not use a spoon. Indeed, only 20 per cent of Stage V children used a spoon, most spilling food from it. Stage V appears to be the transitional stage and given that none of these children could use spoon or cup at Stage IV, this has clear implications for the cognitive prerequisites of self-feeding and appropriate training programmes.

Recent studies adopt a more global approach than did Woodward, relating performance of sensorimotor scales to standardised measures of adaptive behaviour (Wachs and De Remer 1978 and Kahn 1983).

The link between cognitive development and adaptive behaviour is clearly of central importance in devising curricula for mentally handicapped people. Of equal significance is the question of language and cognition. A variety of studies have demonstrated that it is necessary for the individual to have reached Sensorimotor Stage V or VI before true language begins to emerge. In addition, enhancement of language acquisition following sensorimotor teaching to those levels has also been shown. (For reviews, see Kahn 1985 and Hogg and Sebba 1986b, Chapter 3.) This important link points to the way in which cognitive development needs not only to be treated as a concern in its own right, but must be seen as an essential prerequisite to curriculum areas that are often wrongly taught in isolation.

Considerations in choosing tests

As my review has indicated, there is a limited number of tests available in the various areas considered, though these can be readily supplemented by more elaborate schemes from experimental studies. Despite different emphases, they present a consistent and often complementary picture. Their applicability to people who are severely and profoundly mentally handicapped has been amply demonstrated. Even where multiple handicaps exist their adaptation has been shown to be feasible (Fieber 1977; Stephens 1977). Here questions of positioning and choice of materials are central issues on which these authors have a number of suggestions to make. With less impaired people, presentation can typically take the same form as for the nonhandicapped population. Bearing in mind the emphasis on flexibility of presentation, use of objects preferred by the person, including the use of edible items, it is perfectly justified to tailor the assessment to the person involved.

With respect to sensorimotor development, it is likely that the potential user will opt for the original Uzgiris-Hunt Ordinal Scales or Dunst's (1980) modification. Lowe's (1975) assessment of play suggests itself as the best-documented procedure with regard to symbolic play. In the area of Preoperational Assessment, the conditions and material described by Smith (1982) provide a valuable way of looking at more advanced cognition, though her procedures are not yet available in the form of a commercial test battery.

REFERENCES

Bayley, N. (1969) *Manual for the Bayley Scales of Infant Development*, Psychological Corporation, New York

Bricker, W.A. (1970) 'Identifying and Modifying Behavioral Deficits', *American Journal of Mental Deficiency, 75,* 16–21

Chatelanat, G. and Schoggen, M. (1980) 'Issues Encountered in Devising an Observation System to Assess Spontaneous Infant Behaviour-Environment Interactions' in J. Hogg and P.J. Mittler (eds.), *Advances in Mental Handicap Research: Vol. 1,* Wiley, Chichester and New York

Corman, H.H. and Escalona, S.K. (1969) 'Stages of Sensorimotor Development: A Communication Study', *Merrill-Palmer Quarterly, 15,* 351–61

Coupe, J. and Levy, D. (1985) 'The Object Related Scheme Assessment Procedure: A Cognitive Assessment for Developmentally Young Children who may have Additional Physical or Sensory Handicaps', *Journal of the British Institute of Mental Handicap, 13,* 22–4

DeVries, R. (1974) 'Relationships among Piagetian, IQ and Achievement Assessments', *Child Development, 45,* 746–56

Dunst, C.J. (1980) *Clinical and Educational Manual for Use with the Uzgiris and Hunt Scales of Infant Psychological Development,* Pro-ed, Austin, Texas

Escalona, S.K. and Corman, H.H. (1971a) 'Object Permanence: A Film', Albert Einstein College of Medicine, Division of Audio-Visual Education, New York

Escalona, S.K. and Corman, H.H. (1971b) 'Spatial Relationships: A Film', Albert Einstein College of Medicine, Division of Audio-Visual Education, New York

Feiber, N.M. (1977) 'Sensorimotor Cognitive Assessment and Curriculum for the Multihandicapped child' in J. Cronin (ed.), *The Severely and Profoundly Handicapped Child,* State Board of Education, Illinois

Foxen, T. (1977) 'Play Object Schema', Hester Adrian Research Centre, University of Manchester, Manchester

Gouin Décarie, T. (1962) *Intelligence and Affectivity in Early Childhood*, International Universities Press, New York

Gouin Décarie, T. (1969) 'A Study of Mental and Emotional Development of the Thalidomide Child' in B.F. Foss (ed.), *Determinants of Infant Behaviour: Vol. 4*, Methuen, London

Griffiths, R. (1970) *Griffiths Mental Developmental Scales*, Child Development Research Centre, Taunton

Hogg, J. and Moss, S. (1983) 'Prehensile Development in Down's Syndrome and Non-handicapped Preschool Children', *British Journal of Developmental Psychology, 1*, 189–204

Hogg, J. and Sebba, J. (1986a) *Profound Retardation and Multiple Impairment: Vol 1 Development and Learning*, Croom Helm, London

Hogg, J. and Sebba, J. (1986b) *Profound Retardation and Multiple Impairment: Vol. II, Education and Therapy*, Croom Helm, London

Inhelder, B. (1968) *The Diagnosis of Reasoning in the Mentally Retarded*, Day, New York

Kahn, J.V. (1975) 'Relationship of Piaget's Sensorimotor Period to Language Acquisition of Profoundly Retarded', *American Journal of Mental Deficiency, 79*, 640–3

Kahn, J.V. (1983) 'Sensorimotor Period and Adaptive Behavior Development of Severely and Profoundly Mentally Retarded Children', *American Journal of Mental Deficiency, 88*, 69–75

Kahn, J.V. (1985) 'Uses of Scales of Psychological Development with Mentally Retarded Populations' in I.C. Uzgiris and J. McV. Hunt (eds.), *Research with Scales of Psychological Development in Infancy'*, University of Illinois Press, Champaign, Ill.

Lowe, M. (1975) 'Trends in the Development of Representational Play', *Journal of Child Psychology and Psychiatry, 16*, 33–47

Lowe, M. and Costello, A.J. (1976) *Manual for the Symbolic Play Test: Experimental Edition*, NFER, Windsor

Lunzer, E.A. (1970) 'Construction of a Standardised Battery of Piagetian Tests to Assess the Development of Effective Intelligence', *Research in Education, 3*, 53–72

McCune-Nicholich, L. and Hill, P. (1981) 'A Comparison of Psychometric and Piagetian Assessments of Symbolic Functioning in Down's Syndrome Children' in M.P. Friedman, J.P. Das and N. O'Connor (eds.), *Intelligence and Learning: NATO Conference Series III: Human Factors, Vol. 14*, Plenum, London

Nicholich, L.M. (1977) 'Beyond Sensorimotor Intelligence: Assessment of Symbolic Maturity through Analysis of Pretend Play', *Merrill-Palmer Quarterly, 23*, 89–101

Philips, J.L. (1981) *Piaget's Theory: A Primer*, W.H. Freeman, San Francisco

Piaget, J. (1953) *The Origin of Intelligence in the Child*, Routledge and Kegan Paul, London

Piaget, J. (1955) *The Child's Construction of Reality*, Routledge and Kegan Paul, London

Piaget, J. (1962) *Play, Dreams and Imitation in Childhood*, W.W. Norton, New York

Riguet, C.B., Taylor, N.D., Benaroya, S. and Klein, L.S. (1981) 'Symbolic Play in Autistic, Down's and Normal Children of Equivalent Mental Age',

Journal of Autism and Developmental Disorders, 11, 439–48

Sheridan, M.D. (1969) 'Playthings in the Development of Language', *Health Trends, 1,* 7–10

Sinclair, H. (1971) 'Sensorimotor Action Patterns as a Condition for the Acquisition of Syntax' in R. Huxley and E. Ingram (eds.), *Language Acquisiton: Models and Methods,* Academic Press, London

Smith, B. (1982) 'A Study of Mental Growth in Young Severely Subnormal Children', unpublished Ph.D. thesis, University of Birmingham, Birmingham

Smith, B. (1984) personal communication

Stephens, B. (1977) 'A Piagetian Approach to Curriculum Development for the Severely, Profoundly and Multiply-Handicapped' in E. Sontag (ed.), *Educational Programming for the Severely and Profoundly Handicapped,* Council for Exceptional Children, Reston, Va.

Uzgiris, I. and Hunt, J. McV. (1975) *Assessment in Infancy: Ordinal Scales of Psychological Development,* University of Illinois Press, London and Champaign, Ill.

Wachs, T.D. (1975) 'Relation of Infant's Performance on Piaget Scales between Twelve and Twenty-four Months and their Stanford-Binet Performance at 31 Months', *Child Development, 46,* 929–35

Wachs, T.D. and De Remer, P. (1978) 'Adaptive Behavior and Uzgiris-Hunt Scale Performance of Young Developmentally Delayed Children', *American Journal of Mental Deficiency, 83,* 171–6

Whittaker, C.A. (1980) 'A Note on Developmental Trends in Symbolic Play of Hospitalized Profoundly Retarded Children', *Journal of Child Psychology and Psychiatry, 21,* 253–61

Wing, L., Gould, J., Yeates, S.R. and Brierly, L.M. (1977) 'Symbolic Play in Severely Mentally Retarded and in Autistic Children', *Journal of Child Psychology and Psychiatry, 18,* 167–78

Woodward, W.M. (1959) 'The Behaviour of Idiots Intepreted by Piaget's Theory of Sensorimotor Development', *British Journal of Educational Psychology, 29,* 60–71

Woodward, W.M. (1967) Notes on Techniques Devised for the Assessment of Severely Subnormal and Young Normal Children on the Basis of Piaget's Observations and Interpretation of Sensorimotor Development, University College Swansea, Swansea

Woodward, W.M. (1972) 'Problem-solving Strategies of Young Children', *Journal of Child Psychology and Psychiatry, 13,* 11–24

Woodward, W.M. (1979) 'Piaget's Theory and the Study of Mental Retardation' in N.R. Ellis (ed.), *Handbook of Mental Deficiency, Psychological Theory, and Research,* 2nd edn, Lawrence Erlbaum, Hillsdale, NJ

Woodward, W.M. (1983) 'The Development of Thinking in Young Children: The Problem of Analysis', *International Journal of Behavioral Development, 6,* 441–60

Woodward, W.M. (1984) personal communication

Woodward, W.M. and Hunt, M.R. (1972) 'Exploratory Studies of Early Cognitive Development', *British Journal of Educational Psychology, 42,* 248–59

Woodward, M.W. and Stern, D.J. (1963) 'Developmental Patterns of Severely Subnormal Children', *British Journal of Educational Psychology, 33,* 10–21

4

Adaptive Behaviour Scales

N. V. Raynes

GENERAL CHARACTERISTICS OF THE APPROACH

The concept of adaptive behaviour, initially referred to as 'social competence', has been defined by Heber (1961) as 'the effectiveness with which the individual copes with the nature and social demands of his environment' (p. 61). Its development was in part a reaction to the felt inadequacy of IQ as a measure of human performance and in part a response to the need to find a basis for the overall functional classification of people with mental handicap.

Unlike IQ, adaptive behaviour is assumed to be capable of short-term environmental manipulation. Efforts to measure adaptive behaviour have a long history and have focused on the assessment of a person's current abilities as they are manifest in particular social situations. An inference is made that these measured skills will be applied adaptively in a variety of different social contexts. The products of an adaptive behavioural assessment can be used as the basis for a programme plan for an individual mentally handicapped person. They may also be used, with caution, to explore change in that person's behaviour.

In trying to assess adaptive behaviour we are trying to measure a potential for an adaptive process. To do this it is not enough to measure a single skill, for example, the ability to use a knife. We need to measure and analyse patterns of many skills which characterise an individual in a given setting. There are obviously an infinite number of skills which we could look at. Existing scales vary in the number of skills they cover and items relating to them. Statistically measures have been used to group together a number of items relating to particular skills which appear to be measuring a factor. The skills are then further grouped together to constitute domains. Some scales group many behaviours into huge general domains, in other instruments the domains are quite specific. The domains usually included are communication; physical development; self-help; community orientation; vocational skills; academic skills; and personality and behaviour problems. The domains identified in the many instruments do not necessarily represent independent areas but they are often useful in providing a basis for thinking about adaptive behaviour and for helping in the interpretation of the results of an assessment.

THE DEVELOPMENT OF THE CONCEPT OF ADAPTIVE BEHAVIOUR

In the 1920s Edgar Doll began to work on the *Vineland Social Maturity Scale*. This was first published in 1935 (Doll 1935). Doll was attempting to measure an overall characteristic of human performance which he called 'social competence'. Doll understood social competence in terms of social responsibility and personal independence. These were the products of cultural, physical, intellectual, habitual, emotional, occupational, educational, and other factors.

Doll stressed that 'social competence' was a dynamic phenomenon. Thus it could be quantified in terms of normative scales and deviations from normal maturational development. It reflected in essence progressive self-development and independence. In the construction of his scale, Doll drew from child development data and descriptions of adult behaviour. His measure generated a social age and social quotient score. For a long time his *Vineland Social Maturity Scale* was unique in measuring people's actual abilities as they were manifest in everyday situations. It can be seen to be the first type of the adaptive behaviour scales which are now legion.

Further development of measures of adaptive behaviour were given a boost by the decision of the American Association of Mental Deficiency in 1952 to set up a committee to study nomenclature because of the dissatisfaction of relying on IQ scores alone to classify mentally handicapped people. This committee recommended that levels of retardation should reflect educational, motor, social and other abilities in addition to intelligence. Its work led eventually to the publication of a 'Manual on Terminology Classification in Mental Retardation' (Heber, 1961). This manual was the first to officially incorporate a concept of adaptive behaviour into the definition of mental retardation. In the manual mental retardation is defined as 'sub-average general intellectual functioning which originates during the developmental period and is associated with impairment in adaptive behaviour' (Heber 1961, p. 3). This definition is now familiar to most people working with mentally handicapped individuals. Adaptive behaviour was thought to be an age-related concept which reflected the overall effectiveness with which individuals adapt to the natural and social demands of their environments. Heber suggested that although there was no comprehensive standardised measure of adaptive behaviour at the time the 1961 manual on terminology and classification was published, the Vineland Social Maturity Scale would be the best instrument with which to obtain measures of adaptive behaviour.

The continued development of the concept of adaptive behaviour was very much an American phenomenon. With the exception of Gunzberg in the UK, British psychiatrists and psychologists seemed to be wedded to the power of IQ as a basis for classification of people with mental handicap and the crude performance indicators subsumed in the definitions idiot, imbecile and feeble-minded.

In 1964 the American Association on Mental Deficiency in conjunction with the Parsons State Hospital and Training Center received an NIMH grant to study the function and measurement of adaptive behaviour. A series of special conferences ensued and brought together people interested in the concept of adaptive behaviour (Leland, Nihira, Foster, Shellhaas and Kagin 1966). At this stage emphasis was placed on the development of meaures to predict community adjustment, that is a measure with a diagnostic function rather than the development of measures for the purpose of individual programme planning. The single form for people of any age was developed (Nihira, Foster, Shellhaas and Leland 1974).

Many of the designers of the multiplicity of tests which now exist began by reviewing assessment instruments and adapting items from them which seemed to fit their particular needs. Other researchers have obtained item information from interviews with parents and used the observation of parents and professionals to identify critical behaviour. The selection of items has reflected the need to assess behaviours which are observable and for which the degree of proficiency of performance and the environmental conditions present at the time can be specified. Hence questions are written by and large in behavioural language. The responses can be obtained either by direct observation or (more usually) through an interview with someone who knows the individual being assessed or the completion of a self-administered questionnaire by such a person. The development of measures of adaptive behaviour have involved:

(1) the identification of behaviours in relation to the environment in which they occur;
(2) generating and selecting assessment items;
(3) developing administration procedures;
(4) developing scoring procedures.

When these tasks have been carried out a series of statistical procedures are usually undertaken to determine the degree of meaningfulness of the items in the assessments and the items as a group. The statistical analyses lead to the final selection of items for inclusion in the assessment instrument.

A number of approaches have been adopted to determine which items should be retained in the final versions of the instruments. Items in the *Adaptive Behavior Scale* (Nihira *et al.* 1974) were evaluated and selected on the basis of: (1) their inter-rater reliability; (2) their effectiveness in discriminating amongst mentally handicapped people living in institutions who have been classified as different adaptive behaviour levels; and (3) their effectiveness in discriminating amongst adaptive behaviour levels when variations due to measured intelligence were statistically controlled. Items on other measures have been retained on the basis of:

(1) their ability to discriminate along progressively difficult levels related to age;
(2) agreement among judges as to rank ordering of items along the social competency continuum;
(3) the undimensionality of items in terms of particular skills;
(4) the applicability of items to their sexes; and
(5) the observability of each piece of behaviour in the home and its susceptibility to rating by parents.

Just as there is no one criterion for the final selection of items which have been incorporated in the many adaptive behaviour scales which have been developed, so there is no single criterion in terms of which we may judge the utility and efficacy of a particular instrument.

COMPREHENSIVE LISTING AND DESCRIPTION OF THE MAIN EXAMPLES

In the United States staff of the Individualized Data Base (IDB) Project carried out a survey of existing techniques relating to performance measures of skills and adaptive competences in people who are developmentally disabled. The team identified 132 such measures (IDB Project 1977). The development of measures to test adaptive behaviours has proliferated. As each research worker or clinician has attempted to use an instrument for diagnostic or programme planning purposes it appears as if he or she has felt that these are inadequate or overelaborate for his or her specific purposes. Most of the development in this area has occurred in the United States but some tests have been developed and applied specifically in the United Kingdom. It is not possible within one chapter to review all of these instruments. The majority of American ones are reported in *Performance Measures of Skill and Adaptive Competences in the Developmentally Disabled* (IDB Project 1977). Short descriptions are given below of six English instruments frequently referred to in the literature and five of the many instruments developed and used in the USA. They are listed alphabetically beginning with those instruments which have been developed in England.

Tests of adaptive behaviour

Six English Examples

The Development Team for the Mentally Handicapped Mental Handicap Assessment Form. Initially the Development Team for the Mentally Handicapped following on the work of the National Development Group (1977) used the assessment form developed by the Wessex Health Care Evaluation Research Team, which is referred to below (Kushlick *et al.* 1973). The Development Team, before their visit to the various residential facilities, asked the care team involved in these facilities to complete for each resident the Mental Handicap Register Form which had been developed by the Wessex team. The information obtained was to give the team data about the residents in the establishments they were to study. The form was subsequently revised and the product was different in a number of ways from that now in use in Wessex (Development Team for the Mentally Handicapped 1982). The Development Team's own

Mental Handicap Assessment Form is a short form designed for use in the assessment of mentally handicapped people of all ranges of ability over the age of five years. It is still used by the team to obtain information about the clients in the facilities it continues to visit.

The assessment form has 29 questions grouped in eight sections. The sections are general; continence; mobility; behavioural problems; self-help; sensory abilities; skills; and medical problems. The items are rated to reflect levels of ability and the responses are precoded. It can be completed by care staff in any residential setting, social workers or parents. It is self-adminstered and has accompanying brief notes and it takes a few minutes to complete the form. The form is designed in such a way that the information can be easily processed by computer.

The information from the asesssment can be used to place a person in one of four groupings derived by the Development Team for use with mentally handicapped people in long-term care to determine an appropriate placement for them. These groupings are linked to an opinion concerning the type of care required (Development Team for the Mentally Handicapped 1980). The classification of people in these groupings is seen by the Development Team as an informatory first step which 'should always be followed by a joint assessment by representatives of Health and Social Services using the more detailed "progress profile" ' (Development Team for the Mentally Handicapped 1980, p. 6).

The form can be obtained from the Development Team for the Mentally Handicapped, Department of Health and Social Security, Alexander Fleming House, Elephant and Castle, London SE1. The system of classification is clearly spelt out in the second report of the Development Team for the Mentally Handicapped (1980).

Disability Assessment Schedule (DAS). This instrument was developed from a combination of items in two other measures: the *Wessex Behaviour Rating Scale* (Kushlick, Blunden and Cox 1973 — see below) and the *Children's Handicap Behaviour Skills Structured Interview Schedule* (Wing and Gould 1978). It was developed for use in a study of adults, one purpose of which was to explore the importance of communication, symbolic activity and social interaction as guides to management and placement. Such behaviours have been shown to be a more useful guide to management in children than have overall IQs (Wing and Gould 1979).

In its current form the DAS is designed to obtain information about mentally handicapped adults and children. The authors argue that it is different from other assessments of performance of mentally handicapped people in that it contains items concerning impairment of nonverbal communication, social interaction; and a wide range of behavioural abnormalities.

The instrument has 44 items which are grouped into eight sections. These sections are self-help skills; vision and hearing; communication; literacy; domestic and practical skills; behavioural problems; abnormalities of social and imaginative activities; stereotypes and echolalia. Each of the sections contains two or more items and each item has it own precoded rating. The higher the rating the higher the level of development.

The information is obtained by an interviewer carrying out a structured interview with someone who knows the client well. The interviewer has to make decisions regarding the rating that best describes the client. The Disability Assessment Schedule 'may only be administered by individuals who have been trained by the authors' (Holmes, Shah and Wing 1982, p. 879). The assessment takes a trained interviewer between 20 and 25 minutes to complete for each client.

A profile can be drawn for each client from the information obtained providing a system of sub-classification which it is claimed 'is more detailed than any based solely on self-help skills, physical and sensory handicaps or behaviour problems' (Holmes *et al.* 1982, p. 879). The Disability Assessment Schedule can be obtained from the Medical Research Council, Social Psychiatry Research Unit, Institute of Psychiatry, De Crespigny Park, London SE5 8AF.

Hampshire Assessment for Living with Others (HALO). HALO was developed to provide an aid to decision-making about the type and level of residential services required for an individual and an individual adult's major training needs by Shackleton-Bailey in collaboration with Hampshire Social Services. It is one of four linked assessment tests and is best used for assessments related to residential service needs for adult mentally handicapped people. The other three assessments are HANC2 for use by training centre staff and a handicapped person; HANC-F, a test for use with families; and HANC-S, a test for use in schools.

HALO is designed for use with mentally handicapped adults and children but the authors note that its use is 'limited with those who have the most profound physical and mental handicaps' (Shackleton-Bailey and Pidcock 1983, p. 5).

There are 276 items in HALO which is divided into ten major sections. These are self-care; domestic skills; community living skills; communication; personality; close circle relations; use of leisure; health/physical disabilities; group membership; and employment. Each section has a different number of items. The assessor rates the individual's level of independence indicating whether this rating is observation-based or not. Symbols relate the individual's level of independence and behaviour to the client's service needs within three types of residence. The types of residence reflect the different levels of service offered: high, medium and low. The first level is typified by Social Services hostels, the last by a minimally staffed or unstaffed Group Home.

Information is collected by a person who knows the individual being assessed well. It is recommended that the assessment be based on observation and also discussion with the client. The assessment may be carried out by 'anyone with responsibility for housing, teaching or caring for adults with a mental handicap' (Shackleton-Bailey and Pidcock 1983, p. 5). A companion book of behavioural anchors and a user's book are available. The author also runs an action workshop and a self-teaching tape is being developed to train people in the use of the assessment procedures. The assessment can take up to five hours to complete.

When the ratings are completed a profile of the client's requirements for service within the three types of settings referred to above is obtained by totalling the symbols. Each profile shows graphically 'the number of skills in which a resident requires no more service than is routinely provided' (Shackleton-Bailey undated, p. 4). Once this profile of independence has been completed and a placement plan agreed, the assessor can use the information to inform decisions about training priorities.

Copies of HALO and the other assessment systems related to it can be obtained from Hampshire Social Services, Trafalgar House, The Castle, Winchester SO23 8UQ.

Progress Assessment Chart of Social and Personal Development. A series of Progress Assessment charts have been developed by Gunzberg (1966, 1968a, 1977). There are six of these designed for use with a different age group. They were developed for client assessment and to provide a data basis for individual programme planning. One of them is specifically designed for use with Down's Syndrome clients. All of the others are for use with mentally handicapped people whose abilities range from profound to borderline mental handicap. Here I discuss as an example of these charts the Progress Assessment Chart 1 of Social Development (P-A-C-1). The P-A-C-1 was developed to assess the social development of mentally handicapped children aged 6–16 years and to provide a basis for programme planning and evaluation for them.

The P-A-C-1 has four domains. Three of these are self-help, communication and socialisation. These have 40 items, and the fourth domain, occupation, has 20 items. The items are mainly binary, requiring a yes/no response and the results can be represented visually in a chart of concentric circles. Each circle represents a higher level of skill, the innermost circle representing the very basic level.

The information is best collected by someone familiar with the client's behaviour, e.g. a parent, teacher or primary caretaker; in lieu of this interviewing someone familiar with the handicapped individual and combining this information with direct observation is described as an acceptable procedure for collecting the information.

Completion of the assessment can, as indicated, generate a visual profile of the individual's skill levels and additionally can be used in conjunction with the Progress Evaluation Index which provides information relating to average achievement levels of peers.

Each of the Progress Assessment Charts are available from SEFA Publications Ltd., The Globe, 4 Great William Street, Stratford-upon-Avon.

The Scale for Assessing Coping Skills (SACS). This scale, developed by Whelan and Speake (1979), was designed initially as a tool for use by parents to assess the performance levels of their mentally handicapped sons and daughters. It has subsequently been used by staff working with mentally handicapped adults in a variety of settings to facilitate decision-making about the types of appropriate training.

There are 36 items in the scale grouped under the headings self-help; social/academic and inter-personal skills. Each of the items within these groupings is described at five levels of difficulty. The person completing the scale puts a tick in the box opposite the statement which appropriately describes the individual's performance for each level of the item identified in the scale. There are seven boxes in a row. These are grouped under headings which represent the rating which ranges from 'can do without any help or supervision' to 'cannot yet do' and additionally 'do not know whether the individual can do this'. Boxes 5–7 are concerned with whether the ability is adequately used or not and range from 'uses the ability in adequate amount' to 'there is no opportunity to do this'.

No information is given about the length of time it takes to complete the 36 items in the scale which, having five levels within them, in effect constitute 180 scale elements.

The information is collected by someone who knows the individual mentally handicapped person well. He or she needs no special training to complete the form but the authors encourage the use of observation as a basis for the rating of the items. The questionnaire is self-administered.

Further details are given in the book *Learning to Cope* (Whelan and Speak, 1979). Users of the scale are recommended to obtain a copy of that book for description of the methods, which amongst other things provides advice about the application of SACS. The scale itself contains a set of instructions for its completion.

The scale can be purchased by writing to Copewell Publications, 29 Worcester Road, Alkrington, Middleton, Manchester M24 1PA.

Wessex Behaviour Rating Scale. This was originally developed by Kushlick and Cox (1973) for a survey of mentally handicapped people in the Wessex region carried out in 1963. It was intended for use with people of all ages and all levels of mental handicaps where assessment relating to problems with management was required rather than assessment based on clinical syndromes.

In the latest version there are 21 questions grouped under three headings used for the assessment. These are: incapacities (15 items); speech (1 item); and behaviour problems (5 items). These items are precoded reflecting levels of dependence.

The questionnaire was designed so that information could be collected and recorded quickly and easily by the people concerned with the day-to-day management of mentally handicapped children and adults. Thus it is intended for use by parents, nursing and other direct care staff for those mentally handicapped people who are living in residential care.

The questions are framed in terms of behaviours which could be assessed as objectively as possible. No training is required for completion of the questionnaire. Notes accompany it and it can be completed quickly.

The information derived from the questionnaire has been used to generate a number of sub-scales. Two scales were originally devised. The Social and Physical Incapacity Scale (SPI) is based on the items in the questionnaire concerned with incontinence, mobility and behaviour disorders. The second scale, the Speech, Self Help and Literacy Scale (SSL), is derived from items relating to speech, feeding, washing and dressing and to reading, writing and counting. These sub-scales are intended for use in the planning of services for individually mentally handicapped persons with particular regard to the kind of care they are to receive. More recently a fivefold classification combining the SPI and SSL has been developed. This new classification comprises the following categories: nonambulant (NA); severe behaviour disorder with severe incontinence or severe behaviour disorder alone (SB); severe incontinence (SI); continent, ambulant, no severe behaviour disorder — incorporates mild or no handicap and SSL or speech only (CAN); continent, ambulant, no severe disorder, feeds, washes and dresses self — incorporates people who would have mild or no handicap on the old SPI and who would on the SSL score as self-help only or speech and self-help to literate (CAN FWD).

The Wessex Joint Planning Group introduced a rule determining which agency was to be responsible for the provision of residential care and the assessment data provide enough information to categorise the person as the responsibility of the National Health Service or Social Services. Different criteria were used in the categorisation of the appropriate service agency for children and adults.

In its current form the instrument is still intended to produce data for service planners 'enabling the planners to estimate the scale of provision needed for various kinds of service' (Palmer and Jenkins 1982, p. 2). The ratings are intended to generate lists of mentally handicapped people who according to their age, their area of residence and their disability level may be eligible for a particular type of service. The schedule can also be used for research purposes.

The Wessex Behaviour Rating Scale can be obtained from John Palmer at the Wessex Regional Health Authority, High Croft, Romsey Road, Winchester, Hampshire.

American Examples

The Adaptive Behavior Scale (ABS). This scale was developed by Nihira *et al.* (1974) originally in 1969. It has gone through a number of revisions since then. The most recent of these occurred in 1974. The scale was developed to be used for client assessment and invidiual programme planning and assessing the total programming needs of groups of clients for research purposes.

It can be used to make assessments of mentally retarded, emotionally maladjusted and developmentally disabled persons of all ages from childhood or adulthood.

It is divided into two parts. Part I is concerned with matters described as adaptive behaviour and comprises ten domains with a total of 66 items. The domains are: independent functioning; physical development; economic activity; language development;

numbers and time; domestic activity; vocational activity; self-direction; responsibility; and socialisation. The items in these domains are predominantly ordered from highest to lowest at developmental levels but some are in binary format. Part II of the instrument is concerned with what are called maladaptive behaviours. These are grouped into 14 domains. They include: violent and destructive behaviour; untrustworthy behaviour; withdrawal; stereotyped behaviour; inappropriate inter-personal manners; unacceptable vocal habits; unacceptable or eccentric habits; self-abusive behaviour; hyperactive tendencies; sexually aberrant behaviour; psychological disturbances; and use of medication. There is at least one item within each of these areas. There are a total of 43 items in this section of the assessment instrument. The items in Part II are rated by the frequency of the occurrence of the maladaptive behaviour. (This is discussed more fully in Chapter 5 of this volume.)

The ABS is designed for use by someone who knows the individual being assessed. Thus it can for example be completed by a residential care worker or teacher. The assessor records responses to the item on the questionnaire, and no special training to complete it is necessary. There are related instructions within the questionnaire itself and scoring sheets and profile summary sheets. Additionally a detailed manual about completing ABS and scoring the information obtained from it is available.

The raw scores can be interpreted by percentile ranks relative to national norms and these can provide a profile summary for the client. The percentile ranks are based on national norms established in the USA for discrete age groups for profoundly to mildly mentally handicapped people living in residential institutions.

Copies of the ABS, and the associated manual and scoring sheets, can be obtained from American Association on Mental Deficiency, 1719 Kalorama Road, Washington, D.C., 20009.

Balthazar Scales of Adaptive Behaviour (BSAB): A System for Programme Evaluation and Development: (1) scales of functional independence; (2) scales of social adaptation. These scales were developed by Balthazar (1973, 1976). They were designed to be used for client assessment, for programme planning and for evaluation as well as research.

They are to be used with developmentally disabled, mentally retarded or emotionally disturbed people within the age range 5–57 years.

The BSAB-1 is focused on three domains: eating; dressing; and toileting. It contains 88 items. The BSAB-2 focuses on unadaptive and adaptive self-directed behaviours; unadaptive and adaptive inter-personal behaviours; play activities; responses to instructions; personal care; and other behaviours. There are 71 items in the BSAB-2. (This is discussed fully in Chapter 5 of this volume.)

The BSAB is essentially a sequential weighting scale in which items are grouped serially from low to high. Each item is rated on a 0–10 scale where zero signifies a behaviour which never occurs and 10 signifies a behaviour which happens 10 out of 10 times.

The rating scales can be completed by anyone who knows the client well. Some practice is advised, as is the use of the associated manual. The information is collected using direct observation of the client while he or she is engaged in typical daily activities. A profile of the client can be obtained from the completed scale. The BSAB was standardised on severely and profoundly ambulant institutionalised persons aged 5–57 with IQs of less than 35. Percentile norms are available for each sub-scale (domain) within the BSAB-1 so that an individual's performance on these can be compared with that of his peers.

The scales can be obtained from Consulting Psychologists Press Incorporated, 577 College Avenue, Palo Alto, California 94306. Reference norms are also available from them.

The Behavior Development Survey. The Behavior Development Survey is a modified and short form of the AAMD Adaptive Behavior Scale (ABS). It is therefore very similar to the ABS but a shorter time is required to complete it. The development of such an instrument was requested during the course of the work being carried out by the staff at the Lanterman State Hospital in California for the Individualised Data Base Project. The instrument can be used for assessment of individuals, the development of individual programme plans and for research purposes.

It is designed for use with developmentally disabled people of the same age range and levels of ability as the ABS.

Like the ABS the Behavior Development Survey is in two parts. Part I, the adaptive behaviour section of the instrument, contains 32 items, yielding three domains. The domains are personal self-sufficiency (10 items); community self-sufficiency (15 items); and personal self-responsibility (7 items). The items in each domain are structured along developmental lines and a rating has to be made for each item.

Part II of the instrument contains 11 items relating to personality and behaviour disorders. The response format for these differs from that in the second part of the ABS. Two domains have been identified. These are social adaptation (7 items) and personal adaptation (4 items).

The Behavior Development Survey also contains 19 items which are not added into the scores in the five domains. They are included because they are thought to be significant characteristics of the client and to provide necessary information for planning for care and training. They are grouped into four areas: health and medical; cognitive and communicative; social living; and personal problems requiring special attention.

Anyone who knows the client well can complete the assessment. It can be carried out in a variety of settings. When the rater is familiar with the client he/she should complete the questionnaire. A 'third party' procedure may be used to carry out the assessment where several people are needed to provide the information or the person best able to provide it cannot complete the schedule itself.

A computer scoring service is available for Behavior Development Survey users as well as work sheets for hand-scoring.

There are several uses for the information the Behavior Development Survey provides. It can generate a profile for the purpose of planning individual programmes or for comparing changes in competency over time. Additionally an individual's scores can be compared with those of an appropriate norm/peer group since national norm figures are based on 13,140 institutionalised and 6,145 community-based developmentally disabled people. Additionally percentage factor scores can be obtained (IDB 1979).

The assessment questionnaire and the latest manual can be obtained from the Individualized Data Base Project, UCLA, Neuropsychiatric Institute Research Group at Lanterman State Hospital, Pomona, California.

Cain-Levine Social Competency Scale. This scale was developed by Cain, Levine and Elzey (1963). The information from it can be used for client assessment, individual programme planning and evaluation and total programme planning for a group of clients.

It was intended for use with trainable, moderately retarded children aged 5–13 years.

There are four domains. These are self-help (13 items); initiative (10 items); social skills (10 items); and communications (10 items).

The four or five behaviour descriptions within each item are ordered from the least difficult (i.e. most dependent) to the most difficult (i.e. most independent) level. Although anyone can use the rating system it is recommended that the manual accompanying it is studied first. the scale is then completed by interviewing someone familiar with the client on a day-to-day basis, for example a parent or a residential care worker.

The instrument has been standardised on 716 trainable mentally retarded children aged 5–13 (IQs 25–59). Thus percentile ranks for specified age groups are available to permit comparisons of an individual's performance.

The Social Competency Scale can be obtained from Consulting Psychologists Press, 577 College Avenue, Palo Alto, California 94306.

The Vineland Social Maturity Scale. This was developed by Doll (1935). It has been revised several times since its first appearance, the most recent revision occurring in 1965 (Doll 1965). It was intended to be used for programme evaluation and in research.

The scale was designed to assess the social competence of individuals of all ages from birth to 30 years. It was for use with mentally handicapped and other people such as those who are blind, deaf or physically handicapped.

There are seven domains. These are: self-help general (14 items); self-help eating (12 items); self-help dressing (13 items); self-direction (14 items); occupation (22 items); communication (15 items); and locomotion (10 items). The items of the scale are arranged sequentially in order of increasing average difficulty and represent progressive maturation. Items are scored plus for those items the client does perform and minus for those items not performed. For items that are in transitional or emergent state a half credit is given.

The information has to be collected by a trained examiner through an interviewer with an informant who is familiar with the client on a day-to-day basis, for example, a parent or residential care worker. The examiner has to obtain as much information as is possible about a subject's performance with regard to a particular behaviour. To do this he or she has to use judgement in structuring the question and adapting the order of items until each item can be scored. A manual is available to provide the rater with guidance (Doll 1965).

Scoring the items gives the basis for a Social Age or Social Quotient for the subject. The scale is categorised by age means which are given for each item so an individual's performance can be compared normatively. The scale itself was calibrated on a sample of 620 normal subjects selected by age (from birth to 30 years, and social status (using parental occupation).

The Vineland Social Maturity Scale can be obtained from the American Guidance Service Incorporated, Publishers' Building,

Circle Pines, Minnesota.

MEASURES OF ADAPTIVE BEHAVIOUR: TECHNICAL INFORMATION AND APPLICATION

There should be available information about the reliability, validity and standardisation of any instrument developed to measure adaptive behaviour. (These terms have been defined in the Chapter 2.) However, such a requirement is not always met.

Reliability

Trying to assess the reliability of adaptive behaviour scales is not easy. The content of these scales is rarely homogeneous simply because they sample a wide range of behaviours. Additionally many of the scales use a variety of item formats. For example, yes/no responses are used for some items and rating scale responses are used for others, as for example in the ABS. However, because the assessments by and large are made on the basis of an informed observer's judgement regarding what the mentally handicapped person being assessed can or cannot do, measures of inter-observer agreement within and across different settings and of stability over short periods of time do appear to be the most appropriate means of assessing the reliability of these measures. One should therefore look for the existence of such measures of reliability in assessing whether the test is a reliable one which you can use.

Validity

It is also difficult to establish the validity of measures of adaptive behaviour. The reasons for this have been well summarised by Hill and Bruininks (1977). They state:

(1) definitions of adaptive behavior are general and provide little guidance in clearly defined areas of content; (2) adaptive behavior is likely to be a function of many complex influences such as the characteristics of the setting, the abilities of the person and the social value to the person of expressing behaviors expressed by any given instrument; (3) objective criteria of

adjustment for validating adaptive behavior do not exist. Given these considerations approaches that stress all aspects of validity — concurrent, predictive, content and construct — should be used in developing and researching adaptive behavior scales. (p. 27)

Standardisation

Not all adaptive behaviour scales have been standardised. This is often because they have been developed for particular purposes. Age-related norms for the performance of specified behaviours or domains are thus not always available. This will limit the interpretation you can put on the results when such norms are not available so you are precluded from making any comparison of an individual's performance with that of his age peers.

Below I have provided some information about the availability of such technical information with regard to the assessment instruments already described and I have also indicated some of the uses to which they have been put. The same convention, that of listing first the English and then the American tests, and in both instances listing them in alphabetical order, has been followed.

English Tests

Disability Assessment Schedule (DAS)
Validity: No data are yet available about this. The authors propose to explore it.
Reliability: Extensive studies of reliablity of the DAS have been carried out (Holmes, Shah and Wing 1982). Levels of inter-rater reliability of between 78 per cent and 90 per cent are reported and test-retest levels of reliability of 74 per cent and above.
Standardisation: No information is available about this.
Applications: The instrument is being used in studies of deinstitutionalisation in England (Humphreys *et al.* 1983; Rawlings 1985). It is also used by the Salford Case Register.

Hampshire Assessment for Living with Others (HALO)
Validity: Shackleton-Bailey and Pidcock (1983) report that the validity of the instrument has not yet been examined.
Reliability: Shackleton-Bailey and Pidcock (1983) report test-restest levels of reliability ranging from 0.42 to 0.96 with inter-rater reliability levels 'generally lower' but at levels the authors state 'to

be generally satisfactory' (Shackleton-Bailey and Pidcock 1983 p. 47).
Standardisation: No data are given on the standardisation of the instrument.
Application: This instrument is used by Health and Social Services staff in Hampshire and elsewhere. Since 1980 more than 500 HALO assessments have been made in the Social and Health Services.

The development team for the mentally handicapped mental handicap assessment form
Validity: No information is given about this.
Reliability: No information is given about the reliability of the instrument itself but the Development Team's second report (Development Team for the Mentally Handicapped 1980) states that the system of classification derived from it, the four groupings, are periodically checked for 'inter-observer variations' (p. 5) which is said to be less than 5 per cent.
Standardisation: No information on standardisation is available.
Application: The instrument has been used to collect information about 15,000 adults and 1,400 children in hospital (Development Team for the Mentally Handicapped, second and third reports, 1980 and 1982), and it is known to be in use in several Health Authorities and Social Service Departments (personal communication).

Progress Assessment Charts
Validity: Several studies of the validity of the P-A-C-1 of Social Development have been carried out (Marshall, 1967; Elliot and MacKay 1971). Domain scores were inter-correlated giving coefficients ranging from 0.54 to 0.91. Domain scores were also correlated with Stanford-Binet scores of subjects. Coefficients range from 0.37 to 0.61.
Reliability: No information is available about this.
Standardisation: The P-A-C-1 was standardised on a sample of 337 children aged 6–16 years in training centres in England. The norms are contained in the Progress Evaluation Index.
Application: The P-A-C-1 has been used in several British and American studies (Gunzberg 1968b; Elliot and MacKay 1971) and is used in service settings in England and the USA.

The Scale for Assessing Coping Skills (SACS)
Validity: Content validity was reported as 'achieved by the inclusion of items of high relevance to independent functioning' (Whelan 1984). Concurrent validity is reported by reference to studies

showing differential scores of SACS of individuals performing at different levels of community independence or receiving different levels of training (Whelan 1984).
Reliability: Inter-rater reliability is reported ranging from 71.3 per cent to 68.8 per cent. Test-retest reliability levels achieved are reported as between 79 per cent and 81 per cent.
Standardisation: Nothing is reported about this.
Application: The use of the measure is reported in Whelan and Speak (1979) and it is in use in many Social Education Centres.

The Wessex behaviour rating scale
Validity: Kushlick *et al.* (1973) cite as evidence of validity: (1) the estimate provided by the census data for which purpose the measure was originally used. These estimates 'have been extremely realistic and the management problems presented by those entering the new unit have been much as expected from the data' (p. 471). (2) The mortality of those identified in the 1963 census was studied in 1967 and the result showed that 'proportionately more of those rated as severely handicapped had died by the end of 1967' (p. 472).
Reliability: Levels of reliability between cases are reported by Kushlick *et al.* (1973), giving 67 per cent overall for the SPI sub-scale and 76 per cent for the SSL sub-scale. Palmer and Jenkins (1982) more recently report on an inter-rater reliability study based on systematic investigation using pairs of raters in the same setting for each subject, ensuring adequate representation of different ages and levels of ability. Their examination was of the reliability of the new fivefold classification and they note that the levels of reliability achieved are 'well above chance but not particularly high' (p. 6). They question whether the system should be used in service management for selecting clients as potential recipients of a particular form of care but are more positive about the use of the measure in large-scale surveys.
Application: The instrument has been used in the process of compiling the Mental Handicap Register in Wessex. It is also used in other parts of England in service settings. It has been recently redesigned in such a way that the data can be easily used to generate the original Wessex sub-categories or the categories of the Development Team for the Mentally Handicapped (see above).

American Tests

Adaptive Behavior Scale (ABS)
Validity: Several studies of different aspects of validity including

predictive, concurrent and content validity have been reported (Lambert and Nicoll 1976; Nihira 1976).
Reliability: The reliability reported in the manual was based on the administration of the revised ABS to 133 retarded residents in three state institutions. The reliability for Part I is reported to be 0.86 and for Part II 0.57 between ratings given by ward personnel working morning and evening shifts (Fogelman 1975).
Standardisation: Percentile ranks have been developed based on national norms for profoundly to mildly retarded people in residential institutions in the age range 3–69 years (Fogelman 1975).
Application: the scales have been used in many studies, some of which are reported in the *AAMD Adaptive Behavior Scale Manual* (Fogelman 1975) and have been used in service settings. The measure is widely used in the United States (Eyman and Call 1977; Nihira 1976; Nihira, Meyers and Mink 1983). It has also been used in studies being carried out in the United Kingdom (Hemming, Lavender and Pill 1981; Heron and Myers 1983; Humphreys, Lowe and Blunden 1983; Felce, de Kock, Saxby and Thomas 1984).

Balthazar Scales of Adaptive Behavior (BSAB)
Validity: Concurrent validity ranging between 0.59 and 0.67 using four raters to compare total self-help scores with the Vineland Social Maturity Scale has been reported.
Reliability: Inter-rater reliability for each sub-scale range from 0.59 to 0.97 on the BSAB-1 and 0.42 to 0.95 on the BSAB-2 are reported.
Standardisation: The BSAB was standardised on severely and profoundly ambulant institutional residents aged 5–57 years with IQs of less than 35. The percentile norms are available for each of the BSAB-1 sub-scales but not for the BSAB-2 sub-scales.
Application: The scales have been used in some American studies of people living in institutions (Balthazar and Phillips 1976) and in England and Wales (Felce *et al.* 1984; Humphreys, Lowe and Blunden 1983).

Behavior Development Survey
Validity: The authors cite data relating to the Adaptive Behavior Scale in this area comparing Behavior Development Survey total scores with ABS scores, correlating at 0.94 (Conroy 1980).
Reliability: Inter-rater reliability based on the administration of the measures to two staff for 75 cases in several state hospitals yielded correlation coefficients of 0.95 to 0.84 for the three domains in Part I, and of 0.55 and 0.68 for the two domains in Part II (IDB 1979).

Further work has been done on the reliability of the instrument by Conroy (1980) which suggests that for the purposes of assessing developmental growth, the Behavior Development Survey data appeared to be sufficiently reliable to suggest 'genuine changes among large groups of residents' (p. 5).

Standardisation: Reference is made to ABS data by the authors. Age and sex norms have been derived from a large-scale study of institutionalised and non-institutionalised people using the Behavior Development Survey.

Application: In the United States this test is used to collect data on 20,000 developmentally delayed individuals on a regular basis in California as part of the work of the Indivdualised Data Base Project. It has been used in the work of Conroy and his colleagues in Philadelphia (Conroy and Bradley 1985). In England it is currently being used by Raynes and Sumpton (Raynes and Sumpton, 1985).

Cain-Levine Social Competency Scale

Validity: Validity is reported to be 'based on the criteria of expert judges and of item analysis after tryout' (IDB 1977, p. 28).

Reliability: Levels from 0.88 to 0.97 for the sub-scales are reported, derived from test-retest reliability studies on a random sample of 35 subjects over a period of three weeks (Cain *et al.* 1963).

Standardisation: The scale was standardised on mentally retarded children aged 5–13 years with IQs ranging from 25 to 59. Percentile ranks for ages 5–13 years are available for each of the sub-scales as well as for total scale.

Application: It has been used in a study of communication in the classroom (Semmel, Sitko and Kreider 1973). Its use is not reported in any English studies.

The Vineland Social Maturity Scale

Validity: In two studies of mentally handicapped people, one of 250 and one of 78, Social Age quotients were correlated with independent assessments of Social Age. Correlations of 0.85 were obtained in the first study and of 0.85 to 0.95 in the second.

Reliability: Inter-rater reliability in a study of a sample of 123 mentally handicapped people was reported as 0.92 for Social Age.

Standardisation: A study was undertaken on a sample of people to develop age means for each item. Six hundred and twenty normal subjects selected by age and sex within each year from birth to 30 years were used to calibrate the measure.

Application: The scale has been used in research studies and in clinical settings for the assessment of mentally handicapped people.

COMMENTS ON THE USES AND ABUSES OF ADAPTIVE BEHAVIOUR SCALES

Perhaps the major problem related to the measures of adaptive behaviour which exists derives from their great number. Here only a few of those available have been cited. In determining which instrument you should use it is important to choose a test suited to your purpose. Adaptive behaviour can be measured to permit the data-based construction of programmes for individuals; to facilitate matching of individuals to certain vocational, education or residential settings; to explore change in the development of an individual's performance in given areas; and to describe an individual's performance at a given point in time in a given environment. Once you have identified for which of these purposes you are collecting your information it will be important to bear in mind a number of other factors. These are:

(1) The ease and speed with which the instrument can be administered.
(2) The cost of its administration.
(3) The appropriateness of the test for your clients in terms of age and sex and level of disability.
(4) The number of domains and related items covered.
(5) Evidence of the reliability and validity of the instrument.

The amount of detail you want will depend on the purpose for which you are administering the test. A large number of items is not inherently better than a small number. More information is necessary in developing an Individual Programme Plan than in making diagnostic assessments. The cost of a test will clearly influence decisions about the amount of detail obtainable as will the related issue of the amount of staff time involved in carrying out the test, and the difficulty of obtaining information about a behaviour which is not, for example, normally observed in the settings in which a staff member works with a client.

Look for Evidence of Reliability and Validity

It is hardly worth using tests in which these issues have not been addressed. Without such information, we have no knowledge of the extent to which the differences which are shown as a result of one test and another are due to systematic sources of error related to differences among the persons at the single testing or differences over time in the scores of individual people. Perhaps most important in terms of validity in relation to the use of tests of adaptive behaviour are measures of the concurrent and predictive validity of the test itself.

MEASURES OF ADAPTIVE BEHAVIOUR

For whichever purpose you use measures of adaptive behaviour, they should be used as one of a battery of assessment measures in any decision relating to a change in the placement of a mentally handicapped person. They do not predict success or failure in alternative placements. The evidence is clear that they are no better on this score than are IQ tests in predicting success in community placements (Windle 1962; Eagle, 1967; Cobb 1972). If this is the purpose for which you intend to use them, then it must be remembered that they are not surrogates for information either about IQ, motivation or personality and should not be used as if they were a total statement about a person's abilities, aptitudes and adaptability. As descriptors of an individual's performance characteristics and as the data base for individual programme plans, measures of adaptive behaviour can be used in their own right.

REFERENCES

Balthazar, E.E. (1973) *Balthazar Scales of Adaptive Behavior, Part 1: Scales of Social Adaptation*, Consulting Psychologists Press, Palo Alto, California

Balthazar, E.E. (1976) *Balthazar Scales of Adaptive Behavior, Part 2: Scales of Functional Independence*, Consulting Psychologists Press, Palo Alto, California

Balthazar, E.E. and Phillips, J.L. (1976) 'Social Adjustment in More Severely Retarded, Institutionalised Individuals: The Sum of Adjusted Behavior', *American Journal of Mental Deficiency, 80*, 454–9

Cain, L.F., Levine, S. and Elzey, F.F. (1963) *Manual for the Cain-Levine*

Social Competency Scale, Consulting Psychologists Press, Palo Alto, California
Cobb, H.V. (1972) *The Forecast of Fulfillment*, Teachers College Press, Columbia University
Conroy, J.W. (1980) *Reliability of the Behavior Development Survey: Technical Report 80-1-2*, Temple University Developmental Disabilities Evaluation and Research Group, Philadelphia
Conroy, J.W. and Bradley, V.J. (1985) *The Pennhurst Longitudinal Study: A Report of Two Years of Research and Analysis*, Temple University Developmental Disabilities Center, Philadelphia
Development Team for the Mentally Handicapped (1978) *First Report*, HMSO, London
Development Team for the Mentally Handicapped (1980) *Second Report*, HMSO, London
Development Team for the Mentally Handicapped (1982) *Third Report*, HMSO, London
Doll, E.A. (1935) 'The Vineland Social Maturity Scale', *Training School Bulletin, 32*, 1-7, 25-32, 48-55, 68-74
Doll, E.A. (1965) *The Vineland Scale of Social Maturity: Condensed Manual of Directions*, American Guidance Service Inc., Circle Pines, Minn.
Eagle, E. (1967) 'Prognosis and Outcome of Community Placement of Institutionalized Retardates', *American Journal of Mental Deficiency, 72*, 232-43
Elliot, R. and MacKay, D.N. (1971) 'Social Competence of Subnormal and Normal Children Living under Different Types of Residential Care', *British Journal of Mental Subnormality, 17*, 48-53
Eyman, R. and Call, T. (1977) 'Maladaptive Behavior and Community Placement of Mentally Retarded Persons', *American Journal of Mental Deficiency, 82* (2), 137-44
Felce, D., de Kock, U., Saxby, H. and Thomas, M. (1984) *Small Homes for Severely and Profoundly Mentally Handicapped Adults: Second Annual Report*, Health and Evaluation Research Team, University of Southampton
Fogelman, C.J. (ed.) (1975) *AAMD Adaptive Behavior Scale Manual, 1975 Revision*, American Association in Mental Deficiency, Washington, D.C.
Gunzberg, H.C. (1966) *The Primary Progress Assessment Chart of Social Development*, SEFA Publications, Stratford-upon-Avon
Gunzberg, H.C. (1968a) *Social Competence and Mental Handicap*, Baillière Tindall and Cassell, London
Gunzberg, H.C. (1968b) 'Assessing Social Competence', *Special Education, 57*, 11-14
Gunzberg, H.C. (1977) *Progress Assessment Chart of Social and Personal Development Manual* (2 vols.), SESA Publications Ltd, Stratford-upon-Avon
Heber, R. (1961) 'A Manual on Terminology and Classification in Mental Retardation (2nd Edition)', *American Journal of Mental Deficiency*, Monograph Supplement

Hemming, H., Lavender, T. and Pill, R. (1981) 'Quality of Life of Mentally Retarded Adults Transferred from Large Institutions to New Small Units', *American Journal of Mental Deficiency, 86*, 157–69

Heron, A. and Meyers, M. (1983) *Intellectual Impairment: the Battle Against Handicap*, Academic Press, London

Hill, B. and Bruininks, R.H. (1977) *Project Report No. 1: Assessment of Behavioral Characteristics of People who are Mentally Retarded*, Developmental Disabilities Project on Residential Services and Community Adjustment, University of Minnesota, Minneapolis

Holmes, N., Shah, A. and Wing, L. (1982) 'The Disablity Assessment Schedule: A Brief Screening Device for Use with the Mentally Retarded, *Psychological Medicine, 12*, 879–90

Humphreys, S., Lowe, K. and Blunden, R. (1983) *The Long-term Evaluation of Services for Mentally Handicapped People in Cardiff: Research Methodology*, Mental Handicap in Wales, Applied Research Unit

IDB Project (1977) *Performance Measures of Skill and Adaptive Comptences in the Developmentally Disabled*, Neuropsychiatric Research Group at Pacific State Hospital, Pomona, California

IDB (1979) *Behavior Development Survey User's Manual*, Neuropsychiatric Institute Research Group of the University of California, at Lanterman State Hospital, Pomona, California

Kushlick, A., Blunden, R. and Cox, G. (1973) 'A Method of Rating Behaviour Characteristics for Use in Large Scale Surveys of Mental Handicap', *Psychological Medicine, 3*, 466–78

Kushlick, A. and Cox, G.R. (1973) 'The Epidemiology of Mental Handicap', *Developmental Medicine and Child Neurology, 15*, 748–59

Lambert, N.M. and Nicoll, R.C. (1976) 'Dimensions of Adaptive Behavior of Retarded and Nonretarded Public-School Children', *American Journal of Mental Deficiency, 81*, 135–46

Leland, H., Nihira, K., Foster, R., Shellhaas, M. and Kagin, E. (eds.) (1966) *Conference on Measurement of Adaptive Behavior: II*, Parsons State Hospital and Training Center, Kansas

Marshall, A. (1967) *The Abilities and Attainments of Children Leaving Junior Training Centres*, NAMH, London

National Development Group (1977) *Mentally Handicapped Children: A Plan for Action (Pamphlet No. 2)*, London

Nihira, K. (1976) 'Dimensions of Adaptive Behavior in Institutionalized Mentally Retarded Children and Adults: Developmental Perspective', *American Journal of Mental Deficiency, 81*, 215–26

Nihira, K. (1977) 'Development of Adaptive Behaviour in the Mentally Retarded' in P. Mittler (ed.), *Research to Practice in Mental Retardation'*, vol. II, University Park Press, Baltimore

Nihira, K., Foster, R., Shellhaas, M. and Leland, H. (1969) *Adaptive Behavior Scales*, American Association on Mental Deficiency, Washington, D.C.

Nihira, K., Foster, R., Shellhaas, M. and Leland, H. (1974) *AAMD Adaptive Behavior Scale, 1974 Revision*, American Association on Mental Deficiency, Washington, D.C.

Nihira, K., Meyers, C.E. and Mink, I.T. (1983) 'Reciprocal Relationship Between Home Environment and Development of TMR Adolescents',

American Journal of Mental Deficiency, 88, 139–49
Palmer, J. and Jenkins, J. (1982) 'The Wessex Behaviour Rating System for Mentally Handicapped People: Reliability Study', *British Journal of Mental Subnormality, 28,* 88–96
Rawlings, S. (1985) 'Behaviour and Skills of Severely Retarded Adults in Hospitals and Small Residential Homes', *British Journal of Psychiatry, 146,* 358–66
Raynes, N.V. and Sumpton, R.C. (1985) *Follow-up Study of 448 People who are Mentally Handicapped: Final Report,* Hester Adrian Research Centre and Department of Social Administration, University of Manchester
Semmel, M.I., Sitko, M. and Kreider, J. (1973) 'The Relationship of Pupil-Teacher Interaction in Classrooms for the TMR to Pupil to Gain in Communication Skills', *Mental Retardation, 11,* 7–13
Shackleton-Bailey, M.J. (undated) *An Introduction to Hampshire Assessment for Living with Others,* Hampshire Social Services, Winchester
Shackleton-Bailey, M.J. and Pidcock, B.E. (1983) *Halo Report 1983: Hampshire Assessment for Living with Others — Research and Development Programme, 1981–1983,* Hampshire Social Services, Winchester
Whelan, E. (1984) 'A Note for the RLG Concerning the Validity and Reliability of the Scales Used During the Habilitation Technology Project' (mimeograph), Hester Adrian Research Centre, University of Manchester, Manchester
Whelan, E. and Speake, B. (1979) *Learning to Cope,* Souvenir Press, London
Windle, C. (1962) 'Prognosis of Mental Subnormals', *American Journal of Mental Deficiency,* Monograph Supplement, *66,* No. 5
Wing, L. and Gould, J. (1978) 'Systematic Recording of Behaviours and Skills of Retarded and Psychotic Children', *Journal of Autism and Childhood Schizophrenia, 8,* 79–97
Wing, L. and Gould, J. (1979) 'Severe Impairment of Social Interaction and Associated Abnormalities in Children: Epidemiology and Classification', *Journal of Autism and Developmental Disorders, 9,* 11–29

5

Behaviour Disturbance and its Assessment

I. Leudar and W.I. Fraser

WHAT IS BEHAVIOUR DISTURBANCE?

Behaviour disturbances present varied management problems and prevent the handicapped person from realising his or her full potential (Eyman and Call 1977; Sternlich and Deutsch 1972). Such disorders are frequent in the mentally handicapped individual (Jacobson 1982; Koller, Richardson, Katz and McLaren 1983). Although not attributing the behaviour disturbances directly to mental retardation, Koller *et al.* (1983) found 50 per cent of their cohort to exhibit significant behaviour disturbance by the age of 22 years. A wide variety of behaviours can be classified as disturbed, as shown in the following vignettes:

EC is a 25-year-old mildly retarded woman with a history of suicide attempts. She intermittently refuses to leave her bed for lengthy periods, and refuses to wash or eat. She will not talk to most people but laughs and pulls faces at them behind their backs.

PF is a 40-year-old woman who is severely retarded. She was born after a protracted delivery. In childhood she developed epilepsy. She is solitary, she talks to herself in public but she speaks little to others. Her contributions to conversations are often quite irrelevant. Some of her gestures are bizarre andd seem purposeless to the people around her. She does not express feelings: psychiatrists would say that her mood is 'flattened'.

MS is a 17-year-old adolescent labelled 'autistic'. His lifelong delight has been fiddling with, dismantling and disconnecting electrical appliances. He has now transferred his interest to fire alarms.

IB is a 22-year-old, moderately handicapped man, mild in manner, who has nevertheless been repeatedly 'in trouble' because of vagrancy, stealing chickens, damaging a phone box, running away from a hospital and involvement in car thefts. He spent several years in a maximum security hospital.

AM is a 40-year-old severely handicapped man who spent most of his life in a subnormality hospital. One has to 'watch him' because he frequently bites and otherwise assaults people, unexpectedly and without apparent provocation.

These vignettes exemplify some behaviour disturbances, namely withdrawal; seemingly purposeless aggression; delinquency; idiosyncratic behaviours; and apparently meaningless ways of expression. The list of examples could continue. Two problems are, however, immediately obvious. First, it is meaningful to subsume such wide variety of behaviours under one term, behaviour disturbance? Secondly, what is the appropriate basis on which to classify disturbed behaviours? Clearly, all the disturbances do not have a common cause and the antecedents of one particular disturbed action can vary. Take, for example, withdrawal; this can reflect emotional disturbance, psychotic breakdown, autistic traits or profound handicap (Leudar, Fraser and Jeeves 1984; Leudar and Fraser 1985). Thus, a classification cannot only take into account the causes of behaviour disturbances. What other relevant considerations are there? A useful distinction can be made between factors which lead to the onset of disturbed behaviours (e.g. stress, emotional disturbance, brain damage) on the one hand, and on the other hand the factors that determine which particular actions are considered by people to be 'disturbed'. Behaviours are usually labelled and reacted to as disturbed for two reasons:

(1) The disturbed person behaves in an idiosyncratic manner and the goals or motives of his or her actions are either inappropriate or idiosyncratic. In other words, we have problems in understanding disturbed behaviours.
(2) The person's actions conflict with the smooth functioning and the norms of relevant social groups. Behaviour disturbances create management problems. 'Behavior problems of the retarded [are seen] as deviant behavior patterns, related to impaired current functioning and progressive changes in interactions between the individual . . . and the environment' (Bijou 1966).

The assessment tools which we shall describe do not always take these properties of behaviour disturbances explicitly into account. Their users should, however, be familiar with the concept of behaviour disturbance if they are to conduct assessments effectively, validly and reliably.

GENERAL CHARACTERISTICS OF THE APPROACH

In this section we shall outline in detail the properties of behaviour disturbances which are in the focus of current research, as well as some which are often neglected.

Two important properties of behaviour disturbances emerge from the section above. First, behaviours are disturbed if they violate norms of conduct accepted by a particular social group, or if they are uninterpretable in terms of rules which make ordinary actions meaningful. Secondly, since the norms of conduct may vary between social groups and even from individual to individual, behaviour disturbances are to a certain extent subjective (Isett, Roszkowski, Spreat and Reiter 1983). These two properties may make it difficult to assess whether measurement tools are valid and reliable *in general* (see Wing and Gould 1978; Holmes, Shah and Wing 1982) (see also Chapters 2 and 4) and see below.

Another important point about disturbed behaviours is that their consequences are important: 'consequences . . . requiring medical treatment or which result in exclusion from social and educational programs appropriate to one's adaptive level' (Schroeder, Mulick and Schroeder 1980). Behaviour disturbances may also negatively affect the long-term character of interactions between the disturbed person and others. They result in labelling which sets the occasion and determines the environment for further disturbance. Thus classifications of disturbances should take into account their *consequences*. The relevant research on the organisation of behaviour disturbance is summarised below.

The disturbed behaviours may also vary in seriousness (Clements, Bost, Dubois and Turpin 1980; Holmes and Batt 1980; Searles, Isett and Bowders 1981). Hitting and abusing somebody are both instances of aggression but the former is usually taken as more serious than the latter. An adequate measurement of disturbance should take into account both its structure and the relative seriousness of disturbed behaviours in each class. Some investigations have, however, ordered disturbance only according to their seriousness (e.g. Jacobson 1982).

Finally, behaviour disturbances are better seen as dynamic features of an individual's characteristic ways of acting, rather than simply as instances of static categories. Disturbances may increase or decrease, for example as a function of environmental changes. Additionally, acting in a disturbed manner induces negative and often hostile changes in an individual's social environment. As an individual's disturbance becomes established socially, his or her actions come to have different consequences, and the same goals have to be attained by different means. The actual character of the postulated environmental changes depends on the specific nature of the disturbed actions. Occasional lying, for example, may bring about a lack of trust. The deceivers' environment becomes non-standard, in that their truthfulness is not taken for granted when normally it would be, and other hostile changes are also possible. The liars have to adjust to such changes and the adjustments may further affect the social context. The dynamic character of disturbances thus stems, in part, from mutual adjustments between the individual and the social environment and some features of disturbed behaviours can only be understood from this viewpoint. Other trends may, of course, reflect the neuropsychological deterioration in individuals (e.g. the onset of pre-senile dementia).

So behaviour disturbances are multifaceted phenomena — they are properties of social environments as well as reflections of, for example, an individual's personality or psychiatric disturbance. It may seem counter-intuitive, but disturbances are to an extent encoded 'in the environment' as well as 'in the head' of the disturbed subjects. This conclusion is supported by the finding that there is no simple and consistent relationship between psychiatric disturbances and behaviour disorders (Fraser, Leudar, Gray and Campbell 1985). This relation will be discussed in some detail below.

In this section we have isolated four important properties of behaviour disturbances all of which bear on its measurement:

(1) It is not unidimensional but can be organised into types.
(2) The seriousness and the cost of disturbed actions varies between and within the types.
(3) Behaviours are disturbed because they violate norms and expectations which govern social interactions.
(4) Finally, disturbances are dynamic in character.

All of the available scales take the point (1) into account but the principles on which behaviours are organised into domains are usually intuitive rather than explicitly given. Some scales order disturbed behaviours in each domain according to seriousness, as we shall show below.

THE AVAILABLE SCALES

All of the instruments which we shall describe are rating scales. The assessors, who are usually nurses, instructors or teachers, rate handicapped persons on scales reflecting either (1) frequencies of disturbed behaviours, or (2) the appropriateness of personality characteristics for the person.

Adaptive Behavior Scale, Part II (ABS Part II)

The scale (Nihira, Foster, Shelhaas and Leland 1974) contains 14 domains of disturbance, each of which is divided into sub-domains. The summary of the scale is given in Table 5.1. Each sub-domain consists of several items such as 'Uses threatening gestures' or 'Does not return things that were borrowed'. The rater has to decide for each item whether it is true of the person being assessed and, if so, to rate the frequency of the behaviour on a two-point scale labelled 'occasionally' and 'often'. Thus in effect the ratings are on three-point scales, the implicit point being 'never'. The rater is also able to specify, in each sub-domain, 'related behaviour problems not covered by the examples listed'. What counts as 'related behaviour problems' is left to the raters' judgements. This may in practice be problematic as the bases on which domains are distinguished are not explicitly given and consequently the intuitions may vary. The completed assessment consists of a disturbance profile containing the sums of ratings in each domain. The items are not weighted for seriousness.

Balthazar Scales of Adaptive Behavior Part 2 (BSAB – 2)

Part 2 of Balthazar's scale (Balthazar 1973) contains several domains relevant to behaviour disturbance. These are given in Table 5.2. Each domain contains several items, some of which are completed on the basis of the rater's experience with the behaviour of the rated person and others are scored on the basis of direct observation. The overall score in each domain is simply a sum of the ratings on the relevant items. This means that, as in ABS Part II, the items

Table 5.1: The Domains and Sub-domains of AAMD Adaptive Behavior Scale — Part II

I. VIOLENT AND DESTRUCTIVE BEHAVIOUR
(1) Threatens or Does Physical Violence
(2) Damages Personal Property
(3) Damages Others' Property
(4) Damages Public Property
(5) Has Violent Temper or Temper Tantrums

II. ANTISOCIAL BEHAVIOUR
(1) Teases or Gossips About Others
(2) Bosses and Manipulates Others
(3) Disrupts Others' Activities
(4) Is Inconsiderate of Others
(5) Shows Disrespect for Others' Property
(6) Uses Angry Language

III. REBELLIOUS BEHAVIOUR
(1) Ignores Regulations or Regular Routines
(2) Resists Following Instruction or Orders
(3) Has Impudent or Rebellious Attitude to Authority
(4) Is Absent From or Late for Proper Assignments
(5) Runs Away or Attempts to Run Away
(6) Misbehaves in Group Settings

IV. UNTRUSTWORTHY BEHAVIOUR
(1) Takes Others' Property Without Permission
(2) Lies or Cheats

V. WITHDRAWAL
(1) Is Inactive
(2) Is Withdrawn
(3) Is Shy

VI. STEREOTYPED BEHAVIOUR AND ODD MANNERISMS
(1) Has Stereotyped Behaviours
(2) Has Peculiar Posture or Mannerisms

VII. INAPPROPRIATE INTER-PERSONAL MANNERS

VIII. UNACCEPTABLE VOCAL HABITS

IX. UNACCEPTABLE OR ECCENTRIC HABITS
(1) Has Strange and Unacceptable Habits
(2) Has Unacceptable Oral Habits
(3) Removes or Tears Own Clothing
(4) Has Other Eccentric Habits

X. SELF-ABUSIVE BEHAVIOUR

XI. HYPERACTIVE TENDENCIES

XII. SEXUALLY ABERRANT BEHAVIOUR

XIII. PSYCHOLOGICAL DISTURBANCES
(1) Tends to Overestimate Own Abilities
(2) Reacts Poorly to Criticism
(3) Reacts Poorly to Frustration
(4) Demands Excessive Attention or Praise

Table 5.1: (Cont.)

(5) Seems to Feel Persecuted
(6) Has Hypochondriacal Tendencies
(7) Has Other Signs of Emotional Instabilities

XIV. USE OF MEDICATION

Table 5.2: The Relevant Domains and Sub-domains of Balthazar Scales of Adaptive Behaviour 2

UNADAPTED SELF-DIRECTED BEHAVIOURS
I. Failure to Respond
II. Stereotypy
III. Non-directed Repetitious Verbalisation, Smiling
IV. Inappropriate Self-directed Behaviour
V. Disorderly Non-social Behaviour

UNADAPTIVE INTER-PERSONAL BEHAVIOURS
VI. Inappropriate Contact with Others
VII. Aggression, Withdrawal

are not weighted for seriousness (see McDevitt, McDevitt and Rosen 1977).

Behaviour Disturbance Scale (BDS)

This scale (Leudar, Fraser and Jeeves) has been standardised and mainly used in Scotland and England. BDS consists of 49 rating items from six domains of disturbance given in Table 5.3. Each item is rated on a five-point rating scale with the points labelled 'never', 'rarely', 'occasionally', 'often' and 'very often'. The completed assessment consists of six scores, one for each domain of disturbance. When these overall scores are calculated, the items are weighted for seriousness — the weights have been validated for a population of 600 retarded Scottish men and women living both in the community and in hospitals. The scale is available in the form of a check-sheet, but a computerised version for use on the BBC microcomputer can also be obtained, both from the first author (see Appendix).

Table 5.3: Behaviour Disturbance Scale

I.	Aggressive Conduct
II.	Emotional Disturbance
III.	Antisocial Conduct
IV.	Communicativeness - Withdrawal
V.	Idiosyncratic Mannerisms
VI.	Self-injury

Goldberg's standardised psychiatric interview

This psychiatric assessment schedule (Goldberg, Cooper, Eastwood, Kedward and Shepherd 1970) was originally developed for community surveys and, in its modified form, is more sensitive to neurotic than to psychotic symptoms. The symptoms measured include depression, anxiety, sleep disturbance, somatic symptoms, etc., and are given in detail in Table 5.4. The scale has been widely used in psychiatric community surveys and has been adapted for use with mentally handicapped individuals by Ballinger, Armstrong, Presley and Reid (1975) and Reid, Ballinger and Heather (1978). In its original form, the rating scale consists of two parts:

(1) ratings of psychiatric symptoms based on verbal information elicited from subjects during an interview; and
(2) ratings of 'manifest symptoms'.

The interviewer (and the rater) is a psychiatrist and the symptoms are rated on five-point, unlabelled scales. Ballinger *et al.* (1975) observed that there were problems with the scale where the less verbally able or willing individuals were concerned. They therefore focused on the second part of the scale, which they expanded to record the following features: slow; suspicious; histrionic; depressed; anxious or agitated; elated; flattened (i.e. emotional withdrawal); delusions; misinterpretations and thought disorders; hallucinations; intellectual impairment; overactivity; distractability; sterotypy; hostile irritability; lability; pica; and self-injury. In this adaptation, the information about some behaviours is obtained from the primary caretakers. A diagnosis is made by the psychiatrist on the basis of the ratings of manifest symptoms.

Table 5.4: The Symptoms Rated on Goldberg's Clinical Interview Schedule

Part 1:
1. Somatic Symptoms
2. Excessive Concern with Bodily Functions
3. Fatigue
4. Sleep Disturbance
5. Hypnotics
6. Irritability
7. Lack of Concentration
8. Depression
9. Anxiety
10. Phobias
11. Obsessions and Compulsions
12. Depersonalisations

Part 2:
1. Slow and Lacking Spontaneity
2. Suspicious and Defensive
3. Histronic
4. Depressed
5. Anxious, Tense, Agitated
6. Elated, Euphoric
7. Flattened, Incongruous (Affect)
8. Delusions, Thought Disorder
9. Hallucinations
10. Intellectual Impairment
11. Overall Severity Rating

The Disability Assessment Schedule (DAS)

This scale has been compiled for screening purposes by Lorna Wing and has been briefly described by Holmes, Shah and Wing (1982). The scale consists of two parts; the first one measures physical and development skills; the other, behavioural abnormalities. Raynes has discussed the first part (Chapter 4). It is the second part which is relevant here. DAS is 'completed by conducting a structured interview with an informant who knows the mentally retarded person well'. The second part of the scale contains 23 items summarised in Table 5.5. These items are not explicitly organised into domains of disturbance but the scale nevertheless enables one to draw a disturbance profile for a mentally handicapped person. The items of the scale are rated on three- to eight-point scales which express the frequency and importance of behaviours in question. It is stated that the interviewer needs to be trained in the use of the scale.

Table 5.5: The Relevant Items of the Disability Assessment Schedule

Wanders and runs away
Screams
Temper tantrums — verbal abuse
Disturbs others at night
Difficult or objectional personal habits
Scatters or throws objects around
Antisocial, delinquent
Sexual delinquency
Others
Quality of social interaction
Imaginative pretend play or other symbolic activities
Repetitive symbolic activities
Choice of activities
Simple stereotypes
Elaborate routines
Immediate echolalia
Delayed echolalia
Repetitive speech

The Aberrant Behaviour Checklist

This scale is a checklist developed for research purposes by Aman, Singh, Stewart and Field (1985a, b). The given purpose of the scale is the assessment of effects of drug treatments on severely and profoundly retarded individuals. The scale has been constructed by means of factor analysis in samples of 418 and 509 severely and profoundly retarded individuals in New Zealand. The scale consists of 76 items which are organised in five domains, given in Table 5.6. Each item is scored by a member of nursing staff on a four-point rating scale, with the extremes (0 and 3) labelled 'not at all a problem' and 'the problem is severe' respectively. The scores for each domain are obtained by simply summing the scores on the relevant items. Thus the items are not weighted for seriousness.

Psychopathology Instrument for Mentally Retarded Adults

The scale reported by Senatore, Matson and Kazdin (1985) focuses on the assessment of psychiatric problems. It can be presented in two forms, informant and self-report versions, in which the sources of information are (1) primary caretakers or clinicians, and (2) mentally handicapped individuals respectively. Both versions of the

Table 5.6: The Domains of the Aberrant Behaviour Checklist

I.	Irritability, Agitation and Crying
II.	Lethargy and Social Withdrawal
III.	Stereotypic Behaviour
IV.	Hyperactivity and Noncompliance
V.	Inappropriate Speech

instrument contain 56 matched items derived from the third edition of *Diagnostic and Statistical Manual of Mental Disorders* (American Psychiatric Association, 1980). The items in both versions have been grouped by the authors into eight corresponding domains, given in Table 5.7. Each item is measured on a four-point Likert scale. In the self-report version, the rating scales are presented as labelled bar-graphs to which the patient points to express their ratings. The wording of the items in the self-report version has been simplified to suit mentally handicapped clients. Both versions of the scale have been shown to be internally consistent, reliable and scores relatively stable over time (Senatore *et al.* 1985). Senatore *et al.* (1985) have, however, reported only low correlations between the corresponding items on the two versions of the instrument.

Table 5.7: The Domains for the Psychopathology Instrument for the Mentally Retarded Adults

I.	Schizophrenia
II.	Affective Disorder
III.	Psychosexual Disorder
IV.	Adjustment Disorder
V.	Anxiety Disorder
VI.	Somatiform Disorder
VII.	Personality Disorder
VIII.	Mental Adjustment Disorder

Source: Senatore, Matson and Kazdin (1985).

PAST RESEARCH ON BEHAVIOUR DISTURBANCE

All of the above scales have been extensively used in research. We summarise below the relevant studies, but for the sake of completeness we also include the studies which did not use standardised assessment tools, but rather tailored them specifically for the research in question.

Types of disturbance

The empirical studies we consider in this section were concerned with (1) the organisation of behaviour disturbances and (2) the factors possibly influencing such organisation (i.e. age, institutionalisation, the degree of mental retardation and sex). The term 'organisation of behaviour disturbances' simply refers to which disturbed actions go together. The data used in all the relevant studies were the ratings of the frequency with which disturbed actions are produced by handicapped individuals. These ratings were subjected to factor analysis. The obtained organisations of behaviour disturbances therefore reflect the manner in which disturbed behaviours typically co-vary. In other words, some behaviours are commonly produced by the same individuals, others are not.

Nihira (1969a) had ABS Part II (see Table 5.1) completed for a sample of 919 adult institutionalised residents and factor-analysed the averaged domain scores. Disturbed behaviours loaded on two factors: (1) Social Maladaptation (subsuming violent actions, rebellious behaviour, antisocial and untrustworthy behaviour) and (2) Intra-maladaptation (subsuming behaviour stereotypies, self-abusive behaviour and peculiar and eccentric habits). In a further study of younger retarded subjects, Nihira (1969b) obtained the same two factors together with two additional ones: Withdrawal and Sexually Aberrant Behaviours. A further large-scale study has been conducted by Lambert and Nicoll (1976). ABS ratings have been obtained for 2,618 seven- to thirteen-year-old children. The factor structure has been studied separately in different age and school classification levels. The factors obtained matched Nihira's (1969a, b) inter-personal and intra-personal adjustment; this factor structure was the same for retarded and nonretarded children and neither did it vary with age.

There are, however, two problems with these important studies. First, the inputs into factor analyses were in each case the averages for ABS domains. This means that the division of behaviours into such domains was taken for granted and not tested. Secondly, the frequencies of adaptive and maladaptive behaviours were factor-analysed together. It is likely that this mode of analysis led to the relatively finer aspects of behaviour disturbance structure being missed. This conclusion is supported by the results of studies by Lorr and Jenkins (1953), Conners (1969) and Leudar, Fraser and Jeeves (1984) who factor-analysed the ratings of frequencies of actual behaviours. The factors obtained by Lorr and Jenkins (1953) were: socialised delinquency, internal conflict, aggressiveness, brain injury and schizoid patterns. The factor structure was relatively uninfluenced by sex. Conners (1969) studied a sample of 103 children with behaviour problems, excluding, however, those with IQ less than 80, 'who were psychotic, grossly brain damaged or markedly antisocial'. The factors obtained were aggression, withdrawal, overactivity and inattentiveness. Leudar *et al.* (1984) conducted two studies of behaviour disturbance in 600 and 250 adult retarded subjects living in hospitals or in the community. The disturbed actions were selected on the basis of their salience to nurses and caretakers; they were not organised into domains before being factor-analysed. Six factors were obtained: aggressive conduct, emotional disturbance, withdrawal, antisocial conduct, self-injury, and idiosyncratic mannerisms (Table 5.2). The structure was not affected by the place of residence and seemed to correspond closely to that proposed by Koller, Richardson, Katz and McLaren (1983).

To summarise, behaviour disturbance clearly has a structure, which is relatively unaffected by age, sex or institutionalisation. (This, of course, does not mean that these factors do not affect the *frequency* of disturbed behaviours — see below.) The recurring categories seem to be aggression, antisocial conduct, emotional disturbance, withdrawal, autistic-like behaviours and self-injury.

The prevalence of behaviour disturbance, institutionalisation, age and sex

Jacobson (1982) reported that the rates with which disturbed behaviours are produced seems to depend on whether handicapped persons reside in the community or in an institution, and the quality of the institution matters.

Scanlon, Arick and Krug (1982) compared the rates of behaviour disturbance in institutionalised and community-placed samples matched in sex, age, linguistic age, and diagnosis. They found that the 'institutional' residents exhibited higher rates of aggression, mood disturbance and destructiveness. Taylor (1976) used discriminant analysis to differentiate between hospitalised and nonhospitalised retarded individuals on the basis of their ABS scores. The residents in hospitals scored higher on rebellious, untrustworthy behaviour and were more hyperactive. The higher rate of disturbed actions by the individuals residing in institutions has been further confirmed by several other studies, using ABS Part II (e.g. Eyman and Call 1977; Thiel 1981). Leudar, Fraser and Jeeves (1984) reported that individuals in institutions exhibited only higher rates of aggression, antisocial conduct and self-injury. The institutionalisation, however, did not affect the rate of *change* in these behaviour characteristics.

The term 'institutionalisation' is, however, coarse and does not reflect accurately the range of residential options becoming available. These also include hostels, sheltered housing and lodgings. Each of these has its own stressors which may lead to behaviour disturbances (see Nihira, Mink and Meyers 1984). Janicki, Jacobson and Schwartz (1982), for example, reported a relatively higher proportion of psychiatric disturbance in mentally handicapped subjects living in sheltered housing while confirming that most *severe* disturbances were to be found in institutions. The assessment of the effect of living arrangements on behaviour disturbance is further complicated because the differential rates of disturbance in different environments may reflect the selection of individuals for those environments. The extent to which behaviour problems are *recognised* in different contexts may also vary.

There does not seem to be any clear relationship between Chronological Age (CA) and disturbance. Salagaras and Nettleback (1983) have found that in a sample of 550 mentally retarded young people, 13 to 20 years old, the age and ABS Part II scores were unrelated. In the Leudar, Fraser and Jeeves (1984) study of 16 to 45 year olds, the relationship between age and the disturbance rates was also not significant. Similarly, Koller *et al.* (1983) have reported a lack of any relationship between CA and disturbance in 16 to 22 years age range. Francis (1970), however, observed an increase in idiosyncratic mannerisms and withdrawal in ageing Down's Syndrome subjects. These changes were, however, attributed to progressive institutionalisation rather than to age *per se*. Jacobson (1982), however, reported that young children and the elderly handicapped subjects were more likely to display disturbed behaviours.

The frequency with which disturbed behaviours are produced can be affected by sex. Koller *et al.* (1983) have found that in childhood the most common type of disturbance among boys was aggression and antisocial conduct whereas among girls emotional problems prevailed. A similar relation, however, does not so clearly obtain in adulthood, as Leudar, Fraser and Jeeves (1984) have shown. Leudar *et al.* (1984) have observed that placing women in an institutional setting was likely to increase their emotional problems more than it did for men.

Finally, some studies (e.g. Eyman and Call 1977; Jacobson 1982; Freeman, Ritvo, Schroth, Tonick, Guthrie and Wake 1981) have found that the rate of disturbed actions is higher in the more severely retarded individuals than in those less handicapped. The significance of this finding has, however, been disputed (by e.g. Leudar *et al.* 1984). The problem is that the validity of assessment scales may be different in populations which vary in Mental Age. One reason for this is that the manner in which disturbances manifest themselves may depend on a person's Mental Age. The behaviours which express disturbance in one group of individuals (say, the mildly handicapped ones) may be beyond the competence of another group (say, the severely retarded ones). Some verbal or strategic expressions of aggression are an example. These are usually judged less serious than, say, hitting somebody. Thus, the expression of disturbance in a more severely handicapped person may be limited to more primitive, noticeable and serious actions. In addition, of course, the absence in a severely retarded person of disturbed behaviours observed in mildly handicapped individuals cannot be taken to indicate that the disturbance is also absent. This interesting possibility has not yet been empirically investigated.

Behaviour disturbances and psychiatric problems

It has been repeatedly observed that psychiatric problems are relatively common in mentally handicapped individuals (see e.g. Rutter, Tizard, Yule, Graham and Whitmore 1974; Phillips and Williams 1975; Matson and Barret 1982). The reasons for this are as yet unclear and the exact relationship between mental illness and mental retardation is controversial. The research in the area is hindered by the lack of suitable assessment tools. Their development is difficult for several reasons. First, the manner in which mentally handicapped individuals manifest psychiatric symptoms may differ from nonretarded individuals and the constellations of the symptoms may also be specific to the retarded population (Fraser *et al.* 1985; Senatore *et al.* 1985). The second problem is that the expressive abilities of many handicapped individuals are limited, and many are withdrawn and refuse to disclose information about their problems (Leudar and Fraser 1985). This poses particular problems for psychiatric interviews which are usually an important source of information towards a diagnosis. In pratice the interview information is supplemented by reports on behavioural problems, elicited from primary caretakers (Ballinger *et al.* 1975; Senatore *et al.* 1985). Thus sometimes a clear distinction between the terms 'psychiatric disorder' and 'behaviour disturbance' is not made and disturbed behaviours are treated as symptoms of psychiatric disorders. In fact, the relationship between behaviour disturbances and psychiatric disorders and mental retardation is complex (see Wing and Gould 1979). Fraser *et al.* (1985) observed that particular psychiatric disorders were not expressed consistently by specific behaviour disturbances. Psychiatric and behaviour assessments are complementary and have different goals. Psychiatrists' approach to disturbance is one of pattern recognition: they fit individuals into syndromes which are parts of International Classification of Diseases (ICD) medical labelling, the purpose of which is to classify and determine the appropriate treatment procedures. In other words, psychiatric assessments focus on signs of mentally treatable syndromes.

Dynamic properties of behaviour disturbance

King, Soucar and Isett (1980) used the ABS to investigate the changes in behaviour disturbance in response to the changes in living arrangements. No decrease in the overall frequency of disturbed behaviours was found. Eyman, Borthwick and Miller (1981) also failed to detect temporal changes in behaviour disturbance with change in placement. The studies concluded that behaviour disturbances are relatively persistent characteristics of an individual's behaviour repertoire. This conclusion is, however, not warranted. It is possible that the environmental changes decreased the rate of some behaviours and increased the rate of others, the overall result being apparent stability. Leudar *et al.* (1984) have investigated the stability and temporal changes of discrete classes of behaviour disturbances using the Behaviour Disturbance Scale (BDS) (see Table 5.3). The results obtained suggest that in the absence of intervention, each disturbance is significantly stable (thus confirming the results of the above studies); the stability being highest for aggressive conduct and antisocial conduct and lowest for mood disturbance. In addition, however, the following temporal trends were detected: (1) high aggression scores were predictive of eventual overt mood disturbance; (2) the temporal changes in withdrawal depended on whether it was associated with high levels of idiosyncratic mannerisms or with mood disturbance (in the former case the withdrawal was likely to get worse, in the latter case better); and (3) the changes in antisocial conduct and in aggressive conduct went hand in hand. The authors concluded that not only the classes of disturbance are important, but the disturbance *profiles* also matter. There is as yet no precise guidance available as to which particular disturbance profiles deserve highlighting (but see Leudar *et al.* 1984).

PROBLEMS OF MEASUREMENT

These problems stem from some of the characteristics of behaviour disturbance outlined above. The first one is how to collect the empirical data. The available scales (ABS Part II, Nihira *et al.* 1974; BDS, Leudar *et al.* 1984 and BSAB, Balthazar 1973) use caretakers' ratings of conduct. These are either ratings of the frequency with which particular disturbed behaviours (e.g. hitting somebody) are produced or of the extent to which disturbance traits (e.g. 'aggressiveness') are typical of the rated person. The exclusive use of behaviour ratings may seem to have negative implications for the validity and reliability of assessments but there are strong reasons for using them. First, behaviour disturbances do not have known predictors strong enough to be used in psychological tests (see Halpern, Irvin and Landman, 1979). Secondly, objective behaviour observations are not always practical because of their labour intensiveness, intrusiveness and because of the intermittency and infrequency of some disturbed actions (which are nevertheless salient). Assuming the truth of our previous conclusion (the social consequences of disturbed actions are their crucial defining characteristics and they also determine some of their dynamics), *the ratings by caretakers, nurses or parents are, in fact, precisely the right sort and source of evidence.* In fact, these ratings have been found to be highly reliable in most studies (e.g. Jacobson 1982; Salagaras and Nettlebeck 1983). This applies to all the scales described above. When using the scales to assess problems and progress of a particular individual, however, it may be advisable to obtain ratings by several assessors, averaging the profiles, but also taking note of clear discrepancies between the assessments.

The other problem reflects the relativity of disturbed behaviours. Should just one assessment schedule be used or should different schedules be adapted for particuar contexts and populations? The organisation of disturbance into types seems to be relatively stable over populations but exactly which actual behaviours realise such types, and their relative seriousness, probably depends on a variety of factors such as group specific norms, age and Mental Age. Therefore the general validity of a given assessment scale cannot always be taken for granted. The assessment tools we have summarised have not been validated to this extent. The user's decision should be partly pragmatic and will reflect the reasons for the assessment. If these are practical (such as assessing the response to relocation) and concern a particular person or a specific group of individuals, the stress should be on validity and the appropriateness of the schedule. In the assessment of 'relocation shock' the timing of testing is crucial. Alternatively, the assessment may be a part of a scientific investigation with the added emphasis on the comparability with other studies. The available research suggests that the organisation of behaviour disturbance is relatively invariant. With this proviso it is possible (and advisable), to tailor assessment scales to given contexts and populations, structuring them aroung the generally valid disturbance types (Leudar *et al.* 1984), the actual behaviours under each type being chosen to reflect behaviour repertoires of the given population and ranked according to their seriousness.

Further problems may arise if one focuses on one aspect of disturbance and measures that aspect only. As we have shown above, this is inappropriate, especially where the temporal changes in disturbance are of interest. We have seen above that the decrease in one aspect of disturbance may be associated with an increase in another aspect. It is also the case that a particular disturbance score may have different significance, depending on the remaining profile scores, as we have shown for withdrawal. For similar reasons, averaged overall disturbance scores may not be particularly meaningful. The point is that one should always obtain the full disturbance profile.

On the whole, the main problems in assessing behaviour disturbances are caused by (1) their social-relativity; and (2) the dependence of the manner in which the disturbances are manifested on the subjects' Mental Age. It may be necessary to adjust assessment scales to relevant norms and behaviour repertoires of different populations.

CONCLUSIONS

We have summarised the scales most frequently used in the assessment and research on behaviour disturbance in mentally handicapped individuals. Our survey makes it clear that the scales basically count frequencies of the behaviours that their authors feel intuitively to be deviant, or they quantify the rater's perceptions of the handicapped person's personality traits relevant to disturbance. The Behaviour Disturbance Scale is an exception in this sense, because the expressions of disturbances included in the scale were those salient to the caretakers of mentally handicapped individuals. The problem of how valid the assessments are in general, however, remains. This is so because, as we pointed out, behaviours are disturbed relative to social and group norms (which can vary) and the levels of abilities must also be taken into account. We have suggested that the assessment scales should be used with some flexibility, and have given some indications as to how this can be done.

ACKNOWLEDGEMENT

This work was supported by SHHD grant K/MRS/50/C330.

REFERENCES

Aman, M.G., Singh, N.N., Stewart, A.W. and Field, C.J. (1985a) 'The Aberrant Behavior Checklist: A Behavior Rating Scale for the Assessment of Treatment Effects', *American Journal of Mental Deficiency*, 89, 485–91

Aman, M.G., Singh, N.N., Stewart, A.W. and Field, C.J. (1985b) 'Psychometric Characteristics of the Aberrant Behavior Checklist', *American Journal of Mental Deficiency*, 89, 492–502

American Psychiatric Association (1980) *Diagnostic and Statistical Manual of Mental Disorders*, 3rd edn, American Psychiatric Association, Washington, D.C.

Ballinger, E.R., Armstrong, J., Presley, A.S. and Reid, A.H. (1975) 'Use of Standardised Psychiatric Interview in Mentally Handicapped Patients', *British Journal of Psychiatry*, 127, 540–4

Balthazar, E.E. (1973) *The Balthazar Scale of Adaptive Behavior. II: The Scales of Social Adaptation*, Consulting Psychologists Press, Palo Alto, California

Bijou, S. (1966) 'A Functional Analysis of Retarded Development' in N.R. Ellis (ed.), *International Review of Research in Mental Retardation*, vol. 1, Academic Press, New York

Clements, P., Bost, L., Dubois, Y. and Turpin, W. (1980) 'Adaptive Behavior Scale, Part II: Relative Severity of Maladaptive Behavior', *American Journal of Mental Deficiency, 84*, 465-9

Conners, C.K. (1969) 'A Teacher Rating Scale for Use in Drug Studies with Children', *American Journal of Psychiatry, 126*, 884-8

Eyman, R.K., Borthwick, S.A. and Miller, C. (1981) 'Trends in Maladaptive Behavior of Mentally Retarded Persons Placed in Community and Institutional Setting', *American Journal of Mental Deficiency, 85*, 473-7

Eyman, R.K. and Call, T. (1977) 'Maladaptive Behavior and Community Placement of Mentally Retarded Persons', *American Journal of Mental Deficiency, 82*, 137-44

Francis, S.H. (1970) 'Behavior of Low-Grade Institutionalized Mongoloids: Changes with Age', *American Journal of Mental Deficiency, 75*, 92-101

Fraser, W.I., Leudar, I., Gray, J. and Campbell, I. (1985) 'Psychiatric and Behaviour Disturbance in Mental Handicap', *Journal of Mental Deficiency Research, 30*, 49-57

Freeman, B.J., Ritvo, E.R., Schroth, P.C., Tonick, I., Guthrie, D. and Wake, L. (1981) 'Behavioral Characteristics of High- and Low-IQ Autistic Children', *American Journal of Psychiatry, 138*, 25-9

Goldberg, D.P., Cooper, B., Eastwood, M.R., Kedward, H.B. and Shepherd, M. (1970) 'A Standardised Psychiatric Interview for Use in Community Surveys', *British Journal of Social and Preventive Medicine, 24*, 18-23

Halpern, A.S., Irvin, L.K. and Landman, J.T. (1979) 'Alternative Approaches to the Measurement of Adaptive Behavior', *American Journal of Mental Deficiency, 84*, 304-10

Holmes, C. and Batt, R. (1980) 'Is Choking Others Really Equivalent to Stamping One's Feet? An Analysis of Adaptive Behavior Scale Items', *Psychological Reports, 46*, 1277-8

Holmes, N., Shah, A. and Wing, L. (1982) 'The Disability Assessment Schedule: A Brief Screening Device for Use with the Mentally Retarded', *Psychological Medicine, 12*, 879-90

Isset, R., Roszkowski, M., Spreat, S. and Reiter, S. (1983) 'Tolerance for Deviance: Subjective Evaluation of the Social Validity of the Focus of Treatment in Mental Retardation', *American Journal of Mental Deficiency, 87*, 458-61

Jacobson, J.W. (1982) 'Problem Behavior and Psychiatric Impairment Within a Developmentally Disabled Population I: Behavior Frequency', *Applied Research in Mental Retardation, 3*, 121-39

Janicki, M.P., Jacobson, J.W. and Schwartz, A.A. (1982) 'Residential Care Settings: Models for Rehabilitative Intent', *Journal of Practical Approaches to Developmental Handicap, 6*, 10-16

King, T., Soucar, E. and Isett, R. (1980) 'An Attempt to Assess and Predict Adaptive Behavior of Institutionalized Mentally Retarded Clients', *American Journal of Mental Deficiency, 84*, 406-10

Koller, H. Richardson, S.A., Katz, M. and McLaren, J. (1983) 'Behavior Disturbance Since Childhood among a 5-Year Birth Cohort of all Mentally Retarded Young Adults in a City', *American Journal of Mental*

Deficiency, 87, 386-95
Lambert, N.M. and Nicoll, R.C. (1976) 'Dimensions of Adaptive Behavior of Retarded and Nonretarded Public-School Children', *American Journal of Mental Deficiency, 81,* 135-46
Leudar, I. and Fraser, W.I. (1985) 'How to Keep Quiet: Some Withdrawal Strategies in Mentally Handicapped Adults', *Journal of Mental Deficiency Research, 29,* 315-30
Leudar, I., Fraser, W.I. and Jeeves, M.A. (1984) 'Behaviour Disturbance and Mental Handicap: Typology and Longitudinal Trends', *Psychological Medicine, 14,* 923-35
Lorr, M. and Jenkins, R.L. (1953) 'Patterns of Maladjustment in Children', *Journal of Clinical Psychology, 9,* 16-19
Matson, J.L. and Barret, R.P. (1982) *Psychopathology in the Mentally Retarded.* Grune & Stratton, New York
McDevitt, S., McDevitt, S. and Rosen, M. (1977) 'Adaptive Behavior Scale: Part II. A Cautionary Note and Suggestions for Revisions', *American Journal of Mental Deficiency, 82,* 210-11
Nihira, K. (1969a) 'Factorial Dimensions of Adaptive Behavior in Adult Retardates', *American Journal of Mental Deficiency, 73,* 868-87
Nihira, K. (1969b) 'Factorial Dimensions of Adaptive Behavior in Mentally Retarded Children and Adolescents', *American Journal of Mental Deficiency, 74,* 130-41
Nihira, K., Foster, R., Shelhaas, M. and Lelland, H. (1974) *AAMD Adaptive Behavior Scale,* American Association on Mental Deficiency, Washington, D.C.
Nihira, K., Mink, I.T. and Meyers, C.E. (1984) 'Salient Dimension of Home Environment relevant to Child Development', *International Review of Research in Mental Retardation, 12,* 149-75
Phillips, I. and Williams, N. (1975) 'Psychopathology and Mental Retardation: I. Psychopathology', *American Journal of Psychiatry, 132,* 1265-71
Reid, A.H., Ballinger, B.R. and Heather, B.B. (1978) 'Behaviour Syndromes Identified in a Sample of 100 Severely and Profoundly Retarded Adults', *Psychological Medicine, 8,* 399-412
Rutter, M., Tizard, J., Yule, P., Graham, P. and Whitmore, K. (1974) 'Isle of White Studies', *Psychological Medicine, 18,* 313-32
Salagaras, S. and Nettlebeck, T. (1983) 'Adaptive Behavior of Mentally Retarded Adolescents Attending School', *American Journal of Mental Deficiency, 88,* 57-68
Scanlon, C.A., Arick, J.R. and Krug, D.A. (1982) 'A Matched Sample Investigation of Nonadaptive Behavior of Severely Handicapped Adults across Four Living Situations', *American Journal of Mental Deficiency, 86,* 526-32
Schroeder, S.R., Mulick, J.A. and Schroeder, C.S. (1980) 'Management of Severe Behavior Problems of the Retarded' in N.R. Ellis (ed.), *Handbook of Mental Deficiency,* 2nd edn, Lawrence Erlbaum Associates, Hillsdale, NJ
Searles, E., Isett, R. and Bowders, T. (1981) 'Examination of Item Weighting on the Adaptive Behavior Scale Part II', *Perceptual and Motor Skills, 53,* 654

Senatore, V., Matson, J.L. and Kazdin, A.E. (1985) 'An Inventory to Assess Psychopathology of Mentally Retarded Adults', *American Journal of Mental Deficiency, 89,* 459–66

Sternlich, M. and Deutsch, M.R. (1972) *Personality Development and Social Behavior in the Mentally Retarded,* D.C. Heath, Lexington, Mass.

Taylor, J.R. (1976) 'A Comparison of the Adaptive Behavior of Retarded Individuals Successfully and Unsuccessfully Placed in Group Living Home', *Education and Training of Mentally Retarded,* February, 57–64

Thiel, G.W. (1981) 'Relationship of IQ, Adaptive Behavior, Age and Environmental Demand to Community-Placement Success of Mentally Retarded Adults', *American Journal of Mental Deficiency, 86,* 208–11

Wing, L. and Gould, J. (1978) 'Systematic Recording of Behaviours and Skills of Retarded and Psychotic Children', *Journal of Autism and Childhood Schizophrenia, 8,* 79–87

Wing, L. and Gould, J. (1979) 'Severe Impairments of Social Interactions and Associated Abnormalities in Children: Epidemiology and Classification, *Journal of Autism and Developmental Disorders, 9,* 11–29

6

Assessments of Physical Development, Hearing and Vision that can be used by Educational and Care Staff

J. Sebba

INTRODUCTION

This chapter considers the approaches for assessing physical and sensory functioning in people with a mental handicap. Some general points are made about the need for nonspecialist assessments and their role *vis-à-vis* specialist assessments. Some of the assessment procedures used by specialists are briefly introduced to enable comment on their role relative to nonspecialist procedures which focus on particular areas of functioning such as vision or hearing. The chapter does not include general assessments covering all areas of functioning which have been specifically adapted for people with visual, physical or hearing impairments.

GENERAL CHARACTERISTICS OF THE APPROACH

The prevalence of additional impairments such as hearing or visual problems among people who have a mental handicap is far greater than in the general population (see for example Fryers 1984). Furthermore, the occurrence of these problems becomes more likely with increasing severity of mental handicap. Studies in hospitals and in the community (e.g. Kropka and Williams 1980) have indicated that many people with a mental handicap suspected of having hearing or visual problems have not received specialised assessment and have therefore not received available prosthetics such as glasses or hearing aids. One factor contributing to the paucity of assessment services received by this population is the difficulties they present in terms of testing.

For these reasons it is essential to regard the assessment of people with a mental handicap as an inter-disciplinary process. The term 'inter-disciplinary' is deliberately chosen in preference to 'multi-disciplinary' as it describes an interactive process in which professionals from different disciplines conduct assessments together, or at least, discuss fully their findings in each area of functioning before decisions are made regarding intervention. 'Multi-disciplinary' assessment, on the other hand, can consist of each specialist carrying out procedures independently and writing reports which are filed away without ever having been properly co-ordinated.

There has been a shift in recent years from assessment by the psychiatrist or psychologist to assessment by the teacher, nurse, parent or residential staff member. This has been accompanied by a move from the use of psychometric assessment, employing tests often available only to those with medical or psychological qualifications, to criterion-referenced assessments, such as checklists (see Kiernan, Chapter 7 of this volume). This trend is, in part, indicative of the changing requirement of assessments to provide information more clearly related to intervention strategies, which psychometric testing is unable to provide. The same process has occurred in relation to specialist assessments, teachers, parents and residential staff wanting to make their own observations and records of physical, auditory and visual behaviour to provide a basis for their teaching. This has led to the production of checklists in these areas which complement the more specialised procedures carried out by physiotherapists, audiologists and ophthalmologists.

A further factor contributing to the increased use of less formal, criterion-referenced procedures has been the view that assessing clients in the context of their daily routine is more relevant and likely to yield observations of typical behaviour. For example, it may be possible to observe certain motor skills during the dressing and washing routines. Related to this is the possiblity inherent in criterion-referenced approaches, of staff devising their own checklists containing items most pertinent to their own setting and clients. Many examples of such checklists in the areas of physical, auditory and visual development exist, but this chapter does not describe them since they are not readily available. Obvious factors such as availability, portability and low cost have further led to a proliferation in the use of criterion-referenced procedures in this area.

This picture of the increasing popularity and availability of checklists begs the question of whether assessments carried out by specialists are required at all. In the description of some of these procedures below, the vital role played by the specialist will become apparent. Only their procedures can provide the necessary information about the intactness or internal functioning of the eye, ear and limbs. Furthermore any possibility of surgical remediation or use of aids can only be ultimately determined by the specialist. It is the specialist who can help those in daily contact with the client to provide a programme of intervention and management to minimise the limitations to development that might be imposed by additional impairments.

The nature of the relation between specialist and direct care personnel in the area of assessment will vary depending on such factors as the local resources and services and the nature of the impairments which the client may have. However, it is suggested that all people with a mental handicap should be entitled to specialist assessments of vision, hearing and physical development. Recognising the possible delay in assessing the backlog of all those clients who are no longer young children, the direct care personnel can contribute useful observations which indicate urgent priorities. Furthermore, the specialist can contribute a detailed technical report of the individual's functioning while the direct care staff provide observations of the use being made by that individual of their vision, hearing and physical functioning, impaired though he or she may be.

The ultimate responsibility for devising and implementing the intervention rests with the direct care staff. Furthermore, once a programme has begun, it is their responsibility to monitor the progress and suggest possible modifications. The feedback that direct care staff can provide specialists, regarding progress and difficulties encountered, may assist in the specialist's reassessment at a later stage. The specialists transfer some of their skills to direct care staff in order to ensure intervention has continuity. Moreover, it may be possible for direct care staff to observe the specialist working with the client and vice versa, from time to time to ensure that skill transferral has occurred accurately.

THE ASSESSMENT OF PHYSICAL DEVELOPMENT

Specialist assessment

It is essential to involve physiotherapists as early as possible in the inter-disciplinary assessment of people with a mental handicap in order to limit the effects of impairment on development. Methods of handling and positioning appropriate to each individual can inhibit the development of abnormal postural reflexes or of normal postural reflexes beyond the stage at which they usually disappear. For example, the persistence of the Asymmetrical Tonic Neck Reflex beyond the age of four months restricts the development of rolling over, prevents the child bringing the hands together in midline and inhibits mobility. Detailed physiotherapy assessment can identify joint stiffness and muscle weakness which may enable steps to be taken to avoid deformities.

The physiotherapist can also assist the nonspecialist to identify realistic limitations on physical development. Neuromuscular restrictions may impose such limitations even though handling, positioning and the use of aids have been carried out correctly. Without this identification of the limitations, there is always the danger that direct care staff may unwittingly undermine the confidence of the client by persisting in teaching inappropriate physical skills.

The assessments most commonly used by physiotherapists include assessment of general physical ability, range of joint movement, muscle strength and reflex reactions. These procedures are described fully by Holt (1965) and Levitt (1982) and their application to a group of children with profound retardation and multiple impairments is described in detail in Sebba (1978).

Physical ability charts (e.g. Holt 1965, Holle 1976 and Levitt 1982) list functional gross motor skills in the order of normal development giving approximate age norms for each item ranging from one week to three years. The items are scored on a rating scale from 'no ability' to 'normal performance' which leads to the identification of the stage reached in prone, supine and upright development. The next step in development is identified and possible restrictions to achieving this step considered.

The assessment of the range of movement in the joints of the neck, spine, limbs and shoulders is carried out and the position of adjacent joints noted. Each movement is scored as full, stiff or limited and right or left sides and passive or active movements are indicated where appropriate. The normal range is given on the rating sheet for comparative purposes.

Holt (1965) describes the assessment of muscle strength based on the Bobath techniques (Bobath and Bobath 1956), involving the measurement of the strength of individual muscle groups. The scoring is done on a rating scale from complete paralysis to contraction against powerful resistance. Molnar and Alexander (1983) refer to a variety of procedures aimed at providing objective measurement of muscle strength using equipment designed to isolate the movements.

Assessment of reflex reactions can be found in both Holt (1965; 1975) and Levitt (1982). Positioning and moving the client enables identification of abnormal postural reflexes and absence of normal ones. Likewise, the persistence of normal postural reflexes beyond the age at which they usually disappear can also be noted.

Nonspecialist assessments

It is apparent that the assessment of physical development in people with a mental handicap is complex and the involvement of a physiotherapist essential. However, it is also noted that the physiotherapist is a scarce resource, usually only available to the client on a once a fortnight basis, leading to the necessity for him or her to transfer his or her skills to those in daily contact with the client. Criterion-referenced assessments can provide a framework from which individual programmes can be evaluated on a continual basis. Most of the general checklists described in Chapter 7 of this volume include sections on motor skills. Three procedures specifically designed to assess motor skills in people with a mental handicap will be described here:

Paths to Mobility in 'Special Care' (Presland 1982)
This book is a guide to teaching motor skills to very handicapped children (although it is applicable to adults as well). It includes a checklist, further copies of which are also available separately, and teaching suggestions. The checklist covers development in lying, sitting, kneeling, crawling, standing and walking. As the title of it suggests, it is aimed at children who are profoundly retarded and multiply impaired. For this reason the skills in each section are analysed into a large number of steps (for example, there are 45 steps on sitting) with only small differences between one step and the

ASSESSMENTS OF ADDITIONAL IMPAIRMENTS

Figure 6.1: Example from the *Paths to Mobility* Checklist

	Criteria	Date tested	Date mastered	Date checked
Section 9. UPRIGHT KNEELING 1. With support, sits on heels. 2. Unaided, sits on heels. 3. With adult support, kneels upright. 4. With arms supported on low table, kneels upright. 5. Unaided, kneels upright and maintains position 2 seconds or more. 6. Unaided, kneels upright and maintains position 10 seconds or more. 7. Kneeling upright, reaches for objects on a table, maintaining balance. 8. Kneeling, rotates body, maintaining balance.				
Section 10. STANDING 1. Held in standing position, extends legs as if to support self. 2. Held in standing position, takes a little weight on legs briefly. 3. Held in standing position, places feet flat on floor. 4. Held in standing position, takes most weight on legs. 5. Held in standing position, takes all weight on legs. 6. Held in standing position, bounces up and down actively. 7. Held in standing position, puts feet flat on floor, with legs straight. 8. Placed in standing position holding adult's hand, maintains position 2 seconds or more. 9. Sitting, pulls self to standing holding on to adult's hands. 10. Kneeling on all fours, pulls self to standing holding on to adult's hands. 11. Kneeling upright, pulls self to standing holding on to adult's hand. 12. Standing holding on to chair or other support, maintains position 2 seconds or more. 13. Standing holding on to adult, chair, or other support, maintains position 10 seconds or more. 14. Unaided, stands for 2 seconds. 15. Unaided, stands for 10 seconds. 16. Stands up without pulling on anything. 17. Standing and pushed slightly forward at shoulders, regains upright position. 18. Standing and pushed slightly backward at shoulders, regains upright position.				

Source: Presland (1982 p. 57). Reproduced by kind permission of the publishers BIMH Publications.

next. An example from this checklist is given in Figure 6.1.

Many of the items included in the physical ability charts used by physiotherapists (described above) are also included in *Paths to Mobility*. However, the latter is geared specifically to nonspecialist staff using nontechnical language with clear statements for each step. It also includes a simple but clear recording system into which the criteria for success on each step for each individual is inserted by the person completing the checklist. This means that comparisons between clients would not be possible unless members of staff inserted the same criteria for all clients. However, the items are linked directly to teaching suggestions which indicate that this checklist is designed for programme planning on an individual basis rather than group comparisons. Furthermore, it encourages the maintenance of skills to be recorded by including a recording column on 'date checked' after the 'date mastered'.

The Glenwood Awareness, Manipulation and Posture (AMP) Scale (Webb, Schultz and McMahill 1977)

The Glenwood AMP Scale is designed to evaluate sensorimotor functioning of children who are multiply impaired. The Awareness Scale covers avoidance, approach and integrating memory with present stimuli, but the Manipulation Scale covers handling of objects, gesture and communication and the Posture Scale covers posture and mobility. Hence, although these scales are not exclusively on motor skills, a substantial part of them is of relevance here. The scale requires a more formal testing procedure than the incidental observations approach implied by Presland's checklist. Another factor making this scale of less use to staff in hospitals, adult day services, schools and other agencies is the need for both an observer and an evaluator. The observer should be familiar to the client and presents the items to him or her while the evaluator should be relatively unknown to the client and records the response. However, not many direct care staff would have sufficient resources to involve two people simultaneously in the assessment of one client which may result in the same person being observer and evaluator.

The Fine Motor Skill Assessment Battery (Hogg 1978)

The Fine Motor Skill Assessment Battery was developed to enable assessment of the fine motor skills of young children with developmental delay, regardless of the nature or degree of impairment. The items are organised into ten sections on postural control, visual function, reaching for objects, object insertion, placement of tubes, using a scoop, placement of flat objects, block stacking, bead threading, and complex sub-assembly. Figure 6.2 gives an example from the Fine Motor Skill Assessment Battery.

Hogg (in Gunstone, Hogg, Sebba, Warner and Almond 1982) describes how assessment on the Fine Motor Skill Assessment Battery can be used to identify potential curricular areas and evolve individual programmes from these, although further task analysis was required to determine the starting points for teaching in each case. Improvements in skills taught were reflected in the retest on the Fine Motor Skill Assessment Battery on completion of training. This assessment is likely to appeal more to psychologists and other semi-specialists in the field of assessment than to care staff, partly because it requires a more formal testing procedure rather than incidental observation. However, it provides the only comprehensive detailed assessment of fine motor skills in people with mental handicap available but less detailed motor assessments do occur in most general assessment procedures.

THE ASSESSMENT OF HEARING

Specialist assessments

The assessment of hearing in people with a mental handicap has developed significantly over the past ten years. Earlier detection of hearing loss has become more probable through the health visitor screening process, although the basis for referral to more detailed audiological assessment is variable. Some audiologists have argued (Tucker and Nolan 1984, 1986) that all people with a mental handicap should automatically receive full specialist audiological assessment because of the high prevalence of hearing losses noted in this population, especially among those with Down's Syndrome (see Cunningham and McArthur 1981) and the difficulties encountered in testing. It is clear from the literature (see for example Hogg and Sebba 1986, Chapter 5) that normal auditory ability is a prerequisite to the normal development of language and communication. In particular, it is also of great concern to identify persons with profound hearing losses whose normal or near-normal intelligence may be concealed by their impairment. Williams (1982) noted that language deficits manifesting themselves as an inability to use a vocal system of communication led to the inclusion in hospitals for

Figure 6.2: Example of an Item from the Fine Motor Skill Assessment Battery

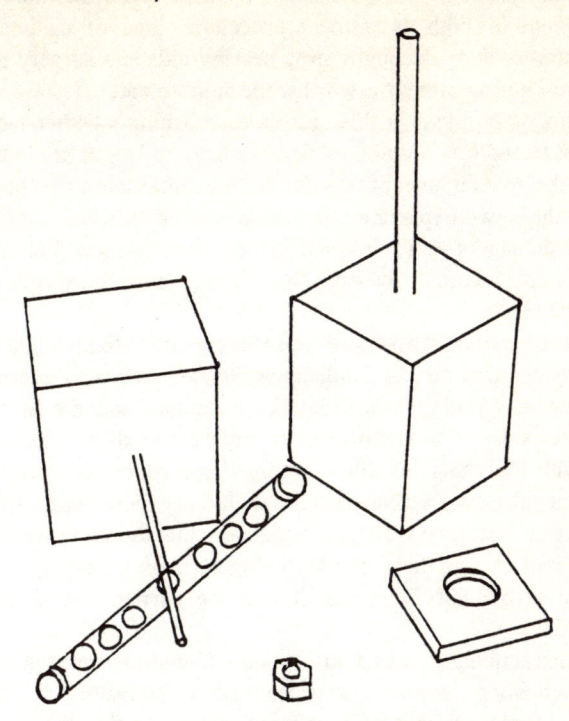

The above materials offer five rod/object combinations. They should be presented in the following order:

Rod	Object (mm)
9	22
4	22
4	10
4	8
9	10

Each combination should be presented twice, once with the rod vertical and once with it horizontal. Present all vertical combinations first. Follow Indicative Sequence.

Target behaviour:

The child picks up the object, locates it over the rod and moves it at least 2 cm down or along the rod.

Record success/failure. Classify grip. Note any use of second hand. Record Indicative Sequence.

Source: Hogg (1978 pp. 31-2).

people with mental handicap of a significant number of people whose main problem was a hearing impairment. Furthermore, the development of both assessment procedures and of methods of remediation such as decongestants, hearing aids and surgery make assessment and treatment a worthwhile investment.

The major problem in this area is establishing whether lack of responses to auditory stimuli are due to a hearing loss or are in keeping with the general level of retardation. It is important to distinguish between these two explanations because hearing aids and amplification may damage a person's ear if inappropriately used. Yet failing to use them where a hearing loss exists may seriously limit development.

The three specialist assessment procedures most likely to be used with people with a mental handicap are those involving distraction, the impedance bridge measurements technique and the auditory evoked response. Co-operative tests and performance tests which require the individual to follow simpler and more complex commands may also be used successfully with older individuals or those who have a less severe mental handicap, but the comprehension required may restrict their use. An otological examination by an ear, nose and throat (ENT) specialist may be carried out if this is suggested.

The distraction test, which in a modified version is used in health visitor screening, involves a tester and a distractor, the latter standing directly in front of the person and distracting him or her, while the former stands slightly behind the person and to one side and presents an auditory stimulus. The timing of the presentation of the stimulus is crucial since the distractor must stop distracting at this point. The intensity of the sound is increased until the person being tested responds with a head turn or other response such as eye movement or startle response. The intensity of sound at the moment the response is given is measured by a sound level meter. The procedure is repeated with sounds covering a range of frequencies and randomising the side on which they are presented.

A number of difficulties arise when using this procedure with people who have multiple impairments, which along with the modifications made to the procedure when used in health visitor screening, may account for the number of infants whose hearing losses went undetected in a study of hearing impairments in infants with Down's Syndrome (Cunningham and McArthur 1981). Physical impairments may result in insufficient head and trunk control to produce reliable head turning. It may also be difficult to position the individual without covering the ears. By about six months developmentally the infant with visual impairments may no longer exhibit locational responses to sound (Freedman 1964). Furthermore, people with a hearing loss may use rapid 'visual checking' to compensate for loss of information. Establishing consistent responses and accurately interpreting them is therefore a highly specialised activity, though this information can be supplemented by that gained from nonspecialist observations such as those suggested below. The distraction test can alert the specialist to a problem and indicate the likely frequencies involved but cannot be used to conclude definitely that a lack of response is indicative of a hearing loss.

The impedance bridge measurement technique involves fitting an ear probe through which a pure sound is passed and measuring the amount of sound passed through the ear and the amount returned. Middle ear hearing losses are indicated by a flatter compliance curve on the tympanogram which uses an automatic recorder. The impedance bridge measurement is relatively simple to carry out requiring little co-operation, which makes it well suited to the detection of middle ear disorders in people who are difficult to test.

One problem with this procedure is that it requires the person being tested to be free from catarrhal problems at the time of testing, since its presence would result in a flatter compliance curve which would be indicative of a fluctuating rather than a continuous hearing loss. Also, this procedure does not distinguish, within those whose compliance curves are normal, between persons with a sensorineural hearing loss and those who are not responding to auditory stimuli due to their general level of retardation. This distinction can really only be established through the use of electrical response audiometry.

Electrical response audiometry (ERA) procedures and some of the limitations of assessing hearing using them are described more fully in Barratt (1980) and Tucker and Nolan (1984). They involve the testing of the functioning of various parts of the neural hearing pathway and are particularly useful for identifying the hearing thresholds in people who are difficult to test. Electrodes are attached to the person's head so that the electrical activity of the brain can be recorded when sounds are presented through headphones. A computer records the resulting activity of the nerves in the hearing system and the responses are visually displayed as a wave form on the screen.

These procedures are of variable reliability and in addition some procedures are affected more than others by drugs or the level of arousal of the person being tested. Furthermore, the equipment is expensive, not readily available, and requires highly trained and experienced testers to interpret the results. However, if used in conjunction with impedance bridge measurements which yield information on low frequency functioning, they provide the only available method of detecting whether auditory stimulation is reaching the brain in people who are unresponsive using more conventional assessment methods.

Nonspecialist assessments

Many of the current population with mental handicaps are beyond the age of routine testing or held up in the backlog of 'difficult-to-test' clients. The contribution that the nonspecialist can make through observations noted during the daily routine is of value to the audiologist, for example, information on the auditory behaviour of the person across a variety of situations in his or her daily environment. Procedures for nonspecialists have therefore tended to be based on observational techniques rather than on any advanced technical equipment. One such technique is described below, but before considering this, the Stycar procedures which fall between the specialist and nonspecialist categories are described.

Stycar Hearing Tests (Sheridan 1976a)

The Stycar Hearing and Vision Tests are available only to psychologists and medical practitioners but may be used by paramedical and nursing staff under the supervision of a physician or psychologist who undertakes to ensure adequate training and periodic checks. In this sense, the procedures are both specialist and nonspecialist but are given here in the latter class as they are not limited to use by audiologists or ophthalmologists. Furthermore, the hearing tests are available to teachers of people who are hearing impaired, visually impaired and physically impaired.

The Stycar Hearing Tests are described as ideal for the assessment of very young (defined as six months to seven years) children with mental handicap. The tests assess children's ability to hear with comprehension in everyday life. They involve showing the child objects and pictures and asking him or her to identify particular items or types of items (e.g. small car, large car) or to follow directions. The Stycar is therefore rather similar to the co-operative and performance tests used by audiologists. It will be likely to have similar drawbacks when used with people who have a severe or profound mental handicap, namely, the difficulty of establishing sufficient verbal comprehension.

Systematic Procedures for Eliciting and Recording Responses to Sound Stimuli (Kershman and Napier 1982)

This procedure presents one of the first attempts to detail a method by which parents, teachers and other staff can make a direct systematic contribution to the assessment of hearing in people with a mental handicap. Two types of observational schedules were used: the Auditory Response Data Sheet and the Auditory Response to Environmental Sounds Sheet as shown in Figures 6.3 and 6.4.

The Auditory Response Data Sheet involved presenting each child with ten noise-making toys selected from readily available items of Fisher Price, Play Skool equipment, etc. The sounds were presented at a distance of four feet at ear level, randomising the side, in a quiet room in each child's home and when the child was quiet and content. Cairns and Butterfield (1975) have shown that the time since an infant's last feed is a critical variable in assessment of auditory functioning. Children with physical impairments were positioned to maximise their relaxation. Observations began at least ten seconds prior to the introduction of the sound and continued for at least ten seconds after it, since it was the change in behaviour that was of crucial importance.

Behavioural definitions for each of the responses given in Figure 6.3 are provided by Kershman and Napier. The category given as Intensity requires a score of the strength of the response from 0 defined as 'no response' (children remained in prestimulus state) to 3 defined as 'high response' (child exhibits an intense response and is completely occupied by responding to the stimulus). Reliabilities were established between teachers, audiologists and parents on these categories despite the difficulties of interpreting responses by children who showed a range of extraneous behaviours such as tremours, seizures, jerks and self-stimulatory behaviours.

Once reliabilities on this schedule were established, parents were asked to note their child's responses to environmental sounds as in the example sheet shown in Figure 6.4. The responses recorded by parents to environmental sounds enabled further information to be gathered which would provide examples of consistent and generalised behaviours.

Finally, the teachers collected further observations using the same behaviour categories as those on the sheet shown in Figure 6.3,

Figure 6.3: Example of a Completed Auditory Response Data Sheet

Child's name: Peter X
Setting: Peter's house

Observers: Mother ✓ & teacher *
Date(s): 4/11 & 4/17/1979

Stimulus	Source of Presentation	Date	No response	Cessation of activity	Quieting	Jerk/startle (extension)	Jerk/startle (flexion)	Increased activity	Vocalization	Crying	Laughing	Smile	Frown	Eye Blink	Eye widening	Eye localization	Head turning	Body localization	Reaching	Intensity	Comments
Jack-in box	Left	4/11										* ✓		* ✓						1	
	Right	4/17		* ✓				* ✓							✓	* ✓				2	
1" cube in can	Left	4/11		* ✓		* ✓	* ✓		* ✓	* ✓					✓	✓	✓	* ✓		3	head turned to left
	Right	4/17		* ✓		* ✓	* ✓		* ✓								* ✓	* ✓		3	
Ping-pong ball in can	Left	4/17		* ✓		* ✓				* ✓		* ✓								2	
	Right	4/11	* ✓																	0	
Cow bell	Left	4/11		* ✓		* ✓	* ✓			* ✓		* ✓					* ✓			3	
	Right	4/17		* ✓				* ✓												2	eye movement

Source: Kershman, S.M. and Napier, D., 'Systematic Procedures for Eliciting and Recording Responses to Sound Stimuli in Deaf-Blind Multihandicapped Children', *The Volta Review*, 1982, *84*, p. 228.

Figure 6.4: Example of a Completed Auditory Response to Environmental Sounds Sheet

Child's name: John

Date	4/21	4/24
Describe sound	portable hair dryer	mother's voice calling "John"
Location of sound (eg. 3 feet from child or next room	one foot from John (no air touched him)	five feet to the right of John
What was the child doing when sound occurred?	lying relaxed in reclining seat	being fed, head held by father
Describe response to sound	head turning, eye turning toward sound, face expressed surprise, eye widening	head turned to right, eyes turned to right, smiled, vocalized
Observer	mother	mother and father

Source: Kershman, S.M. and Napier, D., 'Systematic Procedures for Eliciting and Recording Responses to Sound Stimuli in Deaf-Blind Multihandicapped Children', *The Volta Review*, 1982, *84*, p. 229.

on reponses to prerecorded sounds at a variety of frequencies and intensities. Some audiologists, however, have taken issue with the frequency specificity described in this study (Tucker, personal communication). All the information collected was summarised to enable previously hidden patterns of responses to auditory stimuli to emerge. The information was relayed to the child's audiologist and used to plan an individualised training programme.

One of the strengths of the Kershman and Napier study was that it demonstrated that naturalistic observations can be used in conjunction with the more formal audiological assessment. Furthermore, it showed that parents, teachers and teacher aides can collect systematic observational information with high inter-observer reliability. Similar, but less comprehensive, auditory checklists are described by Sebba (1978) and Jones (1984) and their use with people with profound and multiple impairments reported.

Crossmodal Transfer as a Means of Preparing Individuals for Audiological Assessment (Goetz, Utley, Gee, Baldwin and Sailor 1982)

A systematic method by which nonspecialists can prepare individuals for specialised audiological assessment is described by Goetz *et al.* (1982) and Goetz, Gee and Sailor (1983). As previously noted, those who are difficult to test may not exhibit responses to the conventional procedures described previously under distraction tests. In this innovatory study, it was demonstrated that students with severe retardation and multiple impairments who had previously failed to demonstrate reliable responses to an auditory stimulus, could be taught to do so by pairing the auditory stimulus with a visual one. Once reliable responding had been established the visual cue was systematically faded by delaying it and reducing its intensity.

Training was carried out in the classroom with inexpensive materials and involved nonaudiologists. Once reliable responding had been achieved it was possible for the audiologists to carry out the more formal procedures. The only student who failed to establish a response on the paired visual training was found to have a profound hearing impairment on subsequent audiological testing. The authors suggest that this may be a useful procedure for teaching functional hearing to people who show no auditory responses. They stress that it complements rather than replaces the specialised audiological assessment.

THE ASSESSMENT OF VISION

Assessment of visual functioning in people with a mental handicap is important to the overall development of the individual, since, as with the other impairments discussed above, the limitations imposed on other areas of development by a visual impairment are considerable (see McInnes and Treffry 1982 for a review). Lawson, Molloy and Miller (1977) found that as many as 70 per cent of their sample of children with retardation had visual defects and Wolf and Anderson (1973) noted visual limitations in over 50 per cent of children with cerebral palsy.

The majority of people with significant visual deficiencies retain some functional vision (Langley and DuBose 1976), but if multiple impairments are present, their limited experiential and cognitive abilities may lead to a tendency for their residual vision to remain largely unused. A distinction can be made between 'seeing' and 'looking' (Sheridan 1976b). Seeing refers to the primarily physiological process dependent on intact visual mechanisms, whereas 'looking' is primarily a psychological process involving attention to visual stimuli and meaningful interpretation of them. This suggests the need for assessment of both the structure of the eye and the functional use made of vision, which provides a possible distinction between the roles that might be played by specialists and nonspecialists in the assessment process.

Specialist assessments

The ophthalmologist can carry out a full external and internal examination of the eyes, using an anaesthetic if required. This might include an examination of the contents of the eyeball and the pressure within it. An orthoptist can conduct the full range of refraction tests. Bankes (1975) and Markovits (1975) provide comprehensive descriptions of these procedures.

Full ophthalmological and orthoptist assessments can provide valuable information leading to appropriate treatment and suggestions for the training of any residual vision or appropriate materials for educational programmes. However, if no deficiencies are found, the same difficulty arises as that discussed above in relation to hearing, i.e. whether lack of a visual response is due to general attentional or cognitive deficits or because the visual stimulus is not reaching the cortex. The only method of establishing this is by the use of visual evoked responses. Visual evoked response procedures are similar to the electrical response audiometry described above, only using visual stimuli in a darkened room instead of the auditory stimuli. These procedures have similar disadvantages to the auditory evoked response procedure in that they are expensive, complex, require highly trained technicians to interpret the results and are not readily available.

Much more commonly used is the *Snellen Chart* which is the familiar card of printed letters of decreasing size used to assess visual acuity in the general population. Visual impairments are then expressed in terms of what the individual sees from a specified distance compared to the distance from which a person with normal sight could see the same-sized letters. It is obviously of limited use with individuals whose letter recognition and communication is relatively poor.

Another procedure used by specialists is the *Catford Drum* (Catford and Oliver 1973) which projects a series of spots of light of decreasing size moving across and back through the visual field. The size of spot at which fixation fails to occur is noted and each size corresponds to a Snellen acuity. This provides a routine assessment of visual acuity and this and other procedures measuring optokinetic responses have similarly been used with people with mental handicap (see also Atkinson 1986). However, difficulties arise of distinguishing between failure due to attentional deficits and that attributable to poor vision. Furthermore, the procedure depends on a motor response, making it difficult to distinguish oculomotor defects from problems of visual acuity.

Nonspecialist assessments

Stycar Vision Tests (Sheridan 1976b)

The Stycar Vision Tests like the Stycar Hearing Tests are only available for use by psychologists, doctors and specialist teachers, although clearly with the trend in educational provision towards educating children with sensory impairments in the ordinary school, the range of acceptable users seems likely to be extended. The tests are suitable for children from six months to seven years or people developmentally in this range, except for the 'Panda Test' which is suitable for older children (5–15 years) with visual perceptual problems. The procedures are organised into four distinctive tests, three defined by age and the Panda Test. For the oldest (five to seven years) the test involves matching letters, whereas the preschool children are assessed through object naming in the Miniature Toys Test as well as letter matching. Infants are assessed by the Rolling Balls Test in which balls of decreasing size are rolled across a contrasting surface about three metres from the child. Any visual tracking is then noted.

Langley and DuBose (1976) argue that the Miniature Toys Test and Rolling Balls Test are the most useful for children with additional impairments. Sheridan (1976b) emphasised that the Rolling Balls procedure tests the child's minimal observable distance rather than the minimum discriminatory distance, that is, the child has to observe the object but does not have to find its characteristics, as he or she does with the Snellen letters.

Bax, Hart and Jenkins (1981) report studies using the Stycar procedures to survey visual acuity in both normally developing children and those with developmental delay. They suggest adaptations for the nonverbal child, such as the use of eye-pointing in the Miniature Toys Test and letters test. Hof-van Duin, Mohn and Batenburg (1982) add additional data on the usefulness of the Stycar procedures with children who are severely mentally handicapped, which were employed not only to confirm suspected visual problems but also to suggest programmes of visual stimulation.

However, disadvantages of using the Stycar procedures with people with mental handicaps are also evident. Some of the children who are severely or profoundly mentally handicapped may be functioning below the six-month level considered the earliest age at which the procedure can be used. In addition, Atkinson and Braddick (1982) have argued that the balls in the Rolling Balls test are not the appropriate stimulus for testing visual acuity which should be assessed through pattern recognition as in the 'Preferential Looking' technique described below. Further possible problems include the noise made by the movement of the balls and the motor skills involved in tracking them.

Forced Choice Preferential Looking (Teller 1979)

This technique was developed by Teller (1979) and involves the presentation of a screen which is patterned on one half and blank but of equal luminance on the other half. The side on which the pattern is presented is randomly changed and the child consistently looking at the pattern is taken as evidence of visual acuity. It is called 'forced choice' because the observer who records to which side the child looked cannot see on which side the pattern was presented. Atkinson and Braddick (1982) report use of this procedure with infants of one to six months suggesting its suitability for older children who are severely or profoundly handicapped. This has been demonstrated by Shepherd and Fagan (1981) who showed that the procedure was highly reliable and suggested that observers can be trained in its use to evaluate relatively easily the visual behaviours of children with profound retardation. However, it is clearly a high-resource technique requiring two or more people to administer the procedure and as Nelson, Rubin, Wagner and Breton (1984) point out, it requires an alert and attentive child because of its dependence on a behavioural response.

Frostig Developmental Test of Visual Perception (Frostig, Lefever and Whittlesey 1966)

The Frostig Developmental Test is suitable for children aged four to eight years and older children who have learning difficulties. It provides information on the relation of visual perceptual disabilities to problems of learning and is seen to be testing skills which are prerequisites for reading. The procedures cover eye-motor co-ordination, figure ground, consistency of shape, position in space and spatial relations. Scores for each of these areas are given as well as overall scores which have been standardised on American populations.

The Frostig tests are of limited use with people who are severely and profoundly retarded because of the developmental level at which they start. Furthermore, they take rather a long time to administer which may limit their use in the classroom or on a ward. Moreover, studies (see review by Spache 1976) have shown that completing the related training programme does not necessarily result in increased scores on the reading assessments.

Bell's Observation List (Bell 1983)

This is not a published assessment with a manual, scoring sheets or test materials but a description of the information that should be recorded during observations by a 'significant person' on how the person is using her or his vision. Bell (1983) states that specialist assessments, although necessary to provide information on a child's eye defects, visual acuity and visual field, are unlikely to provide information on the ways in which the child uses vision or about the motivation to do so. Periods of systematic observation during the normal daily routine may pick up on the subtle behaviour changes which may indicate a visual response in a person who is profoundly handicapped. Bell's guidelines for observation are given (Bell 1983, p. 17) as follows:

1. The extent to which he is 'visually curious'. Does he look at desired or new items or does he touch, taste or smell them in preference?
2. The extent of his visual interest in people. Does he look at people's faces? Does he watch people as they move around the room? Is there anyone in particular that he likes looking at?
3. The kind of objects he will look at. Is interest affected by their purpose, size, colour, shape, pattern, or by their appeal to his other senses?
4. The distance at which visual attention is given most readily.
5. The preferred angle of view.
6. The preferred or dominant eye or side.
7. The extent to which vision is used to direct and monitor reach and grasp. The accuracy of the reach in terms of both distance and direction.
8. The speed with which he notices things to the sides when he is looking straight ahead.
9. If mobile, the extent to which he avoids or bumps into

obstacles. Is this related to their size, position, colour or their familiarity?
10. The effect of place or time on his willingness to use sight. Is it related to motivation, lighting, comfort or to the competition from other stimuli? Does he use vision to the same extent at home and at school?
11. The negative signs. The things which he consistently fails to see. The presence of mannerisms, e.g. eye-poking, head-weaving or light gazing which may indicate loss of sight.

From these observations Bell suggests drawing up a 'summary and action sheet' which must include the specification of the conditions under which optimum use of vision occurs and the teaching objective in the area of visual skills. There are no reliability figures reported in Bell's article but this procedure could easily be subjected to a similar attempt to establish reliability between various staff and parents as was reported above in relation to Kershman and Napier's hearing checklist.

Functional Vision Screening for Severely Handicapped Children (Langley and DuBose 1976; Langley 1980) and the Sebba (1978) Adaptation for use with People with Profound and Multiple Impairments

Langley and DuBose (1976) and Langley 1980 devised a functional vision screening checklist for assisting staff to observe systematically basic visual responses in people with severe and profound retardation for whom the more formal testing procedures were considered problematic to administer. It requires no complex materials or procedures and can be carried out in a corner of a classroom without the need to complete all the items in any one session.

The Langley and DuBose assessment covers the presence and nature of the visual response, reaction to visual stimuli, distance and size of objects and pictures, integration of visual and cognitive processing and the integration of visual and motor processing. Examples are given below from the most advanced section of the original Langley and DuBose assessment (Figure 6.5) and of earlier sections of the Sebba (1978) adaptation of Langley and DuBose (Figure 6.6).

It will be noted on the Sebba adaptation that the visual field and tracking items are administered in both sitting and supine (lying on back) positions. The reasons for this are that responses in these two

Figure 6.5: Section of the 'Functional Visual Screening for Severely Handicapped Children'

V.   Integration of Visual and Motor Processing

a.   On activities involving the pegs, stacking cone, puzzles, pounding bench, and beads, watch to see if he directly inserts or applies pieces, overreaches (O) or underreaches (U). Does he look for the recess and the hole or does he tactually approach them?
b.   When shown one colored block, shape, or 2" picture at a time, can he match it, given only two choices? Watch to see which colors, shapes, and pictures he matches and if he attends to color or configuration. Observe the distance from the materials at which he works, then have him match them at a far distance. Note the farthest distance at which he correctly matches each.

V.   Integration of Visual and Motor Processing

a.   Approach
   1. pegs: ___visual___tactual Reach:___O___U
   2. stacking cone: ___visual___tactual Reach:___O___U
   3. puzzles: ___visual___tactual Reach:___O___U
   4. pounding bench: ___visual___tactual Reach:___O___U
   5. beads: ___visual___tactual Reach:___O___U
b.   Matching:
   1. colored blocks:
      ___matches___does not match___near distance___far distance
   2. shapes:
      ___matches___does not match___near distance___far distance
   3. pictures:
      ___matches___does not match___near distance___far distance

Source: Material from 'Functional Vision Screening for Severely Handicapped Children' by Langley, B. and DuBose, R.F. from *The New Outlook for the Blind* is reproduced with kind permission from the American Foundation for the Blind and is © 1976 by American Foundation for the Blind, 15 West 16th Street, New York, N.Y. 10011

positions are sometimes reported as differing. Hisley (1978), for example, has noted that pressure exerted on the back of the head when supine can interfere with vision. Fieber (1977) has noted differences in visual perception in various different positions and Bower (1974) had suggested that infants may not be fully awake when supine. It is therefore of interest to note any differences observed in visual responses in the different positions.

The Langley and DuBose assessment has not been standardised formally and reliabilities are not reported. However, the procedure provides a clear method of systematically observing and recording visual responses which can inform teaching programmes. Teachers, residential and other staff and parents can use this type of procedure to complement the formal specialist assessments described above. They are in a unique position to observe whether the visual

Figure 6.6: Sections from Sebba's 1978 Adaptation of Langley and DuBose (1976), for Children with Profound and Multiple Impairments

1. *Pupil Reaction*
   a) Do the pupils constrict and dilate continually when the person is in constant light?
   If they do, this suggests a visual defect and you should move to question 2.
   If they do not:-
   b) Direct torch light into the eyes from approximately 45 cms
   Do pupils constrict to light?
   Do pupils dilate when light is removed?

	Yes	No

R	L

2. *Muscle Balance* (assessing for a squint)
   Hold light 45 cms from mid point between the two eyes.
   Is the light reflected simultaneously in the centre of each pupil?
   If not, a squint may be observed.

R	L

3. *Blink Reaction*
   From behind the client, move your hand over their eyes from their chin to their forehead approximately 5 cm away from their face. Pause, and repeat 5 times. Tick each time they blink.

1	2	3	4	5	6

4. *Visual Field*
   Flash the light on and off from approximately 45 cms, above, below and to the left and right of the client. Tick if attention is given to the light eg. eyes fix on light, client reaches for light. Repeat.

	Above	Below	Left	Right
1				
2				

5. *Peripheral Vision*
   Bring the light from behind the client, slowly into the left and then the right visual field. Tick if the client turns their head or eyes to the light when the torch is in line with the lateral position of the eye. Repeat 3 times.

	Head or eye turn to right	Head or eye turn to left
1		
2		
3		
4		

6. *Visual Field Preference*
   Present two identical non-sound producing toys simultaneously in the right and left visual fields. Tick the side to which the client looks first. Repeat 5 times.

	1	2	3	4	5	6
Left						
Right						
None						

responses are consistently shown or absent and can relate these observations to the specialist as well as using the information themselves.

COMMENTS ON THE USES AND ABUSES OF THE TECHNIQUES

In the review given above of the various assessment procedures available for nonspecialists in the areas of physical development, hearing and vision, a number of issues have arisen which are general to all three areas. These will be briefly discussed here, in the hope of offering a list of possible criteria from which readers can select those pertinent to their own situations, to use when considering any particular assessment procedure. For example, if the client group of interest is functioning at a very low level, one major criterion must be the level at which the assessment begins.

First then, the issue of the developmental level of assessments is considered. The assessments described in this chapter have tended with notable exceptions such as the Frostig tests to be relevant to very low functioning clients. This is partly because this chapter is dealing with the assessment of additional impairments, which, as stated, occur more in people with profound mental handicap than in those who are more able. It is only in recent years, as can be seen by the dates of the publication of these assessments, that suitable procedures for assessing this population have emerged. Hence, it is not surprising that many of the procedures have not been formally standardised. The problems of standardisation on such a heterogeneous but relatively widely dispersed population are clear. The developmental level at which the procedure begins is likely to be one criterion of relevance, although DuBose and Langley (1977) have demonstrated that criterion-referenced assessments can correlate significantly with the more formal standardised assessments.

A second consideration is the flexibility of the procedure for use with people whose impairments are multiple. The Presland checklist, for example, has sections on walking with crutches, walking with sticks and using a wheelchair. Another example of adaptations to physical impairment is provided by Bax *et al.*'s (1981) suggestion that eye-pointing can be used in the Miniature Toys Test of the Stycar Vision Tests. Hence, for some parents and staff, procedures which either suggest, or at least allow for, adaptations to be made to overcome the restriction imposed by additional impairments, will be of relevance.

A related problem, is the verbal comprehension, and in some cases speech, required by the client in order to demonstrate skills in areas of development other than communication. In the physiotherapist's assessment of muscle strength, the client was expected to follow commands and be able to isolate movements requiring precise comprehension of the labels of parts of the body. In the assessment of hearing, the distraction tests involve both a motor response in terms of head turning and a visual response in terms of location of a sound. Another example was provided by Sheridan's Miniature Toys Test which requires the child to comprehend the difference between the verbal labels 'knife', 'fork' and 'spoon' in order to be able to demonstrate his or her ability to discriminate visually between them. Procedures must offer staff a method of assessing skills in one modality without the procedure necessarily demanding a high level of skills in other modalities.

An important area of concern when considering an assessment procedure is clearly the issues surrounding who is to administer the assessment. Some of the procedures, such as the Stycar Vision and Hearing Tests are stated to be 'Closed tests' available only to the professionals defined. Others, such as the Kershman and Napier hearing checklist and the Langley and DuBose visual checklist, are deliberately attempting to encourage parents and staff, not conventionally responsible for assessment, to become so. It is not only the regulations stipulated by the publisher or distributor that decides who is able to use a procedure. Another important factor determining this is the resources demanded by the assessment. The Preferential Looking technique requires at least two people to administer it as does the Awareness, Manipulation and Posture Scale which involves an observer and an evaluator.

One criterion on which an assessment is considered may be the setting in which it is administered. The checklists which give items that can be incidentally observed within the context of daily living routines are becoming increasingly regarded as more relevant and acceptable. Staff are concerned that testing procedures requiring a one-to-one session in a separate room are of little interest if the client is unable to use the same skills in the context of their daily routine.

Another drain on staff resources concerns the time taken to complete the procedure in one sitting. In the description of the Frostig test, given above, the long time (approximately one hour) taken to carry it out was mentioned, which is both unrealistic in terms of the client's attention span and in terms of the staff time available. A further consideration is how far the items are detailed enough to provide a clear indication of suitable teaching objectives or how much further work needs to be done by the member of staff to move from assessment to intervention. A contrast could be drawn, for example, between the Presland checklist which has so many steps the teacher is required to do no additional work and the Fine Motor Skill Assessment Battery in which further task analysis is used to enable staff to devise a teaching target in relation to each client's individual needs. Hence, more staff time invested at the assessment stage may have the advantage of leading to more individually tailored teaching targets.

The final issue which arises is the reliability of the procedures considered. Kershman and Napier (1982) have demonstrated that observational procedures may be less formal but should still be systematically applied, with an attempt to establish reliability between observers. The rating scale on the physical ability charts used by physiotherapists seems too dependent on the subjective judgement of the observer. This type of rating scale is always more problematic in the middle scores since there tends to be more agreement about the total absence of a skill or normal performance, which would be indicated by a score at either end of the scale.

In this chapter, an attempt has been made to review some of the procedures available to nonspecialists in the assessment of physical development, hearing and vision in people with mental handicap. General features of the approach which combines specialist and nonspecialist assessments to complement one another were outlined, and specialist procedures explained before briefly reviewing some examples of nonspecialist assessments. Finally some general points which arise in relation to the use of these assessments were discussed in order to provide a possible list of criteria on which such assessments might be selected. Throughout the chapter the importance of the distinctive, yet complementary, roles to be played by specialists and nonspecialists in assessing physical, hearing and visual development in people with mental handicap was emphasised.

REFERENCES

Atkinson, J. (1986) 'Methods of Objective Assessment of Visual Functions in Subjects with Limited Communication Skills' in D. Ellis (ed.), *Sensory Impairments in Mentally Handicapped People*, Croom Helm, London/College-Hill Press, San Diego

Atkinson, J. and Braddick, O. (1982) 'Assessment of Visual Acuity in Infancy and Early Childhood', *Acta Ophthalmologica Supplement, 157*, 18–26

Bankes, J.L.K. (1975) 'The Ophthalmologist's Role in Multidisciplinary Assessment of Developmentally Handicapped Children', *Child: Care, Health and Development, 1*, 325–33

Barratt, H. (1980) 'Electric Response Audiometry and its Application to the Assessment of Hearing in Children', *Journal of the British Association of Teachers of the Deaf, 4*, 4–6

Bax, M., Hart, A. and Jenkins, S. (1981) 'Clinical Testing of Visual Function of the Young Child', *Developmental Medicine and Child Neurology*, 23, 92–100

Bell, J. (1983) 'Assessment of Visual Ability in the Profoundly Handicapped', *National Association of Deaf Blind Rubella Handicapped News Letter*, 29, 16–17

Bobath, K. and Bobath, B. (1956) 'The Diagnosis of Cerebral Palsy in Infancy', *Archives of Disease in Childhood*, 31, 408–14

Bower, T. (1974) *Development in Infancy*, Freeman, London

Cairns, G.F. and Butterfield, E.C. (1975) 'Assessing Infants' Auditory Functioning' in B.Z. Friedlander, G.M. Steritt and F.G.E. Kirk (eds.), *Exceptional Infant*, vol. 3, Brunner/Mazel Inc., New York

Catford, G.V. and Oliver, A. (1973) 'Development of Visual Acuity', *Archives of Disease in Childhood*, 48, 47–50

Cunningham, C. and McArthur, K. (1981) 'Hearing Loss and Treatment in Young Down's Syndrome Children', *Child: Care, Health and Development*, 7, 357–74

DuBose, R.F. and Langley, M.B. (1977) *The Developmental Activities Screening Inventory*, Teacher Resources, Boston

Fieber, N. (1977) 'Sensorimotor Cognitive Assessment and Curriculum for the Multihandicapped Child' in J. Cronin (ed.), *The Severely and Profoundly Handicapped Child*, State Board of Education, Illinois

Freedman, D.G. (1964) 'Smiling in Blind Infants and the Issue of Innate versus Acquired', *Journal of Child Psychology and Psychiatry and Allied Disciplines*, 5, 171–84

Frostig, M., Lefever, W. and Whittlesey, J.R.B. (1966) *The Frostig Developmental Test of Visual Perception*, NFER, Windsor

Fryers, T. (1984) *The Epidemiology of Severe Intellectual Impairments: The Dynamics of Prevalance*, Academic Press, London

Goetz, L., Gee, K. and Sailor, W. (1983) 'Crossmodal Transfer of Stimulus Control: Preparing Students with Severe Multiple Disabilities for Audiological Assessment', *Journal of the Association for Persons with Severe Handicap*, 8, 3–13

Goetz, L., Utley, B., Gee, K., Baldwin, M. and Sailor, W. (1982) *Auditory Assessment and Programming Manual for Severely Handicapped and Deaf-Blind Students*, Association for the Severely Handicapped, Seattle, Washington

Gunstone, C., Hogg, J., Sebba, J., Warner, J. and Almond, S. (1982) *Classroom Provision and Organisation for Integrated Preschool Children*, Barnardo Publications Ltd, Barkingside

Hisley, T. (1978) 'Classification and Assessment of the Special Care Child', unpublished paper presented at the Royal Manchester Children's Hospital to a meeting on 'Education of the Special Care Child', 31 January 1978

Hof-van Duin, J. Van., Mohn, G. and Batenburg, A.M. (1982) 'Simple Tests of Visual Function in Multiply Handicapped Children', *International Journal of Rehabilitation Research*, 5, 239–40

Hogg, J. (1978) 'The Development of a Fine Motor Skill Assessment Battery for Use with Mentally Handicapped Preschool Children', unpublished report, Hester Adrian Research Centre, University of Manchester, Manchester

Hogg, J. and Sebba, J. (1986) *Profound Retardation and Multiple Impairment: Vol. 1. Development and Learning*, Croom Helm, London

Holle, B. (1976) *Motor Development in Children: Normal and Retarded*, Blackwell, Oxford

Holt, K.S. (1965) *Assessment of Cerebral Palsy*, Lloyd-Luke, London

Holt, K.S. (1975) (ed.) *Movement and Child Development*, Heinemann, London

Jones, L. (1984) 'Curriculum Evaluation for the Profoundly Retarded Multiply Handicapped Child', unpublished manuscript, Lea Castle Hospital, Kidderminster

Kershman, S.M. and Napier, D. (1982) 'Systematic Procedures for Eliciting and Recording Responses to Sound Stimuli in Deaf-Blind Multihandicapped Children', *The Volta Review*, 84, 226–37

Kropka, B.I. and Williams, C. (1980) 'The Deaf and Partially Hearing in Mental Handicap Hospitals: The Disadvantaged Minority?', *British Journal of Mental Subnormality*, 26, 89–93

Langley, M.B. (1980) *Functional Vision Inventory for the Multiple and Severely Handicapped*, Stoelting, Chicago

Langley, M.B. and DuBose, R.F. (1976) 'Functional Vision Screening for Severely Handicapped Children', *The New Outlook for the Blind*, 70, 346–50

Lawson, L.J., Molloy, J.S. and Miller, M. (1977) 'A Technique for Appraising the Vision of Mentally Retarded Children', in P. Mittler (ed.), *Research to Practice in Mental Retardation. Vol. II. Education and Training*, University Park Press, Baltimore

Levitt, S. (1982) *Treatment of Cerebral Palsy and Motor Delay*, Blackwell, Oxford

McInnes, J.M. and Treffry, J.A. (1982) *Deaf-Blind Infants and Children: A Developmental Guide*, Open University and University of Toronto Press, Milton Keynes and Toronto

Markovits, A.S. (1975) 'Ophthalmic Screening of the Mentally Defective', *Annals of Ophthalmology*, 7, 846–8

Molnar, G.E. and Alexander, J. (1983) 'Strength Development in Retarded Children: A Comparative Study on the Effect of Intervention' in J. Hogg and P.J. Mittler (eds.), *Advances in Mental Handicap Research*, vol 2, Wiley, London

Nelson, L.B., Rubin, S.E., Wagner, R.S. and Breton, M.E. (1984) 'Developmental Aspects in the Assessment of Visual Function in Young Children', *Pediatrics*, 73, 375–81

Presland, J. (1982) *Paths to Mobility in 'Special Care'*, British Institute of Mental Handicap, Kidderminster

Sebba, J. (1978) 'A System for Assessment and Intervention for Preschool Profoundly Retarded Multiply Handicapped Children', M.Ed. thesis, University of Manchester, Manchester

Shepherd, P.A. and Fagan, J.F. (1981) 'Assessment of Visual Pattern Detection and Recognition Memory in the Profoundly Retarded Child', in N.R. Ellis (ed.), *International Review of Research in Mental Retardation*, vol. 10, Academic Press, New York

Sheridan, M.D. (1976a) *The Stycar Hearing Test*, NFER, Windsor

Sheridan, M.D. (1976b) *Manual for the Stycar Vision Tests*, NFER,

Windsor
Spache, G.D. (1976) *Investigating the Issues of Reading Disabilities*, Allyn and Bacon Inc., Boston
Teller, D.Y. (1979) 'The Forced Choice Preferential Looking Procedure: A Psychophysical Technique for Use with Human Infants', *Infant Behavior and Development*, 2, 135–53
Tucker, I. (1985) personal communication
Tucker, I. and Nolan, M. (1984) *Educational Audiology*, Croom Helm, London, Sydney and Dover, NH
Tucker, I. and Nolan, M. (1986) 'Methods of Objective Assessment of Auditory Function in Subjects with Limited Communication Skills' in D. Ellis (ed.), *Sensory Impairments in Mentally Handicapped People*, Croom Helm, London/College-Hill Press, San Diego
Webb, R.C., Schultz, B. and McMahill, J. (1977) *The Glenwood Awareness Manipulation and Posture Scale*, Glenwood State Hospital School, Iowa
Williams, C. (1982) 'Deaf Not Daft: The Deaf in Mental Subnormality Hospitals', *Special Education: Forward Trends*, 9, 26–8
Wolf, J.M. and Anderson, R.M. (1973) *The Multiply Handicapped Child*, Charles C. Thomas, Springfield, Ill.

7

Criterion-referenced Tests

C. Kiernan

INTRODUCTION

Definition

Criterion-referenced tests can be defined as procedures in which items represent 'achievements' which are of importance in the individual's adjustment to his or her environment or which reflect the outcome of teaching or training. If a teacher sets out to teach basic mathematical operations then, after teaching each operation he/she will want to check that the pupil has acquired the skill. So a lesson on addition may be followed by a 'test' in which pupils are given a series of addition problems. The teacher will probably have the hope that all of the pupils will achieve the criterion of 100 per cent success, but will probably build in some flexibility to allow for simple 'mistakes'. He/she may however use errors as a way of deciding which pupils need more teaching or what kind of sub-operations within addition need to be revised.

The example has all of the main characteristics of a criterion-referenced test. It assesses an individual's performance in a specified area of concern. Interest in assessment centres on whether the individual can or cannot perform at a level which, in this case, indicates that he or she can do something. The teacher is not primarily interested in seeing whether one pupil is 'better at adding' than another. The goal of teaching has been to teach the operation. The teacher wants all of the pupils to be able to add so he/she is interested in all of them achieving 100 per cent success in the test. The achievement, being able to add, is seen as being important in itself, it is not an index of something else, like reasoning ability. Finally, the achievement is seen as part of an overall scheme of teaching mathematics. In this case the achievement is also one which has to be reached before the pupil can go on to acquire other skills, such as multiplication or division.

The notion of criterion-referenced tests was first introduced by Glaser (1963) although clearly its logic was not new even then. Tests are concerned with the person's ability successfully to complete items which reflect some explicit criterion. What makes this approach different from most others is that tests are *not* concerned with comparing individuals with each other. Reference is to an absolute standard rather than to norms derived from a group of individuals.

Use with people with mental handicap

The last 20 years have seen the widespread acceptance of the idea that the central problem for people with mental handicap is their difficulty in learning relevant skills. Mental handicap has been seen increasingly as an educational rather than a medical problem. If people with mental handicap are to be helped then the most direct route is to teach them the skill which they have failed to acquire through normal childrearing and experience. In other words, we need to specify which skills or capabilities such people lack and then teach them those skills.

These ideas originated with behaviour modification and indeed represent the basic credo of behaviour modification (see Bijou 1966). Over the years they have provided the impetus for numerous successful teaching programmes (Kiernan 1985a). These programmes have followed a number of familiar basic rules. Responses to be taught are clearly specified in terms of actual behaviour, setting or discriminative conditions, and consequences, often externally provided rewards. This process gives descriptions of performance which are of the same form as those expected from a good criterion-referenced test. Indeed many teaching programmes consist of a series of statements of criterion performances with a breakdown of these performances into steps for teaching.

Given this basic technology the central problem for the educator of people with mental handicap is 'What should be taught?' Two basic sources have been used for this curriculum content. The first is developmental tests and developmental theory. (See Chapters 2 and 3 of this volume.) Bricker (1972) was one of the first to argue explicitly that behaviour modification techniques could provide methods for teaching and developmental research, the content. The second source of content has been the analysis of demands placed by the living environment on the individual. The tasks which a person needs to be able to do in order to function as a member of society are listed and represent the content of teaching.

Norm-referenced tests as bases for curriculum content

The first of these approaches begs the obvious question. Can developmental tests, such as the Griffiths (1954) or the Bayley Scales of Infant Development (1969), provide the curriculum content for teaching programmes? (For discussion of those tests see Berger and Yule, Chapter 2.) Similarly, can norm-referenced tests in specific areas, for example Reynell tests of language development (see Berger and Yule, Chapter 2) provide a curriculum for language teaching? If they can, then all that we need to do is to use their items as criterion tests and we have our bases for teaching.

This logic has certainly been explicit in the thinking of many practitioners. Very often psychologists and speech therapists will advise that 'the next goal in teaching' is the next item of a developmental or language test. Similar suggestions have also been made by researchers, Bricker's work (1972) already having been mentioned. Kiernan (1984) has argued that other researchers in the behavioural tradition took their goals from Chomsky's developmental work in teaching language.

At a very simple level, norm-referenced tests may be an unsuitable basis for a curriculum because the test constructors have explicitly avoided 'trainable' items. Alternatively scales may be deliberately brief. If their main purpose is to place children at age levels then they would, ideally, consist of a few very good items rather than a large number. This means that many developmental tests give very little potential guidance on curriculum.

Norm-referenced tests are typically constructed from sets of items which are assembled from other tests or derived from theory. They are then administered, refined, and finally selected. A good item will discriminate among individuals and relate to whatever criterion underlies the test. A good item for the assessment of language in two year olds will discriminate among the children, ideally splitting the tested groups in two, and correlate with other items showing language development. Items which do not discriminate are not of interest and would be excluded from the test.

Because the emphasis is on measuring differences any behaviour which all, or nearly all the children show, it taken for granted and not assessed. In terms of our curriculum this would mean that such behaviours would not be presented as in need of teaching. As we will see, later, this has led checklists of language targets to place very little emphasis on the function of language as opposed to syntax.

Another consequence follows from item selection aimed at showing differences between age groups. Three behaviours may follow each other in development and may be dependent on one another. Behaviour 'A' may occur reliably in children between 12 and 15 months, behaviour 'C' in children between 28 and 30 months. Behaviour 'B' may, however, emerge any time between 13 and 29 months. However, 'B' may not occur until after 'A' and be a necessary and sufficient condition for the emergence of 'C'.

Norm-referenced item selection is, as we have seen, concerned with items which discriminate age groups. In our example Behaviour 'B' certainly does not do that, it may occur any time between 13 and 29 months, depending on the individual child. As a consequence it would not be selected as a good item. If the test is then used as a basis for teaching we would teach 'A' and then try to teach 'C'. We would not even know about 'B' and the pupil would have to rely on chance conditions to acquire the behaviour.

Items for norm-referenced tests are also selected in terms of their reliability. Items may be eliminated if two observers cannot agree that a particular performance represents an example of tested behaviour (inter-rater reliability). For example, raters may disagree on whether a child is able to imitate his own sounds when they are played back to him on a tape recorder. Try as they might, test constructors may find it impossible to devise a clear enough criterion. Consequently, the item would be deleted despite the fact that this may be an important step in development. Alternatively, a test sample of children may show great variation over time. Individual children may be responsive to approaches from adults one day and not on another. If this occurs then relevant items will be excluded on the grounds of poor test-retest reliability. Again, the behaviour may be important, it may just be difficult to assess in the way required by norm-referenced procedures.

The way in which reliability is assessed can have other consequences. Let us assume that we have four skills which are crucial in development and need to follow each other. We will call these A, B, C and D. These skills may be accompanied by other behaviours, which depend on them but which are not, in themselves, of any significance, A', B', C' and D'. It could well be the case that the items devised for a norm-referenced test tap all eight areas. If the items testing B' and C' were more reliable than those testing B and C, those testing A and D better than those testing A' and D' the following sequence would be included in the test, A, B', C', D. If we then use this as a teaching sequence we may well begin by teaching A, but then teach two irrelevant skills which do not prepare the child to learn D.

This example may seem rather abstract but points to the central dilemma in teaching activities such as block stacking or doing jigsaw puzzles. This is, that such items in developmental tests are highly reliable, but not necessarily of value in teaching activities.

This points us to the central problem with many norm-referenced tests. Although overall item selection may be guided by a broad theory, items are selected on an empirical basis, i.e. on the bases described above. Criterion-referencing, on the other hand, requires a reason for inclusion of an item. There must be a clear logic which dictates the reason for including items and, for some uses, a clear logic which dictates the sequencing of items.

In other terms criterion-referenced tests assume a theoretical framework to dictate item selection which is frequently absent in item selection in norm-referenced tests. However, theory is not always absent. The most obvious examples are tests based on Piagetian theory, the most notable example of which is the Uzgiris-Hunt Scales (Uzgiris and Hunt 1975) (See Chapter 3 of this volume).

Characteristics of good criterion-referenced tests

I have argued that norm-referenced tests do not provide a good basis for curriculum content, mainly because the procedures which they use in item selection may well exclude behaviours which are important in development and because of their generally 'atheoretical', empirically based approach to assessment. On the other hand, I am suggesting that criterion-referenced assessments are built from theories of what represents 'crucial' behaviours. These may be defined as behaviours without which the individual will not develop other behaviours, in a developmental sequence, or without which he/she will not adapt successfully to the environment.

What then would represent a good criterion-referenced test? The first requirement would be that it specify the range of behaviours which it was intending to cover. This may be the whole of early development, as is the case with two of the examples which I will discuss later, the Portage checklist (Bluma, Shearer, Frohman and Hilliard 1976) and the Behaviour Assessment Battery (Kiernan and Jones 1982), or community living for adults like the Bereweeke assessment checklist (Jenkins, Felce, Mansell, Flight and Dell 1983).

The second requirement is that the test should specify the range of achievements which are felt to be relevant to the goal of teaching. In other words, if the aim is to provide a test related to community living, a curriculum for teaching the person to adapt successfully, the rationale for selection and exclusion of areas should be made clear.

By implication this selection represents the test constructor's theory of behaviour relevant to the overall goal. If a test constructor leaves emotional expression out of a test of community adjustment, without saying that it is felt to be important but excluded for specific reasons, then we can reasonably infer that, so far as he/she is concerned, emotional expression is not important as an aspect of community adjustment.

Similarly, the way in which items are arranged in sequences or sections within tests reflect how constructors theorise about the inter-relations of items. Division of discussion of development under a set of section headings implies relative independence of those sections. Ideally their inter-relation would be clearly stated if the constructor felt such connections existed.

Having specified a range of achievements relevant to a goal, the next step in test development should be to specify the criterion levels which are believed to be appropriate. This is a more complex activity than it would appear at first. Let us take a simple example, filling a washbasin. At a broad level this achievement involves blocking the outflow, allowing water to flow into the basin to a particular level, while monitoring and regulating the temperature of the water, and stopping the water flow. A moment's thought will show that this can require an extensive knowledge base. There are at least two commonly used types of plug, there are at least four comonly used types of tap, with numerous variants, water temperature needs to be monitored in at least two different ways, for dual and mixer taps, water level has to be varied to provide adequate depth depending on the type of basin, there are at least two main methods of switching taps off, and one tap which keeps running for several seconds after pressure is released.

Are we to state a criterion which covers all of these conditions?

If so, it would be extremely tedious and yet it is obvious that, if the individual's experience has been restricted to one basin in one bathroom, crediting the item will mean something radically different from a credit for someone with wide experience. More seriously, the latter person may have his or her achievement qualified by the person scoring the test because he/she is known *not* to be able to deal adequately with certain types of fixture. So he/she will end up getting only a qualified 'yes', whereas the person with restricted experience may get an unqualified 'yes'.

Clearly this will only happen if the staff or parents completing the simple criterion-referenced question are unaware of the possible complexities of the items they are dealing with. This brings us to a central point about these procedures. Criterion-referenced tests are often seen as a concrete and practical way of presenting a curriculum to people not trained in theoretical aspects of the areas concerned. The Behaviour Assessment Battery (Kiernan and Jones 1982) contains sections which reflect Piagetian theory in terms of criterion behaviour without any attempt to give the user insight into the underlying theory.

The example of learning to turn on taps may seem relatively atheoretical. Yet it is clear that the item, simply stated, assumes that the user will appreciate the need to explore the generalisation of learned skills. In planning teaching programmes, the user will also be familar with the need to analyse the stimulus and response sets necessary to achieve the generalised skills of 'filling the washbasin'. This might imply learning the skills of 'general case methodology' (Colvin and Horner 1983).

The central point is that, if criterion-referenced tests are to be employed successfully with particular users, we need to know what those users bring to the interpretation of items which will allow them to establish satisfactory teaching programmes. Tests which contain simple items with poorly specified criteria may be attractive because they appear simple, but can be grossly misleading.

The point may be made more clearly with an example. Nursing staff in a mental handicap hospital were asked, using a checklist, to rate the language development of a girl who was severely mentally handicapped. They responded positively to the item 'uses two words together'. The child was in fact nonverbal and, over a period of several weeks, had never been heard to utter any single words, let alone two-word phrases. On further checking it emerged that the child did have a two-word phrase, 'you bitch', which she uttered, occasionally, when very upset. However, she never used either word separately and appeared therefore to produce the phrase as a single unit.

This example may seem simplistic but it emphasises an important point — without adequate understanding of the implications of items, intepretation can be grossly misleading. It raises the question of whether criterion-referenced tests should be used as means through which teaching prescriptions should be formulated.

The final points about construction relate to specific tests of behaviour. Part of the problem in the example quoted was that the nurses were left to interpret the item rather than being asked to test the child, or to observe the range of instances of behaviour. Clearly it is more satisfactory to say: 'Here is the criterion and here are a number of specific ways in which you can examine the person's behaviour to see if the criterion is achieved. If he or she passes all of the items then we would credit him or her with the achievement'.

For example, filling the washbasin as an achievement may involve three specific tests, one with the basin normally used; one with a basin which uses radically different taps and plug system, but again familiar; and one with a novel basin, possibly using a mixture of the filling and plugging mechanisms which he/she has experienced in the other two settings. This approach would overcome some of the problems which were discussed above but would clearly involve a much longer test procedure.

The relation of items to criteria raises questions of validity. In the Behaviour Assessment Battery (BAB), Kiernan and Jones (1982) include items related to Piagetian concepts. One such concept, object permanence, is tested in a series of items of different levels of difficulty (Search Strategies Section). The basic notion of object permanence is that the individual shows awareness of the continued existence of an object or person despite their not being in continuous sensory contact. The way in which this basic notion is assessed in the BAB is by selecting an object which the person is known to like, showing it to him or her and then covering it with a cloth. If he or she then reaches out, removes the cover and takes the object, he or she is credited with the criterion behaviour of achievement of object permanence.

The question is straightforward, and very much like that asked about the extent to which one instance of successful filling of the washbasin can be seen as representative of the skill. Is the one test a valid reflection of what the concept of object permanence means? In this case it probably is, the item is lifted fairly directly from Piaget's writings. However, we can ask a more difficult question.

Does passing this item mean that the individual will have object permanence for all objects under the circumstances?

The answer to this question could be given only if the test constructors had assessed a large number of individuals on a large number of related items and shown that the particular item included predicted performance on all or nearly all others. This, of course, is a formidable task and not one accomplished by Kiernan and Jones, or, for that matter, by other test constructors. However, without such tests the validity of items as reflecting 'achievements' is seriously in question. We need to ask, for each criterion-referenced item, whether evidence of validity has been provided.

Similarly, criterion-referenced tests should provide evidence of the reliability of their items, especially whether any two qualified observers would rate behaviours in the same way, i.e. inter-rater reliability. Low inter-rater reliability may stem from two main sources. Either items may be so poorly specified as to be open to misinterpretation, this was the case with our 'two word' example, or the behaviour assessed by the item may be just difficult to categorise. Items such as 'tends to be attention-seeking' often cause trouble in this way because what may to one person be normal friendliness and a wish to be with you, may to another person be an irritating presence. The other possibility is that two people may differ because they have seen different aspects of an individual's behaviour, as when a child talks at school but does not talk at home.

Of the two problems low inter-rater reliability stemming from ambiguous wording is the greater. Here, when two observers get together, they may spend hours just trying to work out what the test means. In practice, where behaviour is genuinely variable from one setting to another exchange of experiences can be very productive in indicating ways in which programmes can be developed.

We will return to this and related points later in this chapter. For the moment we need to register the notion that demonstration of inter-rater reliablity, where this derives from two people observing the same behaviour at the same time, is important for criterion-referenced tests. However, where reliability estimates rely on the consistency of an individual's behaviour over time, i.e. test-retest reliablity or inter-rater reliabiliy where two raters test independently on different occasions, I would suggest that they are less important.

CRITERION-REFERENCED PROCEDURES

So far this account has defined criterion-referenced tests as being concerned to provide ways in which individuals can be assessed against a clear standard in order to evaluate an achievement. I have suggested that criterion-referenced tests can apply either to development, or ranges of skill related to particular settings, e.g. living in the community. I have argued that norm-referenced tests, especially tests of development, cannot by the nature of their construction satisfy the needs of a criterion-referenced test.

I have also argued that a good criterion-referenced test should have a number of features. These are:

(1) The test should specify the range of behaviours which it is intending to cover.
(2) The test should provide a rationale for selection of behaviours, i.e. should state the theoretical grounds on which it is based.
(3) The test should provide a rationale for the sequencing of test items, since this represents the constructor's theory of development of behaviour.
(4) The test should provide statements about inter-relations of items across sections, if there is evidence to lead one to anticipate cross-linkages.
(5) Appropriate criterion levels should be stated and amplified to the degree necessary to prevent ambiguous interpretation by specified users.
(6) Items should be related to criterion statements in such a way that they can be seen to be valid tests of the criterion.
(7) Items should themselves be reliable, at least at the level of inter-rater agreement of individual test items.

The items which we will look at are all commercially available in the United Kingdom. They are the Portage checklist (Bluma, Shearer, Frohman and Hilliard 1976); the Wessex Revised Portage Language Checklist (White and East 1983a); the Bereweeke Skill-Teaching System assessment checklist (Jenkins, Felce, Mansell, Flight and Dell 1983) and the Behaviour Assessment Battery (Kiernan and Jones 1982). These tests have been selected because all are marketed as procedures which can be used as a basis for programme development. They are also tests which are fairly commonly used by various groups of practitioners and parents.

In what follows I will describe the tests and then discuss each in relation to the above seven questions. I will then try to suggest what safeguards should be employed when using the tests.

Portage guide to early education

By far the most commonly used published criterion-referenced procedure is the checklist associated with the Portage scheme. The Portage scheme was developed initially as a method of guiding parent teaching in Portage, Wisconsin, in the early 1970s (Shearer and Shearer 1972).

The scheme represents a general intervention procedure. A home teacher, who may be a professionally qualified worker or a specially prepared nonspecialist, approaches parents to see if they wish to be involved in a programme to assist their child's development. If they agree, the home teacher and parent complete the checklist as a means of assessing the child and suggesting targets for teaching. These are selected from items on which the child may not succeed, or where performance is uncertain in the context of the child's perceived needs, and on the basis of parental preferences and professional advice if this is available.

Having selected a target the parent and home teacher work out a programme of teaching which is judged to be achievable in a week. The activity is written down in terms of steps, with criteria for achievement, and, if necessary, the activity is tried out. Selection of activities to facilitate achievement of goals is guided by a pack of Activity Cards, one per item of the checklist, which each give a number of suggested teaching activities. These can act as a basis for specific tasks or as a source of ideas from which new activities can be devised.

After a week or so the home teacher visits the parent again, reviews progress, and if necessary, revises targets or agrees new targets. Home teachers themselves report to managers who review their programmes and who may make suggestions on new or alternative activities.

Portage programmes have become very common in the United Kingdom. Bendall, Smith and Kushlick (1984) identified 64 Portage-type services in England, Scotland, Wales and Northern Ireland. There was evidence in their survey of rapid growth in the establishment of the schemes. Indeed around half of the schemes identified had been established within the two years prior to the survey. There is now a national Portage group and a recent

Department of Education and Science grant has been made to foster the establishement of Portage schemes.

Successful use of the scheme has been reported very commonly in the United Kingdom, the United States and developing and Third World countries, often with relatively untrained staff (e.g. Thorburn, Brown and Bell 1979). Success is normally evaluated through the achievement of behavioural targets by children and sometimes through the satisfaction of parents and others participating in the scheme.

The Checklist

It should be clear from this brief description of the scheme that the checklist represents only one element in a total package. Arguably the checklist is also a relatively unimportant part of the package, the provision of a rich source of teaching suggestions and the Portage management system may be more crucial. None the less the checklist represents a framework in terms of which teaching is planned. It therefore represents a curriculum in terms of which development is conceputalised. Therefore the checklist should be appropriate and relevant.

The checklist is divided into six sections. These are Infant Stimulation, Socialisation, Language, Self-help, Cognitive and Motor. Sections include between 45 (Infant Stimulation) and 140 items (Motor). The items are stated fairly briefly, for example 'Imitates movements of another child at play' (Socialisation, 28), 'Prepares own sandwich' (Self-help, 98) or 'Builds tower of 5–6 blocks' (Motor, 70).

The Infant Stimulation section covers visual, tactile and auditory stimulation, general orientation to people and objects, reach and grasp, and early stages of movement, orientation to others and motor development. The items are a mixture of those which might be facilitated or trained, such as 'Follows an object, visually, moved past midline of body' (20). This item satisfies the broad conditions for a criterion-referenced item. Others do not. For example, items refer simply to 'Smiles' (21), 'Repeats own sound' (38), and 'Laughs' (41). These, and early items concerned with responsiveness, could conceivably be facilitated but the mechanism for such facilitation is not clear.

The Socialisation section of the checklist contains 83 items ranging in 'age level' from 0 to 1 year to 5 to 6 years. Early items relate to smiling, vocalisation, imitation and other basic social responses, for example 'Hugs, pats and kisses familiar persons' (23). Since later items in the section refer to play, the first year items include some which are marginal as evidence of socialisation. These include 'Holds and examines offered object for at least a minute' (12), 'Shakes or squeezes object placed in hand, making sounds unintentionally' (13), or 'Plays unattended for 10 minutes' (14). Later levels amplify the play theme with social play with peers, dressing-up, rule-following in group games led by adults, co-operative play and acting out stories being covered.

Co-operation with adults and the development of socially acceptable behaviour represents another thread, as does the evolution of understanding of the feelings of others. The authors have also included several items in the Socialisation section which relate to the development of communication. These include 'Pulls at another person to show them some action or object' (38), 'Says "please" and "thank you" when reminded' (47). It is clearly reasonable to say that these items do reflect the development of social behaviour but it is equally reasonable to see them as a reflection of developing communication skills. Another item 'Withdraws hand, says "no-no" when near forbidden object with reminders' (39) reflects the verbal regulation of behaviour through internalised warnings.

As with other sections the occasional item seems to be a poor fit. For instance, 'Plans and builds using simple tools (inclined planes, fulcrum, lever, pulley)' (81) would seem more sensibly placed in the Cognitive section.

The Language section of the checklist concentrates on hearing and on the development of spoken English. Again the section is fairly long, containing 99 items from the 0 to 1 to the 5 to 6 year old levels. Early items relate to repetition of sounds with very little emphasis on babbling and on vocal imitation. Preverbal communication is indeed covered in only around nine items. Similarly the section as whole places little emphasis on the development of comprehension. Only around 15 or so items cover this aspect of language development.

The Language section of the checklist has been the most heavily criticised by users. In fact the Revised Portage Language Checklist, to be discussed in the next section, was produced because of problems which were experienced. I will run over these in introducing that test.

The Self-help section of the Portage checklist contains 105 items again ranging in level from 0 to 1 to 5 to 6 year bands. Items relate to development of eating, self-feeding and table etiquette (around 36 items), dressing (35), toilet skills (12), washing (8), teeth cleaning

(3), nose-wiping (3), and hair care (1). Another group relates to safety in and responsibility in and out of the house (10 or so items). This rough count shows where the emphasis of the checklist lies. Its items relate very much to what would be expected of a normal preschool child who is living at home and going out on his or her own at around the age of four to five years. I will discuss later how well this model fits the educational needs of people with mental handicap.

One other feature of the checklist should be noted. Items relating to particular self-help skills are not organised together. For example the toilet items are numbered 17, 'Sits on potty or infant toilet seat for 5 minutes', 32 'Asks to go to bathroom, even if too late to avoid accidents', 34 'Urinates or defecates in potty three times per week when placed on potty', 38, 41, 43, 56, 57, 76 and 85, an age four to five item, 'Goes to bathroom in time, undresses, wipes self, flushes toilet, and dresses unaided'. One item, finding the corret bathroom in a public place, follows at 101, in the five to six range.

Section 5 of the checklist is called the Cognitive section. Again it covers the age range 0 to 1 year up to 5 to 6 years, this time in 108 items. Many of the early items in the section relate to simple sensorimotor co-ordination and matching tasks. One item 'Finds object hidden under-container' (10) relates to object permanence. Later items continue the theme of sorting and matching, often with highly conventional activities, e.g. 57 'Matches sequence or pattern of blocks or beads'. These items may be related to prewriting and prenumber work (this is not made explicit). Groups of items are introduced relating to drawing and matching symbols and counting, the five to six year old level containing items such as 105 'Sight reads 10 printed words' and 108 'Counts by rote from 1 to 100'.

A few items relate to memory for events. Item 46, a three to four year old item is 'Describe two events of characters from familiar story or TV program', 77 'Retells five main facts from story heard three times'. How many facts the story is to have in total and how and with what intervals the story is to be told are not specified.

The Motor section of the checklist is the longest with 140 items. Forty-five of these relate to the 0 to 1 year level. These cover reach and grasp, head control, sitting, standing, crawling, creeping and walking. Subsequent items follow through gross motor development in the form of walking, running, climbing stairs, jumping, kicking, bicycle riding, etc. Other items cover manual skills such as throwing and catching, use of scissors, use of a hammer and others.

Another group of items introduces some confusion. These relate to sensorimotor activities like removing and replacing pegs (items 51 and 52), prewriting activities (e.g. 54, 94, 112 and 117 'Can copy small letters') and other items which appear to overlap with the content of the Cognition section. For instance 'Stacks three blocks on request' is item 17 in Cognition and 'Builds tower of three blocks' is item 26 in the Motor section, a three to four year old item. In the Cognitive section 'Puts together three piece puzzle or formboard' is item 81, a three to four year old item in the Motor section.

Evaluation of the Checklist

We can now examine the checklist in the context of the seven questions which were formulated about criterion-referenced tests. The answers to these questions need to be seen against a background of enthusiastic and apparently successful use of the Portage system.

There are no clear statements about the intended coverage of the checklist but it seems safe to assume that it is intended to cover all early child development. However, there are no statements about the theoretical foundations on which it is based. In practice the checklist seems to have been derived from developmental checklists and, presumably, from developmental tests available in the early 1970s. As such it reflects what were felt then to be important areas of behaviour. The problem with this approach is highlighted by the Language section. Since the early 1970s advances in research on normal language development have revolutionised the field. In particular the importance of the use of speech as a means of communication rather than as encoding reality and the importance of nonvocal communication have emerged as major considerations. Since the list was published prior to these developments, it clearly could not benefit from this work and is correspondingly weak in the Language section.

The checklist is based on developmental sequences. However, no data are available to provide a rationale for the sequencing adopted. What is more important, no rationale is given for division of development in to the six areas, or five if Infant Stimulation is seen as in a separate class. As we have seen, there is a lack of differentiation between the Cognitive and the Motor sections. Similar problems arise between the Language sections and others where a number of items relating to comprehension of speech are included. Many practitioners and theorists would argue that expressive skills should be taught in the context of comprehension, if not following comprehension. Yet the checklist provides no basis for cross-referencing items which could be argued as closely related.

The checklist does not employ criterion statements independent of items except that, by implication, items in each section can be presumed to relate to that area of development. However, the relation of items to the relevant area is not made explicit. So, although the significance of some items is reasonably clear, for example most of those in the sections on Socialisation, Self-help and Motor development, the significance of others is not at all clear. Obvious examples are performance on pegboards and with puzzles and colour naming in the Cognitive section.

Items themselves are very broadly stated and have no quoted reliabilities. These psychometric problems might be offset if the people using the checklist were first of all trained in the interpretation of items and secondly trained to administer the checklist in such a way as to elicit reliable responses from parents or set up reliable test situations. So far as documented schemes go, no such extensive training is given to home teachers. What the checklist can yield is only a rough guide to a child's ability.

The checklist fares poorly when rated as a criterion-referenced test. But is it fair to judge it against these criteria? The developers of Portage emphasise that the checklist should be treated flexibly, that 'no child is expected to precisely follow the sequence as stated on the Checklist' (Weber, Jesein, Shearer, Bluma, Hilliard, Shearer, Schortinghaus and Boyd, 1975, p. 19), that the scheme is 'a guide not a cookbook' (p. 20) and that it was 'designed to give the home teacher a starting point' (p. 20).

On the other hand, the system is 'designed to serve as a curriculum for children, either handicapped or normal, between the mental ages of birth and six years. In addition, older children and adults with behaviours common to preschool children can benefit from [the] activities . . . (p. 18). If this claim is to be taken seriously, and the popularity of the use of Portage with individuals who are handicapped attests to the fact that it is taken seriously, then the defects in the checklist merit consideration.

The Wessex Revised Portage Language Checklist (White and East (1983a))

White and East (1981) and White and East (1983b) report that experience of use of the Portage checklist in a home-teaching scheme led to several conclusions. The Language section did not alway succeed in pinpointing behaviour relevant to language, in fact teachers were often left without a baseline in the Language section.

The 'teaching objectives' indicated by the checklist represented too large steps and the checklist did not cover behaviours believed to be relevant to language development. In addition, it was clear that language-related items were spread through other sections and, as we have already noted, the inter-relation of sections was not made clear. Gaps in the sequences were noted. For example, an item relating to combination of nouns and verbs (Language item 30) was introduced without any previous items relating to the child's use or response to verbs. White says that 'home teachers unaware of this omission had unrealistic expectations of the child whose expressive language behaviour was limited to naming objects' (1983b, p. 69).

The Revised Checklist is divided into four levels: birth to one year, one to two, two to three and three to four. No reason is given for missing out the four to five and five to six year old levels. At each level White and East have gathered together items considered relevant to language development from throughout the original checklist. These are drawn from the Infant Stimulation, Socialisation, Cognitive and, of course, the Language section. Around 70 per cent of the items in the Socialisation section of the original checklist have been included along with just under 30 per cent of items in the Cognitive and Infant Stimulations sections. About a quarter of the items in the Revised Checklist are new.

White and East follow the Portage convention in laying out all items at each age level in what is presumably thought to be a developmental sequence. However, no evidence is provided to indicate why items are placed in particular positions. For instance 'Vocalizes in response to music' (Language item 32 at level 1), a new item, is placed after 'Makes four or more different sounds' and before 'Follows conversation by watching speakers'. No data are provided to support this placement.

White and East re-group items at each age level into sequences reflecting particular postulated skills or areas of activity. These include continuing threads running through all levels concerning listening and attending, imitation and responding to language with other groupings concerning speech structures, principally grammatical structures from level 3 questions, and 'play and picture books'. The majority of new items are introduced in context of listening and attending and play and picture books, with several being added in the responding to language section.

This rearrangement and the additional items inserted by White and East certainly serve to make the structure of the checklist easier to follow, to side-step some of the possible arbitrariness in sequencing, and to offset the relative absence of coverage of comprehension. The addition of the play and picture books grouping broadens somewhat the narrow coverage of imaginative play which was a feature of the Cognitive section of the original checklist.

Evaluation of the Wessex Revised Portage Language Checklist

Unlike many other areas of development the level of theoretical development of the area of language and communication provides a framework against which to assess the coverage of the Revised Checklist. White and East aim to cover language development although, as with the original checklist, it is clear through their selection of items that they also aim to cover communication. As such it is clear that they should be covering phonological development, functional or pragmatic aspects of nonvocal and vocal behaviour including discourse skills, semantic encoding, and syntactic development both in expressive and receptive aspects. A comprehensive programme would also cover problems arising from sensory and motor deficts, and from specific language disorders.

No checklist, or for that matter full programme, could hope to cover this range. White and East sample most areas, although there is a failure to acknowledge the possible impact of sensory and motor deficits. The development of phonology is substantially ignored. Furthermore, their taxonomy makes it difficult to map the checklist on to contemporary theory. The clearest thread is concerned with the development of syntax.

The most obvious deficit is in the failure to make explicit recognition of functional use or pragmatics. Accounts of this aspect of development have been appearing since the early 1970s and, although there is some disagreement among authors on the details of classification, the general categories of emerging functional use are clear (see Dore 1974; Bruner 1974–5; Bates 1976; Atkinson 1982).

We can compare a typical listing of such categories with the White and East Checklist. Cirrin and Rowland (1985) based their analyses on studies of normal development and isolated nine categories of use in a group of people with mental handicap. These were request action, request object, request information, direct attention to self, direct attention for communication (getting the listener's attention prior to another communication), direct attention to object, direct attention to action, answer, and protest. A reclassification of the White and East items in these terms shows first of all a general mismatch of the Cirrin and Rowland classification and theirs. Secondly, the Revised Checklist covers direct attention to self (one item) and several request items, mostly not differentiated by type of request. The other category which is clearly represented, and indeed heavily represented, is answer. Items concerned with direction of attention occur in the play and picture books grouping but even here the vast majority of items tap responsiveness to adult requests, e.g. 'finds specific book on request' or 'points to picture of common object described by its use'. Only an occasional item reflects the child engaging adult attention, communicating something he or she wants to say, e.g. (186) 'Pulls at another person to show him some action or object' or (Language item 83) 'Hands book to adult to read or share with him'. Notably, the Revised Checklist does not include items concerned with protest, the indication that the speaker opposes or disapproves of the listener's behaviour or action. The nearest item is (180) 'Answers yes/no question with affirmative or negative reply'.

This analysis suggests that the Revised Checklist implies a language curriculum in which the child is a passive recipient of 'teaching'. The very heavy emphasis on 'answering' as a functional category, with the correspondingly light emphasis on controlling adult attention, requesting and protest, projects an image of teaching in which the child is controlled by adults.

This type of programme does not take into account the contemporary argument that the child learns language, at least in part, through a developing need to communicate and to encode progressively more complex meanings. This is particularly unfortunate in a programme directed explicitly at children who are handicapped since it would seem that they may experience particular difficulties in developing language use (McLean and Snyder-McLean 1984; Kiernan 1985b). White and East show some concern for this aspect of programming in their general suggestions about programming but here again these are often ambiguous or clearly 'teaching', e.g. 'take him or her out regularly and talk about what you see', or 'reply to short phrases with additional words that make his or her meaning clear'. The latter strategy is likely to have a negative effect, or no effect, unless the amplification helps the child to make his or her meaning clearer when his listener is genuinely confused, not just when he is being corrected.

The Revised Checklist fares little better than the original on the rest of the seven questions. No evidence is provided for sequencing of items, no evidence is provided to support the division of items into groups or guidance given on how they inter-relate: items are no less ambiguous than in the original checklist and no evidence on reliability is provided for the new items.

White and East have in practice produced an alternative structure to the Portage checklist. This structure, as we have seen, reorganises many of the Portage checklist items around the topic of Language and Communication, leaving the Self-help and Motor sections intact.

As a criterion-referenced test the Revised Checklist fares little better than the original. Its theoretical structure is only marginally clearer, but, arguably, an opportunity has been lost in the failure to update its contents. On all other psychometric grounds the Revised Checklist is deficient. This leads us to the suggestion that the Revised Checklist cannot be recommended as a basis for a programme of teaching of language and communication skills. The Revised Checklist, and the associated materials, provide one useful resource for teachers and parents. However, they need to be interpreted and complemented in the light of careful assessment of language problems and of accumulating knowledge of development.

The Bereweeke Skill-teaching System (Jenkins, Felce, Mansell, Flight and Dell 1983)

The Bereweeke System was based on and adapted from the Portage model. It owes its name to the hostel in which it was first tested, Bereweeke House in Winchester, England.

The system involves the use of the assessment checklist, data from which are used, along with others, in setting a goal for a three-month period. The goal is then broken down into weekly teaching targets. An activity chart is written and performance is monitored in much the way that the Portage system operates (Jenkins 1982). The Bereweeke materials consist of the assessment checklist, the programme-writer's handbook and the system administrator's handbook.

As with the Portage system the assessment checklist represents only an element in a larger package. Again it is arguable that the checklist is a relatively less important element than the goal-setting process or the management scheme, but, none the less, for the reasons already rehearsed, it is important that it reach adequate standards.

The system is directed toward teaching adults with severe mental handicap in residential care. It was designed for use with care staff, most of whom would not have had teaching qualifications. The system is designed to cover 'the major areas of everyday behaviour'

(Jenkins *et al.* 1983, p. 1) for people who are profoundly handicapped and more able, and for the very young as well as older people.

The areas covered by the checklist are Cognitive Skills, Receptive and Expressive Language, Self-care, Gross Motor Skills, Social Behaviours and what are called Practical Skills. The latter include clothes' care, kitchen tasks, food preparation and use of household amenities.

Each area is broken down into a number of sections, such as undressing or standing. Each section then comprises up to a dozen or so items. These are expressed much more explicitly than in the two Portage checklists. For example item 5 in eating/drinking, Scoops with utensil, involves a description of materials and procedures used '(Spoon or fork, bowl, portion of food, e.g. stewed apple, ice cream). Present utensil and food. Cue'. The cue in this case is 'Eat the food . . .'. The expected performance is then described, 'Scoops food with utensil and brings to mouth; 5 mouthfuls'. Clearly, this specification is much more satisfactory than that seen in the Portage materials.

Evaluation of the Bereweeke Assessment Checklist

The authors of the checklist state clearly that the range of behaviours covered should be those required of adults living in residential care. However, they do not provide a rationale for their specific selection.

Two areas of assessment are clearly related to the settings, Self-care and Practical. In addition to items already specified the items include eating and drinking, mealtime etiquette, for instance use of napkin, laying table, picking up and carrying laden tray; washing, including hair washing and drying; undressing and dressing; clothes fastenings, grooming and toileting. The last section contains several items which refer to the use of a 'potty', a rather inappropriate term in a schedule directed at least in part at adults.

The system loses focus in dealing with Cognitive Skills. The items used in assessment of grasping and releasing, manipulation and conceptualisation of objects make frequent references to child-appropriate activities such as pushing model cars, hammering with a toy hammer or threading beads. Aside from the obvious problems of deviating from the goal of age-appropriateness, the relevance of these items to the everyday lives of adults with severe mental handicap is unclear. However, I understand that the authors are preparing a revision of the system in which items such as placing a cassette in a tape recorder, putting a key in a keyhole and operating a push-button light switch are to replace those in the current version.

This development is clearly to be welcomed.

The Language section is similarly problematic. It is hard to see direct relevance to day to day living of the ability to point to objects such as ball, spoon, book or comb, to identify different coloured blocks or squares, circles, triangles and rectangles. These and other items, such as 'Show me the *big* car . . .' or '. . . the *soft* ball . . .', appear to have been adapted from child-based procedures without thought about their form or relevance to adults.

The section on Expressive Language has similar problems. The items testing imitation of three-word chains require the adult to say 'boy pet dog', 'girl hug Daddy' and 'big red block'. The section on use of language probes the use of regular and irregular plural forms but does not explore any functional use of language beyond the ability to answer questions. It is hoped that the revised version will correct these problems.

Two areas of functioning are missing from the Bereweeke assessment. These are in-house leisure and any kind of outside activity. As a theoretical statement of what adults with mental handicap should be doing, the system presents a rather grim life!

Many of the areas covered in the system are not sequenced. Where a sequence is presented, for instance in the use of language, no justification is given. Nor are statements made about inter-relations of sections, Is there a relation between ability of manipulate pegs and the ability to fasten buttons?

The Bereweeke checklist scores in clear expression of items where it represents an excellent model. The question of validity of items is dealt with satisfactorily in many cases because the item *is* the criterion behaviour. This is the case with Self-care and Practical Skills. In the case of items in the Cognitive and Language areas, the validity of items cannot be easily assessed because they are not related to any theoretical model except an implied developmental model. In this respect they are very suspect.

Finally no information is presented on inter-rater reliability. This is a surprising omission and one which it is hoped would be remedied in the revised version.

The Behaviour Assessment Battery (BAB) (Kiernan and Jones 1982)

The BAB was developed as a criterion-referenced battery of procedures for use by teachers and others involved with developing teaching programmes for children and young people with severe mental handicap. The BAB was first published in 1977. The 1982 edition includes added test procedures, a revised communication section and a chapter concerned with interpretation of results from the battery. The BAB was designed to 'stand on its own'. It has no accompanying training scheme or sets of teaching tips.

The objectives given for the BAB are to give a broad coverage of behaviour, including self-help skills, cognitive and emotional aspects of behaviour, thereby allowing a 'comprehensive programme to be devised' (Kiernan and Jones 1982, p. 13). The BAB was intended however to co-ordinate with other procedures by extending their coverage downward to cover people who are profoundly mentally handicapped. Finally the BAB was to be a set of standardised testing procedures within a framework which allowed the motivation of the individual tested to be taken into account.

The BAB consists of 13 sections in some of which the individual is tested in a flexible test framework. These are sections concerned with Visual Inspection (2), Visual Tracking (3), Visuo Motor Co-ordination (4), Auditory Responsiveness (5), Exploratory Play (7), Search Strategies, a section covering Piagetian object permanence concepts (9), Perceptual Problem Solving, again relating to Piagetian tasks (10), Social Behaviour (11), and Communication (12). Interviews with parents, teachers or care-givers are used to assess Reinforcement and Experience (1), aspects of Auditory Responsiveness (5), Postural Control, the BAB equivalent of gross motor control (6), aspects of Social Behaviour (11), aspects of Communication (12), and Self-help Skills (13).

Test items are expressed in terms of 'criterion behaviours' each of which is tested by a single test. For example, for item E17 (Exploratory Play) 'The child pats or hits a squeaky toy so that it produces a sound at least three times' the presentation asks that 'A squeaky toy' is given to the child who is allowed to play with it. If the child does not pat or hit the toy, examiner should demonstrate and prompt. Record whether demonstration or prompting is necessary to elicit a reponse', (p. 89). Interview items are laid out as a fairly formal interview, for example C33 (Communication) 'Can he understand phrases like, "man sit", "boy fall", "Peter hit", etc., where a person or animal and an action are put together?' (p. 119).

Items are scored on lattices of the type first used by systems analysts interested in behaviour in the early 1970s. These group items together in sequences which are inter-related. For example

Figure 7.1 shows the lattice for the Search Strategies section of the BAB. The three items SS5, SS6 and SS7 on the third spur from the left were all seen as related together and classifiable as concerned with 'Simple Searching'. The series of boxes above the double diagonal line, called the ridge line, describe the achievements which the items are seen to denote.

In developing the BAB Kiernan and Jones began with a bank of items which were then refined in use with children and young people who were handicapped, or in interviews. Items were then grouped in ways which appeared to make theoretical sense, and which gave manageable groups of items which could be assessed in a single test session. Consequently the division of items into sections was purely 'rational'.

The battery or its components were then administered to 174 children and young people (Kiernan and Jones 1982, p. 17 for further detail). From these data the ordering of items within sections was explored using the Guttman scalogram technique (Green 1956; Edwards 1957). This technique allows one to test whether the order of items within a group, judged by the relative ease with which the items are passed, can have occurred by chance or not. In other words, if there is a sequence of difficulty in a group of items it should emerge using this technique. The Guttman technique was used by Kiernan and Jones in an attempt to establish sequences which could be followed in teaching. Most of the sections to which the technique applied turned out to be scalable, the weakest section being Exploratory Play where the overall sequencing effects were not strongly in evidence.

Kiernan and Jones also established inter-observer reliabilities, inter-interviewer reliabilities and test-retest reliabilities on the various sections. Most of these were quite satisfactory judged by conventional criteria.

Evaluation of the BAB

The BAB aims to cover a sufficient range of behaviours of children with severe mental handicap to lead to a 'comprehensive (teaching) programme', but it also aims to complement other procedures. This gives the battery a distinctly baroque structure without any clear logic. The point emerges most clearly in the contrast between the test sections, which concern themselves very much with a level of severe to profound handicap, and the Communication section which taps some higher-level behaviours. Within this framework one or two sections are clearly inadequate. These include those concerning

Figure 7.1: Example of a Lattice and Some of the Corresponding Test Items from the Behaviour Assessment Battery

Section 9: Search strategies: SS

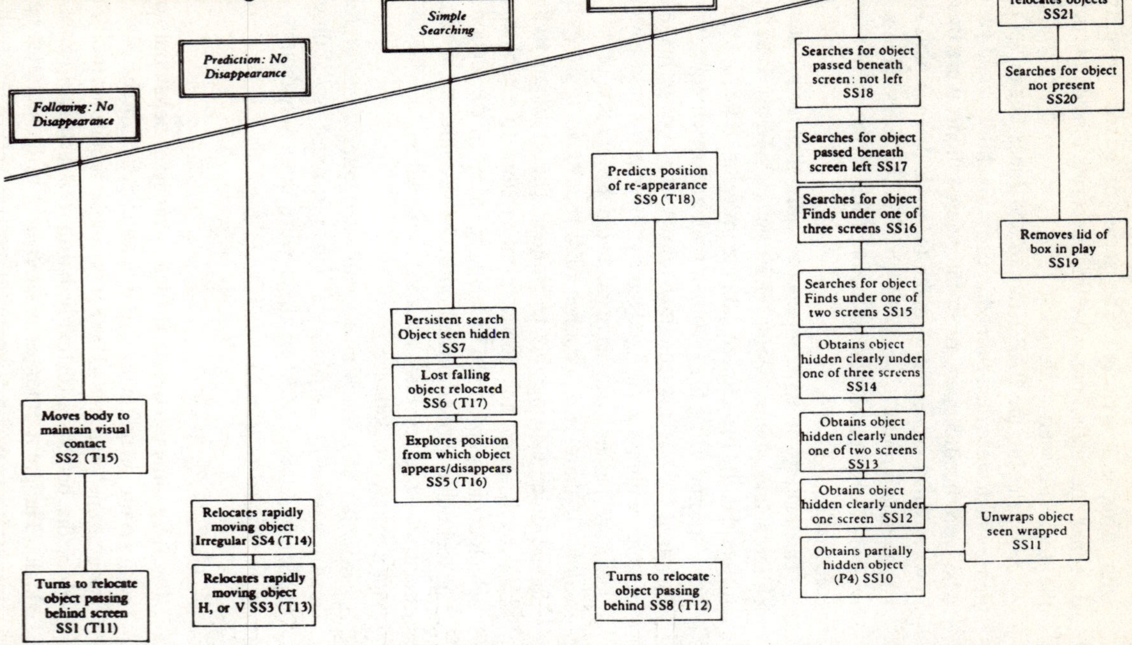

Following: No Disappearance
- Moves body to maintain visual contact SS2 (T15)
- Turns to relocate object passing behind screen SS1 (T11)

Prediction: No Disappearance
- Relocates rapidly moving object Irregular SS4 (T14)
- Relocates rapidly moving object H, or V SS3 (T13)

Simple Searching
- Persistent search Object seen hidden SS7
- Lost falling object relocated SS6 (T17)
- Explores position from which object appears/disappears SS5 (T16)

Prediction of Re-appearance
- Predicts position of re-appearance SS9 (T18)
- Turns to relocate passing object SS8 (T12)

Complex Search Strategies
- Searches for object passed beneath screen: not left SS18
- Searches for object passed beneath screen left SS17
- Searches for object Finds under one of three screens SS16
- Searches for object under one of two screens SS15
- Obtains object hidden clearly under one of three screens SS14
- Obtains object hidden clearly under one of two screens SS13
- Obtains object hidden clearly under one screen SS12
- Obtains partially hidden object (P4) SS10

Search in Spontaneous Play
- Hides and relocates objects SS21
- Searches for object not present SS20
- Removes lid of box in play SS19
- Unwraps object seen wrapped SS11

SS7 *Criterion Behaviour* — When the child has seen an object hidden under two screens he still searches for and obtains the object.

Presentation — The object is put under a half ball cover. A second screen, an orange cloth, is then laid over the ball. The child is not allowed to begin searching for the object for three seconds following the completion of the procedure.

SS8 *Criterion Behaviour* — The child looks at an object and follows
(T12) its movements along a trajectory which passes behind him. The child then turns his head to relocate the object as it reappears.

Presentation — The object should be presented at the side of the child and his attention drawn to it. The object is slowly moved behind the child to reappear to him on his other side. This behaviour may also be seen if examiner walks quietly behind the child.

SS9 *Criterion Behaviour* — When an object which is moving hori-
(T18) zontally passes out of sight behind a screen, the child will shift his gaze to the point where the object would appear if it continued along its original path.

Presentation — The object is shown to the child about 20 cms to one side of the screen. When the child is looking move the object slowly behind the screen. Care should be taken to avoid giving cues by arm movements.

SS10 *Criterion Behaviour* — When an object is partially hidden beneath
(P4) a screen within easy grasping distance of the child, the child obtains the object.

Presentation — The object is put on the table and the child's attention drawn to it. The half ball is then put over the object so that it partially covers it. A delay of about three seconds is imposed between the completion of the presentation procedure and encouraging or allowing the child to respond.

SS11 *Criterion Behaviour* — The child unwraps a cloth that was folded round an object whilst he was watching. He ignores the cloth once it has been removed.

Source: Kiernan and Jones (1982 pp. 92 and 167).

Social Behaviour and of constructive play.

The BAB reflects contemporary interest in the early levels of nonverbal communication and in the use of augmentative systems, sign languages or graphic symbols (Kiernan, Reid and Jones 1982). The 1982 edition provides several procedures specifically relevant to these areas.

If the BAB reflects any specific theoretical orientation it is basically Piagetian. However the precise relation between the tests and Piagetian theory is not discussed. Moreover, the adequacy of the items as representative of Piagetian concepts and the viability of teaching these directly is not explored.

I have noted that Kiernan and Jones used Guttman scalogram procedures to establish sequences. This use represents a test of one aspect of a developmental hypothesis (see also Uzgiris and Hunt 1975). However, the fact that these sequences can be 'inferred' from cross-sectional data does not mean that all individuals follow the sequences outlined.

Secondly, and more important from the point of view of the purpose of this and other tests, the fact that items fall in a sequence does not mean that *all* of the steps in the sequence are represented. Three items, A,C,E, may emerge in order. However there may be missing items, B and D, which may be crucial teaching tasks. Kiernan and Jones tried to forestall this problem by interpolating tasks which appeared to be intermediate. However, in the end, the success of this effort in producing a complete sequence can only be resolved by mounting controlled experimental teaching programmes to explore the necessary and sufficient conditions for emergence of behaviours.

Kiernan and Jones try to deal with the question of inter-relations of sections in two ways. Items which appear to represent two sections are included in both. Consequently the Tracking and Search Strategies sections overlaps on eight items. This strategy was designed to allow smoother administration and readier interpretation. The second edition of the BAB included a chapter in which the inter-relation of sections as they relate to the development of communication and language is explored. There are no empirical tests of the adequacy of these descriptions.

The BAB is about as adequate as the Bereweeke System in specifying criteria and items. As noted, reliabilities were assessed but these are provided for *sections* rather than for *items*. While being a considerable advance, this method of recording still allows the possibility that a proportion of items have poor inter-observer reliabilities. However, in defence of the BAB, the more demanding test-retest reliabilities were computed thereby suggesting a robustness of assessment outcome over time.

Discussion

In this chapter I have concentrated on four criterion-referenced procedures. The conclusions drawn from a critical review of the procedures suggest that none of them meet the requirements for a good criterion-referenced test. In all cases, procedures fall down on either psychometric or logical criteria.

Two possible conclusions follow. Either the procedures are deficient or the criteria are too stringent. It can be argued, for example, that the procedures described were devised to aid programme planning and that, as such, their authors intended that users should interpret them in the light of their own expertise. In other words, the procedures provide a framework; the practitioner provides sophistication in interpreting results.

This is a fair argument, but only if authors include clear indications of how procedures should be used and indications of the level of sophistication required of users. Unfortunately, authors tend not to specify such criteria. As a consequence it is hard to see how deficiencies can be offset. The procedures described could all lend themselves to slavish, unimaginative programme planning.

Furthermore, the argument really cannot be sustained when deficiencies in coverage are extreme. For example I have argued that the procedures described all fall far short of satisfactory coverage of language and communication skills. It would be too generous to excuse these deficiencies on the ground that the user ought to be able to offset them; the procedures are actually misleading.

The extension of this initial argument could be that *some* programme planning is going to be better than *no* programme planning. It is difficult to judge this argument independent of cases. However, there are services in which skills in programme planning and execution are seriously deficient. If such services are presented with the type of procedures described here they may well treat them as a panacea, but in fact fail to teach any new skills. Almost certainly this outcome would result in a discrediting of the procedures and a devaluation of the potential for learning of people with handicaps. These possibilities are by no means remote given the current vogue for seeing packages as providing the solution to staff training problems for direct care staff.

A further level of excuse for shortfall in the technical sophistication of procedures relates to the question of reliability and validity. It is argued that we do not need to establish the reliability and validity of procedures which are simply to be used to guide teaching. At one level this argument makes a reasonable point. If two practitioners scoring the same individual on an item disagree on attainment of a skill this could arise because one has seen it displayed, the other not. Psychometrically this would entail a test-retest problem but, educationally, the discrepancy may indicate a useful starting point for a programme which would ensure display of skills across settings and people.

However, it is hard to see how the argument can be sustained through other instances. Items may be consistently misinterpreted. For example Kiernan (1985c) reports the results of a study in which respondents were initially asked to complete a checklist related to communication skills. They were then interviewed and asked to describe the behaviours which had led them to credit students with particular capabilities. These descriptions were then judged by three raters in terms of the degree to which the score was appropriate in light of the behaviour described. The results showed a high level of discrepancy with some items. For example items concerned with the act of drawing attention, for example 'Shows an object only to draw attention to the presence of an object . . .', were very likely to be misinterpreted as relating to requesting objects. These problems were greatest in respondents who had little relevant training. This aspect of validity, the accuracy of interpretation of items, is not normally formally assessed by the authors of the procedures described. And yet, clearly items may be misleading.

Consistent misinterpretation of items would lead, as in the case just quoted, to high inter-observer reliability. Inconsistent misinterpretation would lead to low inter-observer reliability. However, the disagreements between pairs of practitioners which might arise in programme planning cannot be seen as 'creative' since both would be left wondering who had the correct interpretation of the items!

Absence of estimates of validity relating to the scope of items presents further obvious problems. An item like 'Can turn on taps' which fails to specify the range of taps implied seems so obviously inadequate that it is difficult to see how it can be justified, except possibly, that its inadequacies will be obvious to programme planners! However, other items, relating for example to use of syntactic structures or cognitive skills, may lead directly to narrow and virtually meaningless teaching unless criterion behaviours are specified in more sophisticated terms.

This point leads back to the central reason for development of many criterion-referenced procedures and to the central difficulty in their use. Many procedures have been developed in order to provide assessments within a framework of relevant curriculum content. The procedures have, typically, been developed for use in settings where direct care staff do not have an awareness of required curriculum. In these contexts the procedures specify the goals of teaching. In this application the procedures have made a valuable contribution in distilling knowledge which would otherwise be unavailable to staff. The central difficulty with the procedures is that they are simply not suitable as vehicles for inducing *understanding* of the processes which they may be indicating in test items.

These considerations lead to three fairly obvious conclusions. Authors need to pay more attention to establishing basic reliability and validity of items within procedures. If this is not possible because of time or resource constraints both authors and publishers should insist on making the implications of these deficiencies clear to users. Authors need to be clearer on the theoretical aims of procedures, and again to declare the limits of use of procedures. Finally authors need to specify the characteristics of settings in which procedures can sensibly be used. In the case of the procedures described here users need either skills or guidance on programme planning, and on the development of structured teaching programmes. They also need to be able to interpret test items within broad theoretical frameworks of development or to have such interpretation available.

As noted, the current treatment concentrated on only four procedures. This strategy was adopted in order to allow adequate discussion of each, the aim was not to review all available procedures. The reader is invited to evaluate other procedures in terms of the criteria outlined.

Finally, although much of the discussion here has been negative in tone, the contribution of criterion-referenced tests must be acknowledged. They represent an important component of service delivery, allowing, for all their deficiencies, the development of valuable interventions. The burden of the critique is not to attack their use but to urge authors and practitioners to be more rigorous and critical in the development and use of procedures. The place of criterion-referenced tests in programme development requires that their quality be improved if they are to benefit people with handicaps.

REFERENCES

Atkinson, M. (1982) *Explanations in the Study of Child Language Development*, Cambridge University Press, Cambridge
Bates, E. (1976) *Language and Context*, Academic Press, New York
Bayley, N. (1969) *Bayley Scales of Infant Development*, Psychological Corporation, New York
Bendall, S., Smith, J. and Kushlick, A. (1984) *National Study of Portage-Type Home Teaching Services*, vols. 1 to 3, HCERT Research Reports, The University, Southampton, Hants
Bijou, S.W. (1966) 'A Functional Analysis of Retarded Development' in N.R. Ellis (ed.), *International Review of Research in Mental Retardation*, vol. 1, Academic Press, New York
Bluma, S., Shearer, J., Frohman, A. and Hilliard, J. (1976) *Portage Guide to Early Education*, Cooperative Educational Service, Agency 12, Portage, Wisconsin
Bricker, W.A. (1972) 'A Systematic Approach to Language Training' in R.L. Schiefelbusch (ed.), *Lanuage of the Mentally Retarded*, University Park Press, Baltimore
Bruner, J. (1974–5) 'From Communication to Language: A Psychological Perspective', *Cognition*, 3, 255–87
Cirrin, F.M. and Rowland, C.M. (1985) 'Communicative Assessment of Nonverbal Youths with Severe/Profound Mental Retardation', *Mental Retardation*, 23, 52–62
Colvin, G.T. and Horner, R.H. (1983) 'Experimental Analysis of Generalisation: An Evaluation of a General Case Programme for Teaching Motor Skills to Severely Handicapped Learners in J. Hogg and P.J. Mittler (eds.), *Advances in Mental Handicap Research*, vol. 2, Wiley, Chichester and New York
Dore, J. (1974) 'A Pragmatic Description of Early Language Development', *Psycholinguistic Research*, 3, 343–50
Edwards, A.L. (1957) *Techniques of Attitude Scale Construction*, Appleton-Century Crofts, New York
Glaser, R. (1963) 'Instructional Technology and the Measurement of Outcomes: Some questions', *American Psychologist*, 18, 519–21
Green, B.F. (1956) 'A Method of Scalogram Analysis Using Summary Statistics', *Psychometrika*, 21, 79–88
Griffiths, R. (1954) *The Abilities of Babies*, University of London Press, London
Jenkins, J. (1982) 'The Bereweeke Skill-Teaching System' in R.J. Cameron (ed.), *Working Together: Portage in the UK*, NFER-Nelson, Windsor
Jenkins, J., Felce, D., Mansell, J., Flight, L. and Dell, D. (1983) *The Bereweeke Skill-teaching System*, NFER-Nelson, Windsor
Kiernan, C.C. (1984) 'Language Remediation Programmes: A Review' in D.J. Muller (ed.), *Remediating Children's Language: Behavioural and Naturalistic Approaches*, Croom Helm, London/College-Hill Press, San Diego
—————— (1985a) 'Communication' in A.M. Clarke, A.D.B. Clarke and J. Berg (eds.), *Mental Deficiency: The Changing Outlook*, 4th edn, Methuen, London

────── (1985b) 'The Behavioural Approach to Language Development' in D. Fontana (ed.), *Behaviourism and Learning Theory in Education*, Scottish Academic Press, Edinburgh

────── (1985c) 'Validation of the Preverbal Communication Schedule', Final Report to the Department of Health and Social Security

────── and Jones, M.C. (1982) *Behaviour Assessment Battery: Assessment of the Cognitive, Communicative and Self-Help Skills of Severely Handicapped Children*, 2nd edn, NFER-Nelson, Windsor

──────, Reid, B.D. and Jones, L.M. (1982) *Signs and Symbols: A Review of Literature and Survey of Use of Non-vocal Communication Systems*, University of London Institute of Educational Studies in Education, No. 11 and Heinemann, London

McLean, J.E. and Snyder-McLean, L.K. (1984) 'Recent Developments in Pragmatics: Remedial implications' in D.J. Müller (ed.), *Remediating Children's Language: Behavioural and Naturalistic Approaches*, Croom Helm, London/College-Hill Press, San Diego

Shearer, M.S. and Shearer, D.E. (1972) 'The Portage Project: A Model for Early Childhood Education', *Exceptional Children*, 39, 210–17

Thorburn, M.J., Brown, J. and Bell, C. (1979) 'Early Stimulation of Handicapped Children Using Community Workers', paper to the 5th Congress of the IASSMD, Jerusalem

Uzgiris, I. and Hunt, J.McV. (1975) *Assessment in Infancy. Ordinal Scales of Psychological Development*, University of Illinois Press, Urbana

Weber, J., Jesein, G.S., Shearer, D.E., Bluma, S.M., Hilliard, J.M., Shearer, M.S., Schortinghaus, N.E. and Boyd, R.D. (1975) *The Portage Guide to Home Teaching*, CESA-12, Portage, Wisconsin

White, M. and East, K. (1981) 'Selecting Objectives in Language', *Remedial Education*, 16, 171–8

────── (1983a) *The Wessex Revised Portage Language Checklist*, NFER, Windsor

────── (1983b) 'A New Look at Language Teaching Through the Portage Project', in A. Dessent (ed.), *What is Important About Portage?* NFER-Nelson, Windsor

8

Direct Observation as an Assessment Tool in Functional Analysis and Treatment

G. Murphy

INTRODUCTION

Direct observation techniques essentially involve counting and recording the frequency and/or duration of defined behaviours. In the field of mental handicap, the techniques are most often employed to determine levels of specified behaviours before, during and/or after a treatment intervention (where the intervention may involve behavioural programmes, chemotherapy or a series of other possible treatment methods). In addition, direct observations may be useful in describing facets of the environment and life of handicapped people or the effects of alterations in the environment. Standardised assessments, which are covered in other chapters of this book, do of course involve some degree of direct observation of an individual's behaviour. However, it will be appropriate to resort entirely to direct observation techniques when measurements of levels of behaviour in everyday settings are required (rather than measurements of cognitive skills, for example).

There has been an enormous increase over the last two decades in the use of behavioural methods with mentally handicapped populations, and it is interesting to look at the effect this has had on the development of direct observation techniques. Many of the behavioural methods were adapted from those in the operant learning literature, which concerned itself mainly with the laboratory study of animal learning. Recording techniques in this field were quickly found not to be suitable for human behaviour, consisting, as they did, largely of automatically recorded bar-press or escape responses. Moreover, the associated graphing techniques, such as the cumulative response curve, seemed unsuitable for human behaviour, so that although occasional early studies employed cumulative curves (e.g. Lovaas and Simmons 1969), such methods have since been abandoned in studies of human behaviour.

Ethological methods of observing animal behaviour appeared to provide more appropriate techniques for measuring human behaviour, largely because of their emphasis on the natural environment. This meant that human behaviour could be observed and recorded outside the laboratory, an attractive prospect. Some adaptations were necessary, however, since the categories of behaviour which ethologists employed were often too fine-grained for those interested in measuring behaviour in people with mental handicap. Over the last 20 years, therefore, psychologists have devised techniques to suit their own purposes, combining ethological methods of observation with categories derived from behavioural methods of treatment, applying their treatment interventions in increasingly complex single case experimental designs (Kazdin 1975; Hersen and Barlow 1976).

In this chapter, I begin with a section describing the purposes of direct observation in some detail, with examples from published studies. Following this there is a discussion of the problems of selecting categories of behaviour and situations in which to observe. Then the various different ways of making direct observations are given, with examples of each method. The examples have been chosen from recent mental handicap literature whenever possible. They have been selected so as to represent not only a wide variety of direct observation techniques but also so as to include a number of different kinds of investigation (functional analysis, behavioural treatment procedures, evaluation of the effects of medication and of environmental change) and as many different target behaviours as possible (desirable client behaviours, such as language and self-help skills, undesirable client behaviours such as hyperactivity, stereotypies and self-injury, and a variety of staff or parent behaviours). Following the description of each observation technique one example is given in detail but a number of other references are also provided. Finally, the vitally important topic of validity and reliability in direct observations is presented.

PURPOSES OF DIRECT OBSERVATION

Functional analysis

Professionals and parents working with people who are mentally handicapped are frequently faced with the task of altering the behaviour of a particular individual, either because he or she has developed a behaviour which is unacceptable (such as major tantrums, or aggressive behaviour) or because he or she has not developed the appropriate skills needed for living (such as eating, dressing or more subtle social skills). Before altering someone's behaviour deliberately, ethical considerations, which are not the subject of this chapter, will clearly need to be discussed. Supposing that, after this stage, it has been agreed that the behaviour of the handicapped individual ('target' individual) does indeed need to be changed, then the first step, before embarking on treatment plans, is to complete a proper functional analysis.

Essentially, the term 'functional analysis' refers to the determination of the function of the various stimuli impinging upon the 'target' individual (Kiernan 1973). Normally, it is considered most important when there is a 'deceleration target', i.e. an undesirable behaviour which needs to be reduced, the aim being to discover whether there are discriminative stimuli which 'trigger' the occurrence of the undesirable behaviour and whether there are identifiable stimuli which act as reinforcers, and maintain the undesirable behaviour. Most commonly, this kind of functional analysis is done informally, by merely watching the target individual in settings known to be associated with the undesirable behaviour. It may be possible for those caring for the handicapped person, whether they be teachers, parents, nurses or others, to provide a record to assist in the functional analysis of an undesirable behaviour by completing a very simple chart, which is essentially a continuous event record (see Figure 8.1). Typically, this would require the recording of antecedents (what happened before the target behaviour), the target behaviour itself and consequences (what happened afterwards) for every occurrence of the target behaviour. Jargon can easily be avoided, but the chart would require some explanation if it was to be employed in a setting where staff or parents were unused to behavioural methods. If the target, for example, was tantrum behaviour then a record which provided as the antecedent a description like 'got into a bad mood', or a consequence such as 'calmed

Figure 8.1: Simple Functional Analysis Chart

Date	Time	What Happened Before Target Behaviour	Describe Target Behaviour	What Happened Afterwards

him down eventually', would be almost worthless. Only concrete behavioural descriptions are useful, such as 'asked to sit at a table and do a formboard task' for the antecedents, and 'gave him a cuddle and removed the formboard' for the consequences.

Not everyone finds it easy to provide these kinds of descriptions of behaviour: it requires good powers of observation (and even the best observer will find the task difficult in a crowded schoolroom or hospital ward) and a precise way of thinking. Moreover, it would be important, for the analysis, for all occurrences of the target behaviour to be recorded, something which may be difficult in a busy environment with a low staff:student ratio. Thus, it may be necessary for an outside observer to go in and make the observations, using a similar chart or other observation techniques (see below under the heading 'Techniques of Direct Observation, Recording and Analysis'). Once sufficient records have been collected (i.e. at least 20 occurrences of the target behaviour), then the analysis of the functions of the various stimuli may begin. Table 8.1 (from Swanson and Watson 1982, Chapter 10) provides a guide for this analysis, which may be quite straightforward if there are clear antecedents and frequently occurring consequences which appear to provide a continuous (or almost continuous) schedule of reinforcement.

It may be, however, particularly with well-established undesirable behaviours, that there appears to be a variety of antecedents and a variety of consequences, so that understanding

Table 8.1: Behavioural Contingencies

Operant Concepts – Direction of Target Behaviour	Contingency	Probable Effects	Example of Events
I. Behaviour increases			
A. Positive reinforcement	Behaviour (B) followed ($\rightarrow$) by positive consequence (C+) = B $\rightarrow$ C+	Increase in strength of target behaviour	Teacher praise for math performance
B. Negative reinforcement	= B $\rightarrow$ Reduction ($\downarrow$) in negative consequence (C–)	Same as above: escape or avoidance	Reduction of teacher criticism improves percent correct on math performance
II. Behaviour decreases (punishment)			
A. Presentation of aversive consequence	= B $\rightarrow$ C–	Decrease in strength of target behaviour: escape or avoidance	Presentation of teacher criticism decreases percent of error on math performance
B. Removal of obtained and possessed positive consequences	= B $\rightarrow$ $\downarrow$C+	Same as above: response cost	Removal of tokens or free time decreases math error performance
III. Extinction	= B $\rightarrow$ No C+	Same as above	Removal of teacher verbal attention decreases math error performance
IV. Shaping	= $B_2 \rightarrow$ C+ or $\downarrow$C– = $B_1 \rightarrow$ No C	Increase strength of B_2 and decrease strength of B_1	Teacher only reinforces for 80% correct on math and now provides no consequence for 70% correct

| V. Generalisation | Two stimuli, S_1 and $S_2 \to B \to C+$ or ($\downarrow C-$) | Increase strength of B occurring in S_1 and S_2 | Resource room teacher reinforces math performance: regular classroom teacher reinforces math performance |
| VI. Discrimination | $= S_1 \to B_1 \to C+$ or ($\downarrow C-$)
$= S_2 \to B_1 \to$ No C: $\downarrow C+:C-$ | Increase strength of B_1 occurring in S_1 but weaken strength of B_1 occurring in S_2 | Teacher reinforces correct math performance on school work by having child get answer sheet and correct answers: child is not reinforced for getting answer sheet on standardised math test |

Source: Swanson and Watson (1982).

their functional significance and planning a treatment programme becomes difficult. If this happens, it will probably be necessary to perform a formal functional analysis. This may involve formal direct observations in a natural situation (see Edelson, Taubman and Lovaas 1983, discussed below at p. 224). Alternatively, in very chaotic or complex natural environments, a series of experimental situations can be deliberately set up to present certain putative antecedents or consequences, with direct observations establishing the effect of the conditions on the target behaviour (see Iwata, Dorsey, Slifer, Bauman and Richman 1982, the example discussed below).

The example of formal functional analysis which follows concerns self-injurious behaviour (SIB). Essentially, Iwata *et al.* wished to test the effects of several different settings on the occurrence of SIB, because of evidence that a variety of different stimuli could set the behaviour off (including low sensory stimulus input, high demands and low social attention). Four experimental conditions were deliberately set up to test the function of these different stimuli: a socal disapproval condition, an academic demand condition, an 'alone' condition and an unstructured play condition. The social disapproval condition involved the presence of an experimenter and toys, with social attention (of a mildly disapproving nature) delivered after each self-injurious response. In the academic demand condition, the child was presented with difficult 'academic' or educational tasks and was required to complete them, with prompting as necessary. In the 'alone' condition, the child was alone, without toys or experimenters. The unstructured play condition was a comparison condition, controlling the presence of toys and an experimenter, in which the child had toys available and an experimenter present, delivering reinforcement contingent on the absence of SIB.

Iwata and colleagues discovered, using continuous observation with category coding (see below under the heading 'Techniques of Direct Observation, Recording and Analysis'), that the children tested responded differently in the different conditions (see Figure 8.2). Four of the children showed most SIB in the 'alone' condition, suggesting that the function of their SIB was to provide stimulation (i.e. that their SIB had been reinforced by sensory stimuli). Two other children showed highest levels of SIB during the academic demand condition, suggesting that escape from aversive tasks normally maintained their SIB. One child showed highest levels of SIB during the social disapproval condition which probably meant that his/her SIB had been reinforced in the past by social attention. Finally, for the remaining children, the different conditions appeared to have had no clear effects (a variety of interpretations could be applied to this subgroup, as Iwata *et al.* have discussed). Following this experimental analysis, Iwata went on to design treatment plans, taking into account the function of the SIB, as displayed in the conditions tested (Iwata, Pace, Cataldo, Kalsher and Edwards 1984).

Programmes with deceleration targets like self-injurious behaviour almost invariably employ at least an informal function analysis. Much less commonly is it thought necessary when there are acceleration targets or new behaviours to be taught. This is in many ways surprising, as appropriate behaviours are as bound to their antecedents and consequences as are inappropriate behaviours. Many a programme intended to increase a target behaviour has failed due to an incorrect choice of 'reinforcer'. For acceleration targets, or new behaviours, functional analysis, if completed at all, is most likely to be concerned with the selection of effective reinforcers and thus may employ interview methods (asking the handicapped person or significant other in his/her environment what his/her preferences are), 'cafeteria' methods as Kiernan (1974), has termed them (providing a wide variety of potential reinforcers and seeing which the handicapped person prefers) or the Premack principle, attributed to Premack (1959) (involving the selection of most frequently engaged-in behaviours as reinforcers for less frequent ones). The compatibility of the target behaviour and the reinforcer may also need to be considered, since certain reinforcers appear to be relatively ineffective as consequences for certain target behaviours (Williams, Koegel and Egel 1981; Murphy, Callias and Carr 1985).

The function of various antecedent stimuli may also be important in programmes intended to accelerate desirable behaviours. For example, a boy described by Murphy (1980) with major mealtime misbehaviours was found to have appropriate mealtime behaviour already in his repertoire, once the appropriate antecedent stimuli were presented. Thus for acceleration targets, as well as for deceleration targets, it may prove worthwhile to present a variety of antecedent stimuli, in a formal way, and record the appearance of the desired target behaviour.

Figure 8.2: Percentage of Intervals of Self-Injury for Four out of Nine Subjects Across Sessions and Experimental Settings

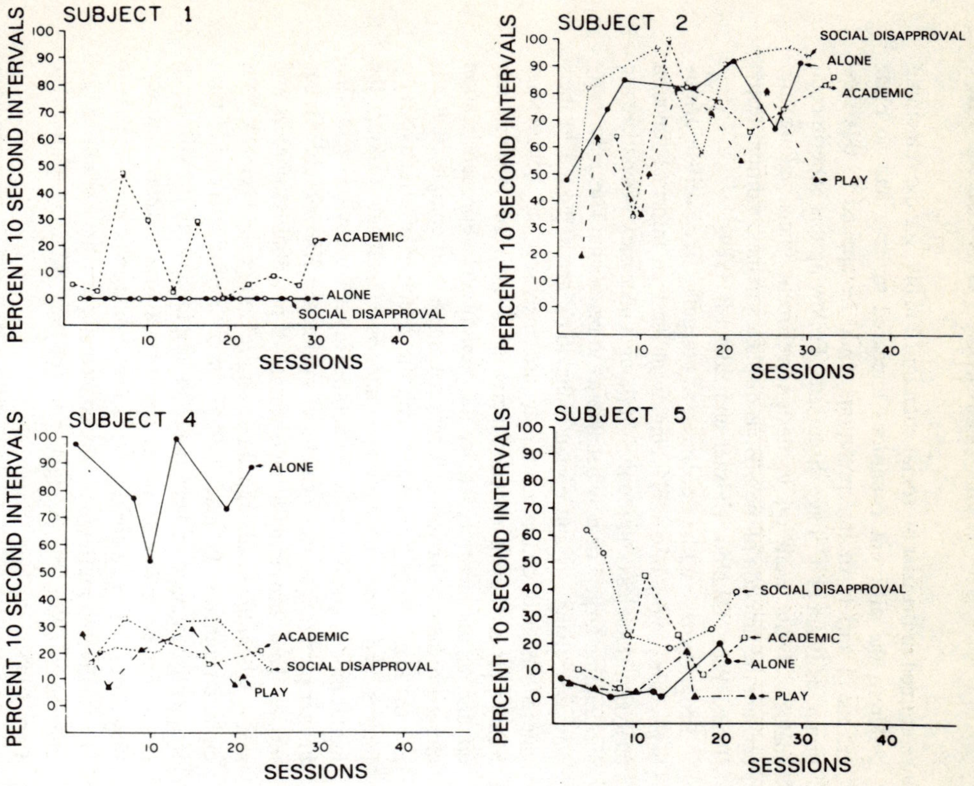

Source: Iwata et al. 1982.

Behavioural treatments

Following functional analysis, it may be decided that a particular treatment or series of treatments should be employed to reduce an undesirable behaviour or to increase a desirable one. Ideally, the treatment(s) should be applied in such a way that the effectiveness of the various treatment component(s) can be identified, using a single-case experimental design (Barlow and Hersen 1984).

Prior to instituting any treatment, the original level of the target behaviour(s) will need to be recorded by one of the methods described below (under the heading 'Techniques of Direct Observation, Recording and Analysis'), to provide a baseline assessment. Following the introduction of the treatment technique, further observations will be required in order to establish the efficacy of the treatment. These latter observations may take the form of the baseline assessment (frequently referred to as 'repeat baselines'), with which they can be directly compared to assess treatment progress provided the conditions of the observation are identical. Alternatively, it may be necessary to make rather different observations during the treatment phase, particularly if the training programme involves teaching new behaviour with the inclusion of techniques such as prompting and chaining. Commonly, a combination of both methods is chosen, with a relatively simple method of data collection during training sessions and a repeat baseline method for periodic use after a number of sessions only (see, for example, Murphy *et al.* 1985).

Precisely how and when direct observations are made in behavioural treatment programmes will therefore depend heavily on the manner in which the treatment is applied. A large variety of single-case designs, with their accompanying scheduling of observations, have been described, including withdrawal, reversal, multiple baseline, multielement and changing criterion designs. They are well reviewed in a variety of texts (Leitenberg 1973; Kazdin 1975; Hersen and Barlow 1976; Barlow and Hersen 1984; Yule 1980; Rusch and Kazdin 1981). They will therefore not be further discussed here, but illustrations of various designs and their accompanying observational strategies can be seen in the examples given in this section (above) and below under 'Techniques of Direct Observation, Recording and Analysis'.

Other evaluations

Direct observation techniques may also be invaluable in programmes or projects which are not simply behavioural functional analyses or behavioural treatments. Thus, if the clinician is asked to evaluate the effectiveness of chemotherapy for reducing the activity level of a hyperactive child, direct observation techniques would certainly be one important evaluative method (as in, for example, Rapport, Murphy and Bailey 1982, described on pp. 216–17). Similarly, in an investigation of whether large group or family group care was superior, in terms of the rates of staff-trainee social interactions and trainee engagement levels, direct observations were the techniques of choice (Munoz 1978). Other examples of direct observation techniques in evaluating service and other treatment facilities can be found in King, Raynes and Tizard (1971), Tizard, Cooperman, Joseph and Tizard (1972), Melin and Golestam (1981), Raynes, Pratt and Roses (1979) and in Felce, de Kock and Repp (in press), some of whose work is described below in the section headed 'Techniques of Direct Observation, Recording and Analysis'.

CHOOSING CATEGORIES OF BEHAVIOUR AND SITUATIONS

Inevitably, not all facets of a person's behaviour can be recorded nor can they be recorded in all possible situations. Consequently, before collecting direct observational data decisions will need to be made, not just about *how* to record the behaviours (see below under 'Techniques of Direct Observation, Recording and Analysis'), but also about *which behaviours* to record and in *which situations*.

Choosing categories of behaviour

It was not unusual, in early behavioural research, for only one 'target' behaviour to be recorded. However, nowadays it is common to see a list of as many as 20 categories of behaviour to be coded. The reason for this change is not simply the advent of new methods of recording, but the discovery that different categories of behaviour are not necessarily independent of each other. Thus, for example, if desirable behaviours are reinforced, undesirable ones tend to reduce, particularly if the desirable behaviour is physically incompatible with the undesirable one (see Russo, Cataldo and Cushing 1981, for example). Other classes of behaviour also appear to be linked functionally. Thus if two, or more, undesirable behaviours have the same function (for example, attracting adult attention), they might both be expected to reduce if a new desirable way of obtaining attention is taught. Conversely, if two, or more, undesirable behaviours have the same function, and one is diminished by a punishment (or other) programme, without teaching a desirable behaviour in its place, the untreated undesirable behaviours might be expected to increase. Examples of this kind of phenomenon can be seen in Young and Wincze (1974), and Rojahn, Mulick, McCoy and Schroeder (1978), both studies of self-injury, and also in Singh, Manning and Angell (1982), in a study of chronic rumination.

The difficulty of predicting in advance which behaviours are functionlly linked has meant that most researchers prefer to record a wide range of behaviours, in case treatment of one behaviour leads to unforeseen alterations in another. Those engaged in research into general levels of behaviour in institutions, hospitals, homes and schools may also wish to record a large variety of behaviours, particularly if the study is exploratory in nature.

A number of approaches can be taken to the problem of which behaviours should be observed. It is possible to find 'comprehensive' lists of behaviour for use in direct observational studies of people with mental handicap. One such list for maladaptive behaviour includes 283 different behaviours (Cantela and Upper 1985 quoted by Swanson and Watson 1982). Ideal though this solution may seem to be at first sight, it may create its own problems. Human observers have a limited capacity and increasing the number of categories of behaviour which they are required to record may simply reduce observer accuracy (see under the headings 'Issues of Reliability and Validity' below). In addition, the data analysis will necessarily become more onerous, the more categories of behaviour are coded, particularly if sequential analyses are planned. Perhaps the best solution is to undertake some pilot observations, using a comprehensive list of behaviours (such as that in Cantela and Upper or one from a study of general behaviour, like Felce *et al.* (in press) as an aide-memoire, with the intention of paring the list down to a manageable size. In addition observers will need to consider precisely what their experimental hypotheses are, i.e. what questions they are asking, since this will determine, as least in part, the classes of behaviour which may be relevant. (See Leudar and Fraser, Chapter 5 of this volume for a discussion of general issues on assesment of behaviour problems.) Observers will also need to be aware of recent theoretical and clinical work, in relation to the problems they wish to tackle. Thus, for example, recent evidence of the links between disproprotionately low language skills and the appearance of undesirable behaviour in both normal and handicapped populations (Richman, Stevenson and Graham 1982; Gould 1976; Ando and Yoshimura 1979) might prompt those examining the effect of language training to record some undesirable behaviours as well.

Choosing situations to observe

A number of factors will influence the observer's choice of situations in which to observe. For those working in schools, social education centres and hostels, the considerations will be largely practical. Since laboratory-type settings will probably be unavailable to them, any observations will need to be made in the natural environment. Those who do have special facilities, such as observation rooms with one-way screens, will almost certainly be working in university or hospital-based environments, and they will need to decide, first and foremost, whether to observe their client's behaviour in the special observation rooms or to observe in the natural environment. In this, they will face a dilemma; in highly controlled laboratory or semi-laboratory settings, with one-way screens, observations can be made without fear that the presence of an observer in the room with the target individuals is affecting their behaviour. On the other hand, the individuals may not display their usual behaviour because they are in a laboratory/one-way screen room. Observers stationed in the individuals' ordinary environments, though, despite the advantages of the 'home situation', may produce alterations in the individuals' usual behaviour, simply because of their presence.

Certainly, there is considerable evidence that individuals being observed are aware of the observer's presence, even over long periods of time (Grimm, Parsons and Bijou 1972; Paul 1963 quoted in Patterson 1982). Whether they alter their behaviour *because* of the observer's presence is more debatable. Both parents and teachers have been shown to be able to make their children 'look good' and 'look bad', if so requested by researchers (Lobitz and Johnson 1975; Weinrott, Jones and Boler 1977). It is, therefore, possible that in observations where parents, teachers, nurses or care staff are present, they may produce alterations (not necessarily deliberate ones) in the behaviour of the people with handicaps by adjusting their own behaviour, to 'fake' good or bad. What is less likely is that people who are profoundly or severely handicapped will alter their own behaviour in any predictable way, as a result of observers' presence (for the mildly handicapped adult, though, faking may be a problem, much as it would be for any other adults). Patterson (1982), in an excellent discussion of these problems, suggests that, even despite a certain amount of faking, observational data may still reflect real (though perhaps attenuated) effects. Thus, as Patterson notes, Reid, Taplin and Lorber (1981) demonstrated that mothers of abused children hit their offspring far more than other mothers, when being observed, even though they knew the purpose of the observation. Similarly, in the study described below (pp. 222–3) Felce *et al.* demonstrated large differences between environments in terms of staff behaviour, despite staff knowing about the data collection.

Despite the problems which possible observer presence effects bring, most clinicians and researchers now feel that observation in the natural environment is preferable to that in laboratories or specially constructed environments. Indeed, in many cases, it may be *essential* to observe in natural environments if, for example, generalisation from training sessions is at issue (as in the study by Hurlbut, Iwata and Green 1982, described below at pp. 206–7). Moreover, the degree to which observer's presence alters individual's behaviour may be at least partially checked, when observers wish, by asking parents, teachers or nurses to record the indivdiual's behaviour in the absence of the outside observer, and cross-checking the data with observer's records (as in the study by Rapport *et al.* 1982, described below at pp. 216–17). It will, of course, be necessary to ensure that the data collected by others is reliable however — see the section headed 'Issues of Reliability and Validity'.

Other decisions regarding the situation(s) in which to make observations will depend largely on the nature of the study. Thus, for example, observers may wish to adopt a 'fly-on-the-wall' position if they are investigating facets of a natural situation. Or they may wish to set up situations if they want to test specific hypotheses (for example, in formal functional analysis, as in the study by Iwata *et al.* 1982, described above).

Frequently, in planning direct observational data collection, a question arises as to how long observation sessions should be and how many sessions should be undertaken. The former decision, regarding lengths of observation sessions, will depend to some degree on the behaviour(s) to be observed. Thus, for persistent, high-rate behaviour, occurring thoughout the day (for example, high-rate stereotypies), the observer would probably be best advised to observe several brief periods (half an hour or less) each day, for several days, unless sequential analysis is intended (in which case samples should be longer). Examination of the variability of the data after observations will provide some indication of the need for further sessions; if very variable amounts of behaviour have been recorded, further sessions will be called for, preferably to tease out the reasons for the variability because otherwise these uncontrolled influences may mask or exaggerate other effects, such as treatment effects. For individual case designs, of course, this will be more crucial than for group designs which, with proper statistical analysis, allow such data variance to be taken into account. However, even in group designs, large variability is a disadvantage, in that it may swamp any interesting experimental effects. For behaviours which are of low frequency and which occur only at particular points in the day (for example, tantrums over toileting), the observer will need to time observations carefully, to coincide with the target behaviour. In other respects, however, the decisions about how many observation sessions are needed can be made as described above. If behaviours to be observed are of low frequency and quite unpredictable in timing, the observer may have to spend all day, for several days, making observations (as in the example of Hurlbut *et al.* 1982, described below at pp. 206–7) or, alternatively arrange for on-site staff or parents to record the observations themselves.

Ideally, then observational data should be collected over a number of days. It is useful to plot the data graphically before deciding whether to proceed to the next stage (for example, a treatment phase). If the data show a consistent rising or falling trend there will need to be continued observations until a stable level is reached (or until the factors producing the trend are identified). Otherwise assessment of the effectiveness of any subsequent treatment procedure will be impossible. Equally, if the graph shows great variability in the levels of behaviour, it will be necessary to determine the reasons. There may be features of the environment, as yet undetected, which are exerting major control over the levels of behaviour observed and these factors, once discerned, may contribute greatly to treatment planning. Suppose, for example, in observing a client's tantrums in a school setting, tantrums are recorded at a much lower rate when teacher A is in class than when teacher B is in class. Clearly, the ways in which the two teachers manage the client and the rest of the class may provide valuable clues for any management programme aimed at reducing tantrums.

TECHNIQUES OF DIRECT OBSERVATION, RECORDING AND ANALYSIS

It is impractical to record *all* human behaviour, except in the briefest of observation periods. The art of direct observation (and recording) consists, therefore, in knowing what to omit. Essentially, different techniques omit different facets of the stream of behaviour and the choice which clinicians, or researchers, make will be dictated by their task.

There are a number of variables to be considered in choosing an observation technique. First, it is necessary to decide whether to *observe* continuously (throughout observation periods) or discontinuously (sampling only at discrete points in the observation period). Second, the manner of *recording* the observations will need to be settled. The simplest recording techniques involve only paper and pencil but a growing number of other possibilities are now available, from audio and video taping to event recorders and sophisticated microcomputers. Third, the *analysis* of the behaviour to be recorded must be considered, since a number of products are possible and not all observation and recording methods lend themselves to all kinds of analysis. Following the description of the various methods of observation, therefore, we will consider the possible methods of recording and analysis and how they relate to the observation techniques.

Observational techniques

Continuous Methods. All continuous methods require observers to both watch and record behaviour throughout observation periods. Omissions consist largely of detail or of nontarget classes of behaviour. Information on the sequences of behaviour is retained.
Descriptive Recording. When experimenters or clinicians are interested in more than a few behaviours, a descriptive recording method can be employed. Essentially, this involves writing (or dictating on tape or filming and then transcribing) a brief description of the behaviour(s) observed, within a time frame. Clearly, this can be an extremely inaccurate method if no decisions are made in advance about which behaviours are of interest, since no one could record every response an active person made. However, the technique may be very useful at the initial stage of an experimental or clinical study, particularly if observers are rather unsure about

precisely which behaviours to observe and how to code them. It is unusual, nowadays, for this technique to be selected except at the pilot stage of a study, but it is occasionally employed with some sophistication (Hutt and Hutt 1964; Tizard, Philps and Plewis 1976).
Event Recording. Once observers are certain which behaviours to record, then rather than describe events as they occur, the behaviours of interest can be listed and the observer may simply record when they occur. In event recording, the observer is simply required to note all occurrences of a target behaviour over the observation period. The occurrences may be recorded on paper or on automatic tally counters (e.g. Jones 1983). The frequency of the target behaviour over the observation period can be calculated, at the end, by dividing the number of occurrences by the number of seconds/minutes/hours for which the target individual was observed.

This can be a very effective method of recording the level of a brief, discrete item of behaviour in an individual's repertoire. Moreover, the use of tally counters means that such recording can be adopted by trainers (whether they be parents or professionals), without disruption of the teaching or training programme. Jones (1983), for example, has described this kind of recording as part of normal classroom procedure in a unit for children with handicaps and behaviour problems.

Event recording is not appropriate, however, for behaviours of variable duration when the total amount of behaviour is to be measured, since a record simply of frequency may be an inaccurate reflection of the total time for which an individual displayed the behaviour. The technique is also inappropriate for recording brief behaviours which are emitted so fast that they are uncountable. Thus, event recording is most often employed for recording brief and relatively infrequent behaviours. The length of the observation period can vary from all day to an hour a day or less, although care must obviously be taken in extrapolating from records of brief periods of the day.

Hurlbut *et al.* (1982), for example, employed event recording to examine the spontaneous use of 'words' by three multiply handicapped students involved in a language training programme. All three students were severely physically handicapped and were taught a series of ten new words in either Bliss symbols or iconic signs (five Bliss symbols and five iconic signs for each student). The students' learning of the new words was tested by probe trials, but the experimenters also wanted a measure of students' spontaneous use of taught and untaught words. Therefore, one experimenter remained in the classroom throughout the day and recorded every spontaneous use of board signs by the student (event recording), also reinforcing them for appropriate sign usage.

In general, the experiment showed that the students learned the iconic signs faster than the Bliss symbols. Moreover, event recording in the classroom demonstrated that iconic signs were more often employed spontaneously than were Bliss symbols, there being some generalisation from taught to untaught iconic signs. As an example, the graph in Figure 8.3 shows the results for one of the three students, Tom. Further examples of event recording can be seen in Morris and Dolker (1974), King, Raynes and Tizard's observation checklist, B2 (1971) and Favell, McGimsey, Jones and Connon (1981).

Duration Recording. For behaviours which last more than a second or two, particularly for those which vary appreciably in length, event recording is clearly inappropriate. In this case, duration methods, which involve recording the total length of responses, are more informative. There are a number of possible ways of obtaining a duration record (see recording techniques below) but all involve some kind of real-time base. The simplest variety, such as the cumulative stop-watch, will result in loss of some information about the behaviour (e.g. bout length, spread of behaviour across the observation interval) but the more sophisticated retain these details (see below).

Harris and Wolchik (1979), for example, examined the effects of three different treatment strategies on stereotyped behaviour in four handicapped boys. The treatments which were compared, DRO (differential reinforcement of other behaviour), brief time-out and overcorrection, were applied in a reversal design and the measure of stereotyped behaviour for the first two boys was a frequency measure only (i.e. event recording, see above). For the second two boys, duration measures were also taken, using a cumulative stop-watch.

In general, the study showed that the abbreviated form of overcorrection was the most effective form of treatment for each of the boys. It transpired that, for the two boys where both measures were taken, frequency and duration were significantly positively correlated. However, the correlation was by no means perfect. Figure 8.4 shows the data from one of the boys, Karl, for whom it can be seen that the level of stereotypies was more strongly affected by some experimental procedures when duration measures were plotted, than when frequency measures were used (compare the

Figure 8.3: Mean Number of Pictures and Symbols Used Spontaneously per Hour per Day for Tom

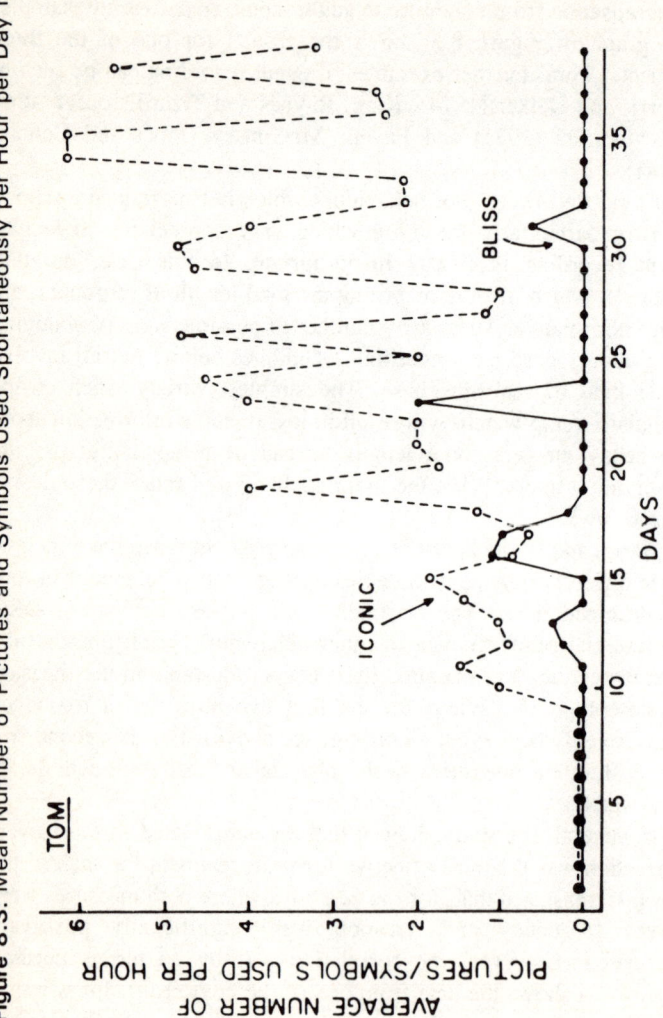

Source: Hurlbut et al. (1982).

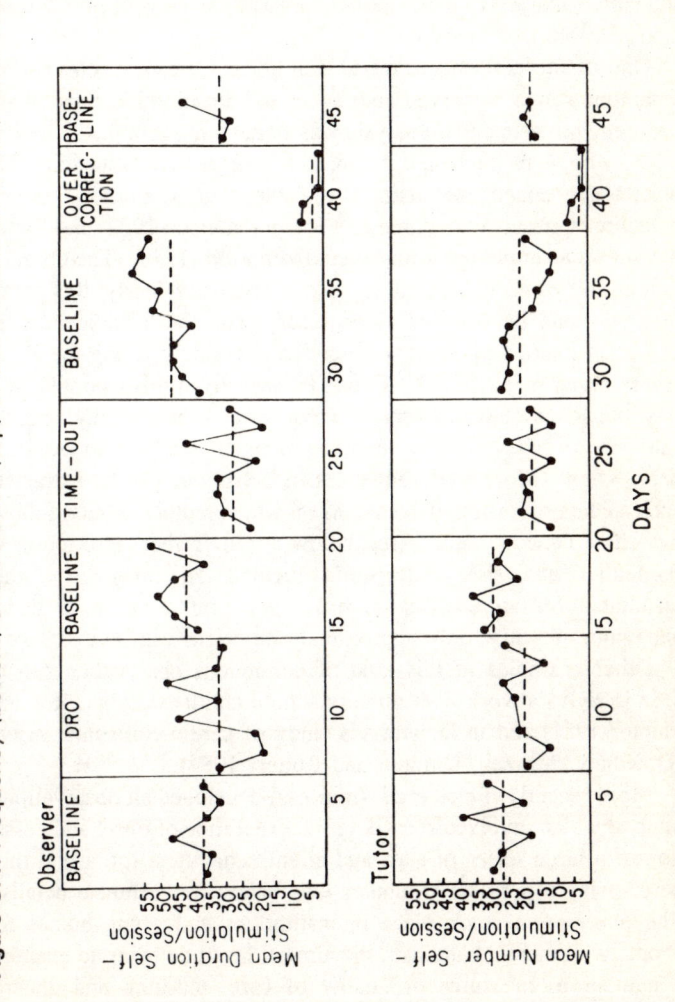

Figure 8.4: Frequency (bottom) and Duration (top) of Self-stimulation in Karl, under Different Treatment Conditions

Source: Harris and Wolchik (1979).

relative levels in adjacent time-out, baseline and overcorrection phases in Figure 8.4).

Sophisticated Continuous Methods. The more sophisticated methods of continuous observation essentially combine event and duration techniques for large numbers of categories of behaviour. The emphasis varies from study to study, some being most concerned to retain sequences of events, others being concerned to keep to a real-time base. Many of these studies employ expensive equipment (e.g. Felce *et al.* in press) but others retain paper and pencil methods (e.g. Patterson 1982). Very often the observations form the basis for a sequential analysis of behaviour but a variety of simpler products are also possible (see below).

One of the earliest groups to employ a continuous observation technique which preserved both event and duration information and proceeded to sequential analysis was Patterson's group, in Oregon, USA, who were interested in children's aggressive behaviour. The behaviours coded are listed in Table 8.2 (definitions of the behaviours are given in Appendix 3.1 in Patterson 1982) and Figure 8.5 shows a simple recording sheet from Reid (1978). The observation period was divided into six-second sections (clearly, this period of time could be adjusted as necessary) and the behaviour of the child and interacting adult were coded alternately, using the coded letters given in Table 8.2. As can be seen from this example, it is possible to extract an event or frequency count for any selected category of behaviour (i.e. number of times a behaviour occurred per session). Moreover, sequences of behaviour can be extracted, such as the proportion of occasions on which mother shouts, following child noncompliance (see below for a further description of sequential analysis). Patterson's method is, however, rather unsuitable for an analysis of exact per cent duration of coded behaviours because only approximate durations can be extracted.

Other examples of this kind of continuous observation can be seen in Sylva's work with nursery school children (Sylva, Roy and Painter 1981) and in Dowdney's study of parent-child interactions (Dowdney, Mrazek, Quinton and Rutter, 1984).

More recently, Felce *et al.* (in press) developed an observational method which involved recording the exact time of onset and cessation of a large series of staff and client behaviours, on a real-time base, using a portable computer (see below for technical details). The observations took place in institutions and group homes for people with mental handicap, the aim of the study being to examine a number of measures of quality of care, teaching and general

Figure 8.5: A Sample Recording Sheet from Studies by Patterson and Colleagues

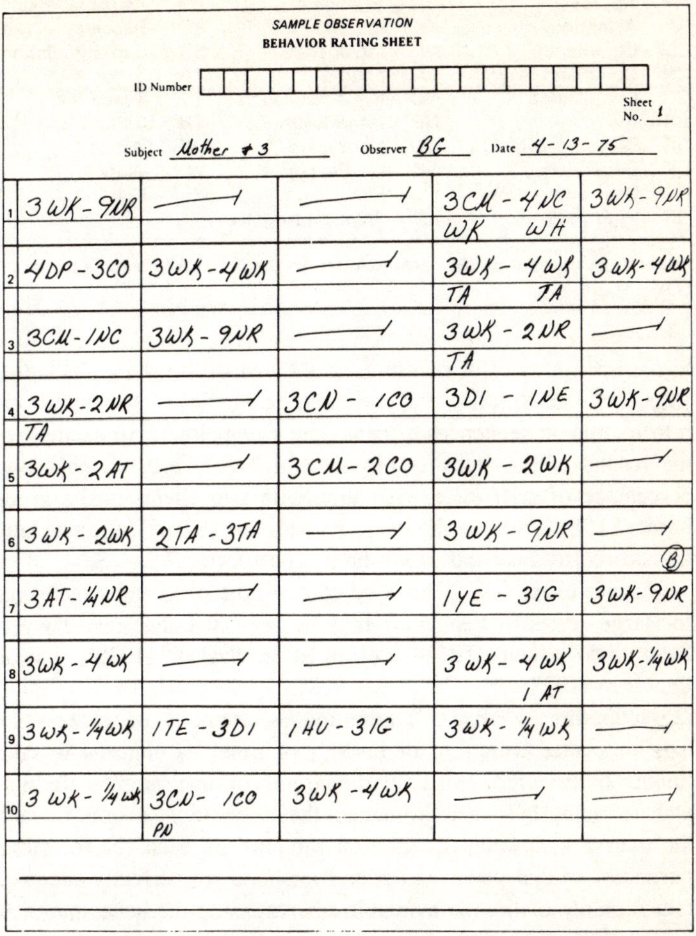

SAMPLE OBSERVATION
BEHAVIOR RATING SHEET

ID Number

Sheet No. 1

Subject Mother #3 Observer BG Date 4-13-75

1	3WK-9NR	——/	——/	3CM-4NC WK WH	3WK-9NR
2	4DP-3CO	3WK-4WK	——/	3WK-4WK TA TA	3WK-4WK
3	3CM-1NC	3WK-9NR	——/	3WK-2NR TA	——/
4	3WK-2NR TA	——/	3CN-1CO	3DI-1NE	3WK-9NR
5	3WK-2AT	——/	3CM-2CO	3WK-2WK	——/
6	3WK-2WK	2TA-3TA	——/	3WK-9NR	——/ (B)
7	3AT-¼NR	——/	——/	1YE-3IG	3WK-9NR
8	3WK-4WK	——/	——/	3WK-4WK 1 AT	3WK-¼WK
9	3WK-¼WK	1TE-3DI	1HU-3IG	3WK-¼WK	——/
10	3WK-¼WK	3CN-1CO PN	3WK-4WK	——/	——/

Source: Reid (1978).

environment in the two types of residential placement. A series of eight appropriate client behaviours, six inappropriate client behaviours and five neutral client behaviours were recorded, together with nine staff behaviours (three antecedent and six consequent ones). Observers coded all the behaviour of the client and all staff behaviour relating to that individual, rather than coding alternate client and staff behaviours (cf. Patterson above). It was possible

Table 8.2: Behavioural Codes used by Patterson (1982) in Studies of Aggressive Behaviour in Children

AP	Approval	HU*	Humiliate	PP	Physical Positive
AT	Attention	IG*	Ignore	RC	Receive
CM	Command	IN	Indulgence	SS	Self-stimulation
CN*	Command Negative	LA	Laugh	TA	Talk
CO	Compliance	NC*	Noncompliance	TE*	Tease
CR*	Cry	NE*	Negativism	TH	Touch
DI*	Disapproval	NO	Normative	WH*	Whine
DP*	Dependency	NR	No Response	WK	Work
DS*	Destructiveness	PL	Play	YE*	Yell
HR*	High Rate	PN*	Physical Negative		

* Indicates categories that are included in the Total Aversive Behaviour (TAB) score.

to extract a variety of measures at the end of the study, including frequency and duration for particular categories of behaviour and information on sequences of behaviour (see below). An example of the results of the study is provided in Figure 8.6, which shows percentage of staff interaction time with two clients in the group home (S1, S2) and two clients in an institution (S7 and S8), who later transferred to a second group home (post-test, S7 and S8).

Further examples of this kind of real-time continuous recording for large series of behaviour may be seen in Landesman-Dwyer, Stein and Sackett (1976), described in Sackett (1978), and in Bakeman (1978).

Discontinuous Methods. Discontinuous methods of observation entail repeated sampling of periods of time, as opposed to continuous observation. Normally the periods of time sampled are brief and are regularly spaced throughout the observation session. Usually the intervals between observation samples are used for recording purposes, so that paper and pencil methods are perfectly adequate (since plenty of time is available for recording the behaviour).

The two main techniques, interval recording and momentary time-sampling, are very commonly employed in behavioural studies. Kelly (1977), for example, reported that 41 per cent of the studies, involving human observers, published in the *Journal of Applied Behavior Analysis* over the previous seven years, involved one or other of these sampling methods.

Interval recording and time-sampling are often poorly differentiated in research reports. Strictly speaking, interval recording involves noting the occurrence or absence of particular behaviour(s) during an observed *interval* of time. In time-sampling, on the other

Figure 8.6: Percentage of Time Spent by Staff in Interactions with Two Handicapped Adults (S1, S2) in a Small Home, and with Two Handicapped Adults (S7, S8) in an Institution (First Block), who then Moved to a Small House (Second Block)

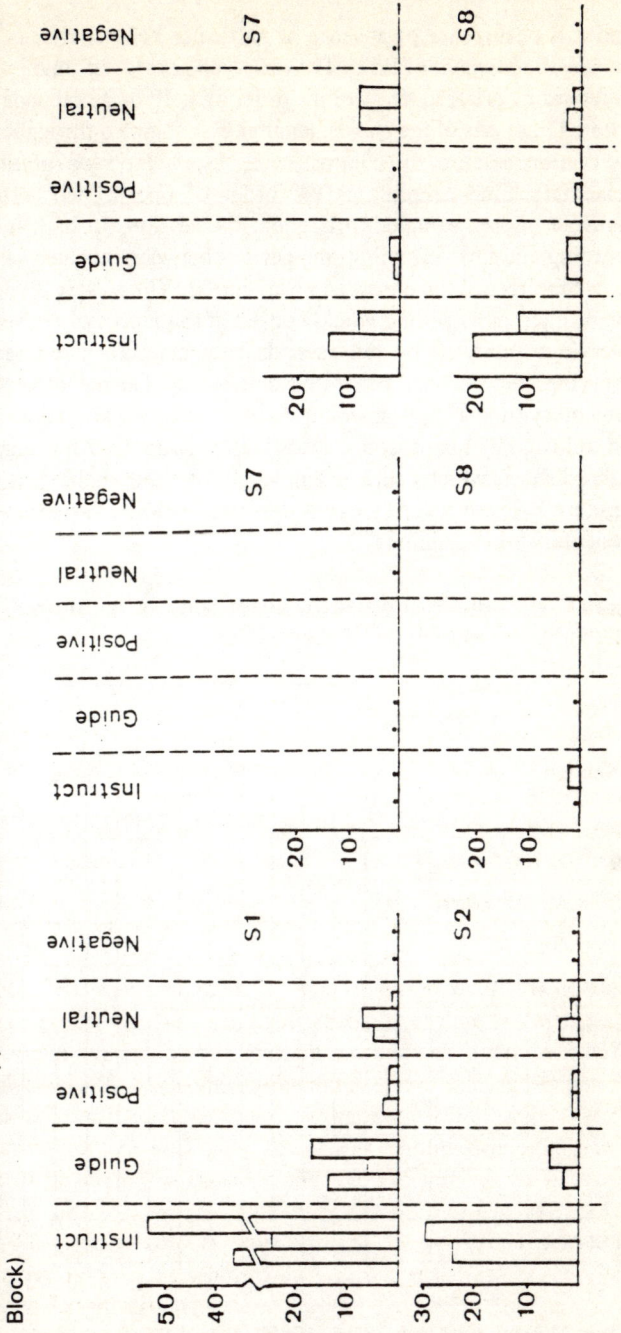

Source: Felce *et al.* (in press).

DIRECT OBSERVATION AS AN ASSESSMENT TOOL

hand, the occurrence or absence of particular behaviour(s) is noted at a specific *moment* of time. The observed periods of time in interval recording are frequently of the order of 5, 10 or 20 seconds long, repeated intervals of the chosen length being sampled throughout the observation session. In contrast, the observed period of time in momentary time-sampling is the order of one second, repeated 'moments' being sampled throughout the session. In both interval recording and time-sampling, the periods between repeated samples are used to record the observed behaviour(s). Thus, typically, a session of interval recording would consist of sequences of ten seconds observing, followed by ten seconds recording, then ten seconds observing, ten seconds recording and so on. On the other hand, momentary time sampling would involve, say, one second observation followed by nine seconds recording, repeatedly. An example of a record sheet, which could be employed for either method, is given in Figure 8.7 (the related study is described below as an example of momentary time-sampling).

Figure 8.7: Example of a Record Sheet Suitable for Interval Recording or Momentary Time-sampling

Date _____ Child _____ Session _____												Time _____ Toy _____ Place _____			
	1	2	3	4	5	6	7	8	9	10	11	12	13	14	15
TOY CONTACT															
TOY MANIPULATION															
MOUTHING TOY															
IMAGINATIVE PLAY															
STEREO-TYPIES															
IN SEAT															

Source: Murphy, Carr and Callias (1986).

One advantage of momentary time-sampling over interval recording is that in time-sampling the target behaviour(s) have either occurred or not occurred at the point sampled, whereas in interval recording the behaviour may have occurred several times in the interval, or continuously, or on only one brief occasion. In one interval method, whole-interval recording, behaviours are coded as present only if they have occurred throughout the observation interval, while in the other, partial-interval recording, behaviours are coded as present if they occur at all in the observation interval.

Until recently, it was thought that both interval recording and time-sampling methods would provide accurate estimates of the 'amount' of behaviour observed, provided sufficient observation samples were taken. Indeed, Hutt and Hutt (1970) preferred interval recording to time-sampling because they considered it to be less likely to produce results unrepresentative of actual rates of behaviour, due to the longer observation interval involved. However, over the last few years, several studies have compared the two methods experimentally, and shown that momentary time-sampling is more likely accurately to reflect the true per cent duration of a behaviour than is interval recording (Powell, Martindale and Kulp 1975; Repp, Roberts, Slack, Repp and Berkler 1976; Powell, Martindale, Kulp, Martindale and Bauman 1977; Green and Alverson, 1978; Murphy and Goodall 1980).

In the earliest study, Powell *et al.* observed the in-seat behaviour of a secretary, who was performing her normal duties. Estimates of the per cent duration 'in-seat', derived from whole-interval recording, partial-interval recording and momentary time-sampling, when compared to a criterion record, indicated that momentary time-sampling was the most accurate. Whole-interval recording consistently under-estimated and partial-interval recording consistently overestimated the true level of behaviour, with shorter duration samples producing smaller errors, as might be expected (Murphy and Goodall 1980). Later studies confirmed this finding and showed that the size of errors could be extremely large (Powell *et al.* 1977 found errors of 80 per cent with long intervals) and that the level of error also depended on response durations (long responses producing smaller errors). It was also clear, from some studies, that observation intervals as short as ten seconds could lead to large errors, if responses were brief, and totally ineffective treatment procedures *could* appear effective if interval recording was the only measure (Murphy and Goodall 1980).

These findings, of the superiority of momentary time-sampling to interval recording, only hold in certain conditions. Thus if the measure required is one of frequency, not duration, momentary time-sampling will not be superior (Repp *et al.* 1976; Powell and Rockinson 1978). Similarly, if response duration is much longer than interval length, then the errors made by interval recording will be negligible (Murphy and Goodall 1980). Finally, it may be that the coding of behaviour viewed only momentarily may be difficult and in this situation it might be advisable to employ either a continuous method (see above) or, if response durations are very long, an interval method.

Descriptive recording has been used occasionally in combination with an interval recording technique (see, for example, Tizard *et al.* 1972, who recorded the first sample of staff speech verbatim in their study of nursery environments). It is more usual, though, to rely entirely on coding categories of predefined behaviour.

An interesting example of the use of an interval method can be found in a study of the comparative effects of behavioural and drug treatments of hyperactivity, by Rapport *et al.* (1982). Two boys, of seven and eight years of age, were both studied. Both had IQs in the normal range and were diagnosed as hyperactive (on the DSM III, the American Classificatory Scheme for Psychiatric disorders).

Each boy received either methylphenidate or a token programme (with points awarded for appropriate behaviour and subtracted for off-task behaviour). The treatments were applied in a reversal design: Baseline assessment phases (A) alternated with drug treatment phases (B) and behavioural treatment phases (C), in a ABACBC design (allowing sufficient time for the drug to wash-out after B phases). Direct observations were made twice a morning, for 20-minute periods and records were made of whether the boys were on task or not in every interval (80 × 10 s intervals). Other measures of behaviour were also taken, including teacher's ratings (on the Connors Scale) and percentage of assignment problems correct.

Figure 8.8 shows the direct observation results for one boy. The other boy's results were similar. Direct observation data indicated that response cost was more effective than methylphenidate (even at the highest dose used) for both boys. Other measures showed identical findings.

Other examples of interval recording can be found in numerous behavioural studies in the *Journal of Applied Behavior Analysis* and many other journals (see, for example, Romanczyk, Diament, Goren, Trunell and Harris 1975, an investigation of social and

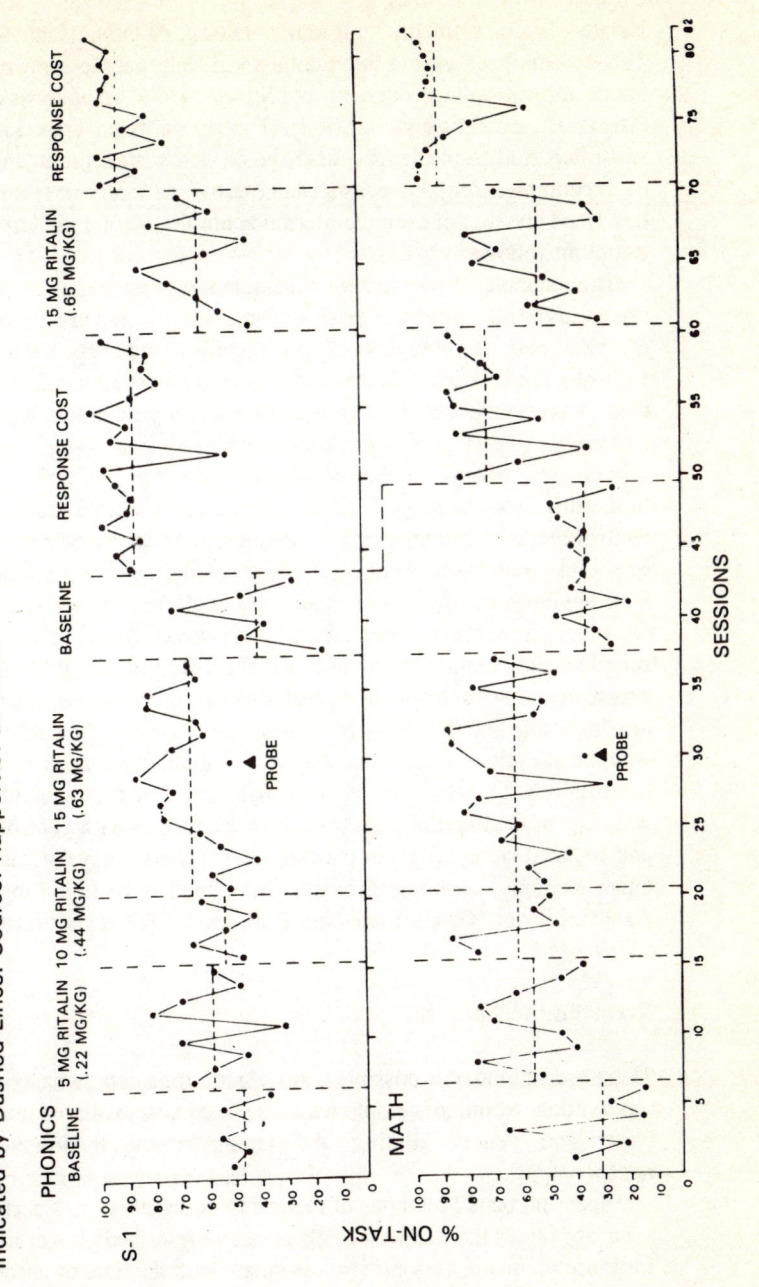

Figure 8.8: Mean Percentage of Intervals of Daily On-task Behaviour for Brian. The Means for Each Condition are Indicated by Dashed Lines. Source: Rapport *et al.* 1982

isolate play in disturbed children; Kleitsch, Whitman and Santos 1983, a study of verbal interaction in elderly people with mental handicap; Marholin, Touchette and Stewart 1979, an analysis of the effects of medication withdrawal). The results from these interval recording studies must, of course, be treated with caution, in view of recent research on measurement error in interval recording, described above. An example of a study employing momentary-time sampling follows:

The example of momentary time-sampling will be taken from a recent investigation of the effects of specially designed toys on the toy-play and stereotypies of profoundly handicapped children (Murphy *et al.* 1986). Children were presented with a single toy and their stereotyped behaviour, toy contact and toy manipulation were recorded in brief sessions, using momentary time-sampling (1 s observe, 9 s record), on the record sheet shown in Figure 8.7. Each of the three toys was available in both an experimental mode and a control mode. Experimental toys delivered stimuli (vibration, light or sound) contingent on interaction, while the control toys did not have any built-in stimulus feedback, although they were identical in all other respects to the experimental toys. Momentary time-sampling data demonstrated that, for the group of 20 children, the experimental toys resulted in significantly more toy contact and manipulation and fewer stereotypies, particularly when vibration was the stimulus in question. Figure 8.9 gives the data for one of the children, D, who showed very high levels of toy manipulation with two of the experimental toys, low toy contact with control toys and reduced stereotypies in parallel with increased toy interaction. Other examples of momentary time-sampling can be found in Hall, Axelrod, Tyler, Grief, Jones and Robertson 1972 (experiment I).

Recording techniques

There are a number of possible ways of recording data, whatever the observation technique employed. The methods available include paper and pencil, filming and taping, event recorders and microcomputers.

Paper and pencil methods of recording observations are perfectly adequate for all the methods of observation described above, except for those requiring very precise information on the time of onset and cessation of behaviour. Some paper and pencil methods will, of course, require some additional equipment, such as audio tapes for

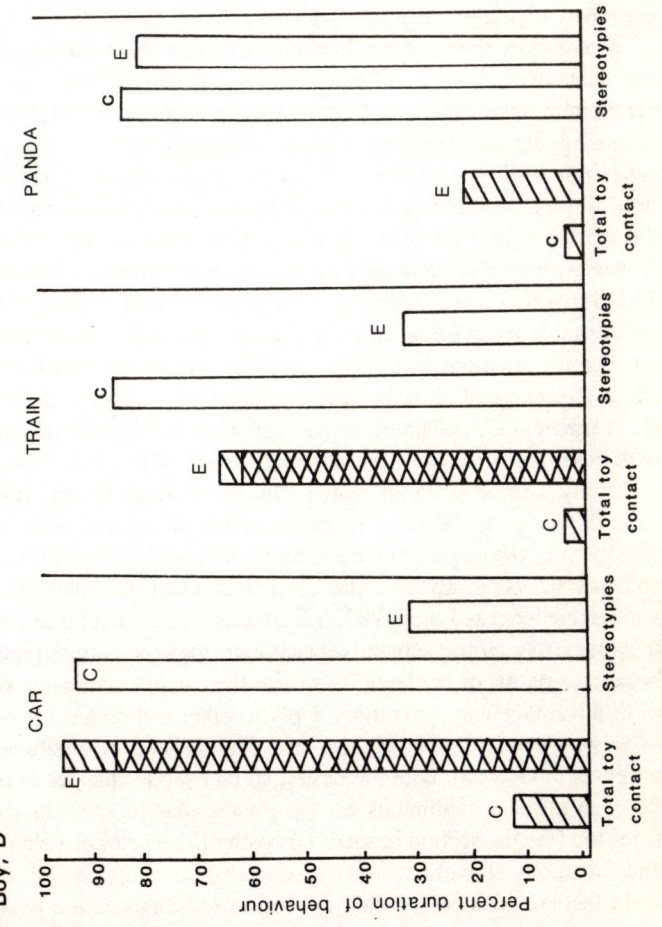

Figure 8.9: Percentage Duration of Toy Contact and Stereotypies with Experimental (E) Toys and Control (C) Toys in a Boy, D

Source: Murphy *et al.* 1986.

cuing intervals or moments to be observed in discontinuous methods of observation, or cumulative stop-watches for simple measures of the total duration of behaviour.

When accurate information is required on the exact timing of series of behaviours, the simplest piece of equipment is a mechanical event recorder, such as the four-channel Rustrak recorder. Essentially, with event recorders, when the target behaviour occurs, the observer is required to depress a key, release of the key occurring when the behaviour ceases. An example of the resultant record is shown in Figure 8.10 (from Murphy and Goodall 1980). The provision of several channels on event recorders means that it is possible to record several behaviours for a single individual or a single type of behaviour for several individuals, something which would be extremely difficult using stop-watches.

Where more than a few behaviours are to be observed, recording can become extremely difficult. This is particularly the case with continuous observation techniques where no time is allocated for recording the observations, so that observers may miss ongoing behaviour while they are in the process of recording. In this situation, filming or video taping may appear to be a perfect solution to the problem in that slowing and repeat viewing are possible. However, the subsequent data analysis may be extremely laborious. Thus Kalverboer, for example, in an extensive study of the relation between minor neurological problems and children's behaviour in a number of situations, took less than 30 minutes of film for each child. Decoding the film, however, took twelve hours for each child (Kalverboer 1975). Patterson has reported similar disadvantages with audio-taped records (Patterson 1982, p. 45).

It may also be difficult, when filming or video taping, for the camera always to be directed to the areas of interest sufficiently rapidly, e.g. the target person suddenly runs out of the camera sight and hits someone. Even if the camera is adequately sited with a wide-angle lens (as Jones 1983, has advised), there will be situations in which the target subject's behaviour may be uninterpretable because, say, his or her back is towards the camera. The same kinds of disadvantage can, of course, apply to other techniques too, such as viewing though a one-way screen. The alternative, of sitting the observer in the room with the target, so that subtle changes of position can allow a continuous adequate view, has its own disadvantages too (see the section headed 'Choosing Categories of Behaviour and Situations above).

In theory, all kinds of data extraction and analysis are possible

Figure 8.10: Example of a Record from a Mechanical Event Recorder

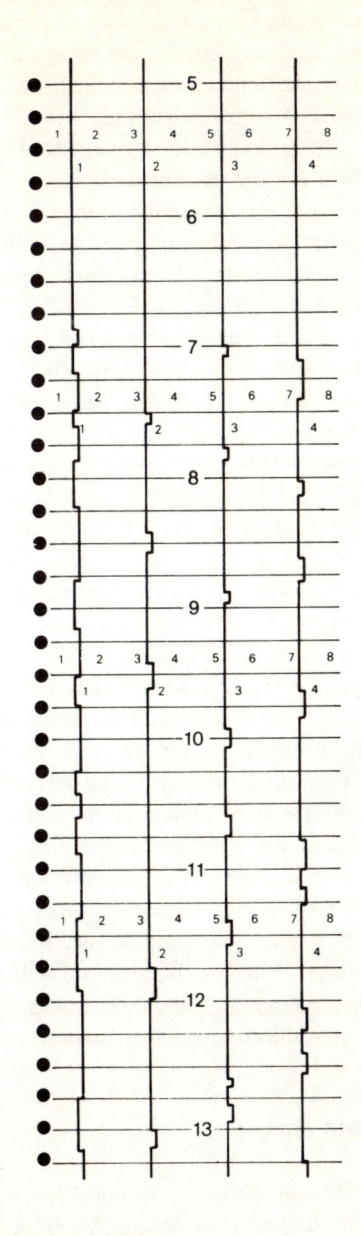

Source: Murphy and Goodall 1980.

from filmed or video-taped sessions. In practice, though, unless there is sufficient time for repeated and lengthy data extraction, most clinicians will use filming or video taping as an initial stage in direct observation. Thus, deciding on the categories of behaviour to be coded and testing out different observational methods on filmed or video-taped samples of target behaviour is probably sufficient for most observers. More rapid and direct methods of data collection are normally necesssary for the main study.

The most recent addition to the list of data recording techniques is the microcomputer. A number of possible devices and programmes are now available, some of which are relatively cheap and portable (see Sackett, Stevenson and Ruppenthal 1973; Stephenson and Roberts 1977; Poole, Sanson-Fisher and Lowe 1982; Browne, Baker and Madeley 1984; Felce *et al.* (in press) for examples). In general the devices have a real-time base and the observer is required to press a predetermined key (or several keys) to indicate the onset of a behaviour. In some cases, cessation of behaviour is also keyed in (e.g. Felce *et al.* (in press)), while in some other cases behavioural categories are designed to be mutually exclusive, so that only onset is required (e.g. Browne *et al.* 1984). One of the advantages of these kinds of devices is that once the position of keys on the keyboard is learnt, observers may concentrate entirely on ongoing behaviour, without looking away for recording purposes. Moreover, some or all of the data analysis can be completed automatically and may be available immediately after the observation sesssion. An example of output from the portable HX-20 computer, using Felce's 'Behaviour' program is shown in Figure 8.11. Identifying information is put in at the beginning of the observation. At the end of the observation there is a print-out option (shown here) which will give identifying information, then a list of the behaviours which occurred with durations as appropriate (keys with no finishing time were here programmed to be 'event' keys for very brief behaviours). Finally, the program will produce a list of behaviours (by key name) with their frequency, rate per minute, duration and per cent duration for that session.

Techniques of data analysis

The simplest possible measures of the amount of behaviour occurring during a set period of time are the number of occasions on which it was observed to occur and the total period of time over

Figure 8.11: Example of an Output from the Portable Computer Used by Felce *et al.* (in press)

Date	:	2.04.85		Beh	Freq	RPM	Dur	%T
Client ID	:	X						
Serial No	:	05		1	0	0.0	0	0
Observer	:	GM		2	0	0.0	0	0
Ending Time	:	32		3	0	0.0	0	0
Tape Date	:	24.04.85		4	0	0.0	0	0
Location	:	HLH		5	0	0.0	0	0
Session No	:	09		6	0	0.0	0	0
Observer No	:	2		7	0	0.0	0	0
				8	0	0.0	0	0
				9	0	0.0	0	0
Beh	Start	Finish	Dur	0	0	0.0	0	0
				-	0	0.0	0	0
M	1	3	2	Q	0	0.0	0	0
N	4	11	7	W	0	0.0	0	0
J	5	12	7	E	0	0.0	0	0
G	5	16	11	R	0	0.0	0	0
B	5	11	6	T	6	11.3		
V	6	9	3	Y	2	3.8	15	47
Y	6	19	13	U	9	16.9		
T	7			I	1	1.9	5	16
T	8			O	0	0.0	0	0
H	8			P	0	0.0	0	0
H	13			@	0	0.0	0	0
H	13			A	0	0.0	0	0
U	14			S	0	0.0	0	0
U	14			D	0	0.0	0	0
N	15	17	2	F	0	0.0	0	0
T	16			G	2	3.8	13	41
H	16			H	8	15.0		
U	17			J	2	3.8	10	31
T	19			K	2	3.8	6	19
U	19			L	0	0.0	0	0
U	19			;	0	0.0	0	0
U	20			:	0	0.0	0	0
U	20			Z	0	0.0	0	0
J	20	23	3	X	0	0.0	0	0
K	21	23	2	C	0	0.0	0	0
I	21	26	5	V	1	1.9	3	9
H	22			B	1	1.9	6	19
H	22			N	2	3.8	9	28
H	22			M	1	1.9	2	6
H	22			,	0	0.0	0	0
T	24			.	0	0.0	0	0
T	24			/	0	0.0	0	0
U	25			\	0	0.0	0	0
U	25							
Y	25	27	2					
G	25	27	2					
K	26	30	4					

which it was observed to be occurring. These are precisely the data which event and duration recording provide, respectively. Since observation periods vary in length, it is usual to convert these measures to frequency (events per unit time) or percentage duration (percentage of the total session during which the behaviour occurred), by dividing by session length. Of course, not all observation methods lend themselves to both kinds of analysis, e.g. event recording cannot produce a duration measure. Moreover, certain behaviours are better described in frequency than in per cent duration terms, or vice versa, i.e. only brief behaviours are suitable for frequency measures.

At times, it may also be necessary to measure other facets of behaviour, such as bout length or the interval between bouts. This kind of information is only provided by continuous observation methods of the more sophisticated type. In addition, observers may sometimes wish to know about the order in which behaviours occurred, so that some form of sequential analysis will be necessary. At times, sequential analysis of observational data can be prohibitively complicated (Macoby and Martin 1983). However, it is possible to answer very specific questions in a relatively simple manner, as the example below demonstrates.

Edelson, Taubman and Lovaas (1983) were interested in the effect of three types of staff behaviour on the appearance of self-injurious behaviour in children who were handicapped. They therefore recorded four categories of behaviour, i.e. staff provision of a demand, a denial, or a verbal punishment, and client self-injury (SIB), over one-hour-long observation sessions. Recorded data were then examined and counts were made of the number of self-injurious responses made in the two minutes preceding and following each of the above staff behaviours. The resulting graph, shown in Figure 8.12, illustrates the effect of the staff antecedents on the appearance of the children's SIB: immediately following demands, denials and verbal punishments the SIB increased rapidly, gradually decreasing over the next two minutes.

This example shows that simple analyses of the sequences of behaviour are possible without major technical innovation. Edelson *et al.* actually obtained their data, perhaps unwisely (since some omissions must have occurred), by using a discontinuous method of observation (see above). Mostly, however, observers engaged in sequential analysis employ continuous methods of observation, either event-based (as in Patterson 1982; Dowdney *et al.* 1984) or time-based (as in Felce *et al.* (in press)), the latter really only being

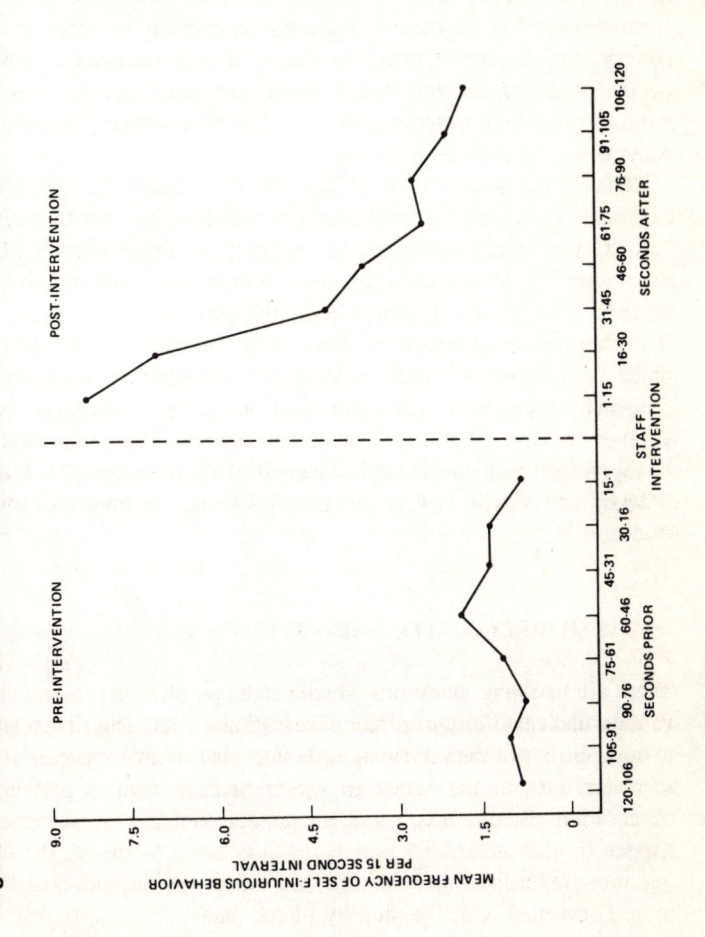

Figure 8.12: Mean Number of Self-destructive Acts for Each 15-second Interval Before and After Staff Intervention

Source: Edelson *et al.* 1983.

possible with the aid of microcomputers if more than a few behaviours are to be coded.

Bakeman (1978) has commented that observational data on more than one individual can be classified as 'concurrent' or 'sequential' in type. In the former case several behaviours can occur together (as in the Felce *et al.* (in press) study) whereas in the latter only one behaviour is coded at a time (e.g. Browne *et al.* 1984). The analysis of streams of behaviour is, of course, much simpler for sequential than for concurrent data. However, certain kinds of behaviour appear to be particularly well suited to certain classes of data, so that, for example, the reciprocal turn-taking of mother-child interactions falls easily into a sequential (as opposed to a concurrent) pattern. On the other hand, for many of the situations in which people who are severely handicapped are observed, there is no natural turn-taking in interactions, so that the concurrent pattern of data collection may be necessary.

Most commonly, the final results of sequential analysis are expressed in terms of conditional probabilities, i.e. the likelihood that, if the target individual is engaged in Behaviour X, then behaviour Y is also occurring (concurrent pattern, with a zero lag) or behaviour Z will follow (sequential pattern, with a lag). As Bakeman had described, these kinds of probabilities can be used to build up pictures of total patterns of behaviour or to describe sequences or chains of behaviour. For the most part, the techniques are more complex than the clinician will require. Those who require further information can consult Bakeman (1978), Sackett (1978) and Macoby and Martin (1983) for descriptions and examples of other studies.

ISSUES OF RELIABILITY AND VALIDITY

There are two main questions which can be posed with regard to the validity and reliability of direct observational data. The first relates to the accuracy of the information: Is that what really happened? The second relates to the extent to which findings from a particular observation session, or sessions, are generalisable; Does that always happen (in that situation)? In general, it is easier to answer the first question, regarding observer accuracy, than the second, which is more concerned with the validity of the data.

Observer accuracy

One way of measuring an observer's accuracy is by comparing his or her direct observational record with a 'criterion' record (i.e. a record known to be accurate) for the same observation session. Such records involve the assumption that there is a 'true' record which can in principle be observed and recorded. Some psychologists would dispute that this is the case (Wiggins 1973, p. 278). Criterion records are either made by the automatic means (such as automatic event recorders) or by filming observation periods, recording from film and checking back repeatedly to ensure that the records are accurate. Alternatively, observer's records can be compared to a second observer's records, thus allowing calculation of inter-observer reliability levels (see below). Clearly observers may make identical errors at times and consequently perfect inter-observer agreement does not guarantee perfect accuracy of observation and recording. However, as the production of a criterion record for every session of direct observation is impractical (and would obviate the need for human observers), it is usual in research and clinical work to keep track of observer accuracy by examining inter-observer reliability levels, taking steps where possible to reduce the likelihood to two observers making identical errors (see below).

Various different indices of inter-observer reliability exist and one of the areas of recent discussion has been the range of reliability levels that different indices give from the same sets of data. There is some controversy, too, over whether the simplest statistics, like per cent agreement, are preferable to the more complex, such as K or Kappa (Baer 1977). Here we shall consider the most useful measures of each type and provide some guidelines for those who need to consider their levels of observer reliability. For more detailed information on the indices available, readers may wish to consult: Wiggins (1973); Hawkins and Dotson (1975); Baer (1977); Hartmann (1977 and 1984); Hopkins and Hermann (1977); Maxwell (1977); Yelton, Wildman and Erickson (1977); Harris and Lahey (1978); Hollenbeck (1978).

The simplest measures of inter-observer reliability are the percentage agreement indices. For discontinuous observational methods (interval recording and momentary time-sampling), the all-interval agreement or total reliability level, R tot, is given by:

$$R\% = \frac{\text{number of intervals observers agreed on}}{\text{total number of intervals}} \times 100$$

Full agreement between observers would produce a figure of 100 per cent, complete disagreement a figure of 0 per cent.

It has been consistently demonstrated, however, that the all-interval agreement can be high (i.e. 70 per cent and over), even when observers are not fully alert, not agreed on the definition of the behaviour to be recorded, and observing rather different events (Bijou, Peterson and Ault 1968; Hawkins and Dotson 1975). The reason for this is that observers may agree simply by chance. The likelihood of chance agreement is highest when the behaviour to be observed is extremely rare (resulting in many possible chance agreements on nonoccurrence) or extremely common (resulting in many possible chance agreements on occurrence). Consequently, it is now accepted that, for low frequency behaviours, a 'scored-interval' or 'occurrence reliability' should be calculated, R occ:

$$R\,occ\% = \frac{\text{number of intervals observers agreed behaviour occurred}}{\text{number of intervals either observer scored behaviour occurred}} \times 100$$

Similarly, for the high frequency behaviours an 'unscored-interval' or 'nonoccurrence reliability' should be calculated, R nonocc:

$$R\,nonocc\% = \frac{\text{number of intervals observers agreed behaviour absent}}{\text{number of intervals either observer scored behaviour absent}} \times 100$$

These indices provide measures of whether observers agree that a behaviour occurred (R occ) or did not occur (R nonocc) and are more sensitive to observer errors and disagreements than the simple R tot measure.

For those who wish to take account of chance agreements, there are numerous formulae available (Hartmann 1977; Hopkins and Hermann 1977; Yelton *et al.* 1977). Probably one of the best known is Cohen's kappa:

$$K = \frac{P_o - P_c}{1 - P_c}$$

where $P_o = \dfrac{B + C}{N}$ $P_c = \dfrac{(A + B)(B + D)}{N^2} + \dfrac{(A + C)(C + D)}{N^2}$

and A, B, C, D are given in the table below. N is the total number of intervals.

For those working with continuous observational records, where data are not conveniently divided into intervals, there are a number of rather similar possible indices. The simplest measure is the ratio measure:

		Observer 1	
		Behav. absent	Behav. present
Observer 2	Behav. present	A	B
	Behav. absent	C	D

$$R = \frac{\text{amount of behaviour observer A records}}{\text{amount of behaviour observer B records}}$$

where 'amount' of behaviour could be the total duration of the behaviour or the number of events recorded. Total agreement would produce a figure of 1.00 and disagreement a figure of 0.00.

When continuous observations are made on a real-time base, then the equivalent indices to R occ and R nonocc may be calculated. For example, the equivalent to R occ would be:

$$R\% = \frac{\text{amount of behaviour (secs) observers agreed occurred}}{\text{total amount seen by either observer (secs)}} \times 100$$

Some observers use rather more stringent methods of calculating reliability for continuous observational data, for example, of only counting an agreement on occurrence if observers differ by less than five seconds on its time of starting (Felce *et al.* (in press)).

Finally, it is important to note that the methods of calculating reliability, described above, confound systematic and random errors. It is, of course, important to distinguish the former from the latter, in that large systematic errors might reflect a disagreement between observers on the definition of a behaviour, one observer perhaps consistently overestimating levels compared to the other. Maxwell (1977) has therefore suggested excluding systematic error altogether and calculating a random error coefficient. A simpler method, however, is for observers to compare the total amount of behaviour each coded over the sessions they observed together. A consistent over-estimation by one observer should then be obvious.

Research into factors affecting observer accuracy has indicated that one of the most important characteristics of observers is that their reliability tends to drop if they are not being overtly checked (Reid 1970; Taplin and Reid 1973; Romanczyk, Kent, Diament and O'Leary 1973; Kent, Kanowitz, O'Leary and Cheiken 1977). With extended practice, pairs of observers can learn to achieve high agreement levels but some of this agreement may be achieved spuriously by observers 'drifting' together, away from the original behavioural definitions (Romanczyk *et al.* 1973). Moreover, observer accuracy levels can be adversely affected by experimenters providing expectations about the behaviour they predict will be seen and/or positive feedback for certain kinds of data (O'Leary, Kent and Kanowitz 1975). The combined effects of these various factors on observer reliability levels are major rather than minor (Kent *et al.* 1977), so that those involved in clinical work as well as those involved in research need to know how to avoid the possible pitfalls.

Ideally, observers should be given clear, concretely defined categories of behaviour, not so numerous that very lengthy training is required, they should work in pairs throughout the experiment to keep observer accuracy up to the 'overt check' level but no two observers should be allowed to work together for long to avoid observer drift. Nor should they always observe the same individuals to reduce the effects of expectation on data gathering. Preferably also, observers should not know who is checking their records to avoid the 'identified assessor' effect.

Such ideal conditions, though, would require considerable resources. At the very least, one-way screen facilities would be necessary and a large pool of observers. Where such ideal conditions cannot be met, the most important factors to be guarded against are those which produce systematic errors in the direction of the experimental hypotheses (Rosenthal and Rosnow 1969). These can be eliminated by keeping observers *un*informed about the direction in which the behaviour is expected to change and ensuring that observers are not given positive encouragement for producing particular kinds of data. If these conditions can be met, then the remaining errors, when they do occur, will be as likely to be in the direction of the experimental hypothesis as in the opposite direction. They will therefore contribute to the data variability but should not increase the likelihood of demonstrating, for example, spuriously positive treatment effects.

Validity and generalisability

The information provided by direct observation techniques is normally very different from that which results from standardised psychometric assessments, so that the two techniques complement one another. Some of the kinds of information which direct observations elicit, however, may also be derived from techniques such as rating scales, questionnaires and interviews. Indeed some studies combine both techniques (for example, the child management schedule of King, Raynes and Tizard 1971). It is therefore important to ask how valid direct observation techniques are and whether the alternative methods of discovering levels of behaviour are superior to those of direct observation.

It is arguable that even information on levels of behaviour derived from interviews, questionnaires and rating scales is dependent originally on direct observation. The difference is, of course, that in the former case the direct observations are made by staff (or parents) in an unplanned way, without written records and are often elicited 'second hand' by the interviewer, whereas, in the latter case, the observations are planned, structured and immediately recorded, without submitting them to the vicissitudes of human memory. It would not be suprising then, if direct observation techniques produced more accurate records of real events than the more indirect methods. Moreover, one would predict that the information elicited in interviews or on questionnaires or rating scales would be likely to be relatively unreliable across different informants, as indeed it often is (Wing and Gould 1978; Bernsen 1980; Holmes, Shah and Wing 1982; Patterson 1982; Rojahn 1984; Oliver, Corbett and Murphy (no date).

On the other hand, it has been argued that, although direct observation methods produce data which accurately reflect the events during the observation sessions (given little or no observer effects — the section headed 'Choosing Categories of Behaviour and Situation' — and adequate observer accuracy, see above) the data are not generalisable to other periods of the day, other days or other environments. This, of course, may be quite true and it is therefore important, as Cronbach, Rajaratnam and Gleser (1963) and Wiggins (1973) have argued, for those planning observations and interpreting direct observational data, to be clear what generalisations they wish to make. Thus, if in a treatment study, the goal is a general reduction in someone's tantrums, then it will be important to record tantrum behaviour in all environments, for example, in various activities at home and at school. If, on the other hand, the goal is simply to reduce tantrums during gym classes at school, then observations could be limited to that situation alone.

The degree to which levels of behaviour observed in one situation or condition can be generalised to that in another can be calculated precisely and is a function of variance across situations (Cronbach *et al.* 1963; Wiggins 1973). A similar method can be employed to examine the extent to which one observer's data are generalisable, using an analysis of variance model. Those who are interested in generalisability theory may refer to Cronbach *et al.* (1963) and Wiggins (1973). The method does have some advantages over the simpler approaches recommended here. However, as others have argued, the more sophisticated the measure, the less easily interpretable it is (Baer 1977). Certainly, for those not involved in research, the more straightforward methods are much preferable.

SUMMARY

Direct observation techniques are often the most appropriate method of assessment to adopt when the information required concerns levels of behaviour in various settings. Most commonly the techniques are employed to provide measures of effectiveness in treatment interventions. However, they are also useful before treatment begins in functional analysis and at other times, such as when measures of quality of care are at issue. These various purposes of direct observation were reviewed, with examples from published literature.

The problems of deciding which behaviours to observe, for how long and in what settings were discussed, prior to describing the two main methods available for making observations (continuous and discontinuous methods). Techniques for recording and analysing data were given, including simple sequential analysis.

Finally, the topic of observer reliability was discussed and simple measures provided for the calculation of reliability levels. The validity of direct observation data was considered, particularly within the context of the generalisability of findings from direct observation sessions.

ACKNOWLEDGEMENTS

I am most grateful to Dr Jackie McGuire of Great Ormond Street Hospital, Dr Janet Carr of St Georges Hospital and the editors of this book for their helpful comments on an earlier version of this chapter.

REFERENCES

Altman, J. (1974) 'Observational Study of Behavior: Sampling Methods', *Behavior, 49,* 227–65

Ando, H. and Yoshimura, I. (1979) 'Speech Skill Levels and Prevalence of Maladaptive Behaviors in Autistic and Mentally Retarded Children: A Statistical Study', *Child Psychiatry and Human Development, 10,* 85–90

Baer, D.M. (1977) 'Reviewer's Comment: Just Because It's Reliable Doesn't Mean You Can Use It', *Journal of Applied Behavior Analysis, 10,* 117–19

Bakeman, R. (1978) 'Untangling Streams of Behavior: Sequential Analyses of Observation Data' in G.P. Sackett (ed.), *Observing Behavior. Vol. II: Data Collection and Analysis Methods,* University Park Press, Baltimore

Barlow, D.H. and Hersen, M. (1984) *Single Case Experimental Designs: Strategies for Studying Behaviour Change,* Pergamon Press, Oxford and New York

Bernsen, A.H. (1980) 'An Interview Technique in Assessing Retarded Children', *Journal of Mental Deficiency Research, 24,* 167–79

Bijou, S.W., Peterson, R.F. and Ault, M.H. (1968) 'A Method to Integrate Descriptive and Experimental Field Studies at the Level of Data and Empirical Concepts', *Journal of Applied Behavior Analysis, 1,* 175–91

Browne, K., Baker, P. and Madeley, R. (1984) 'The Use of a Portable Microcomputer to Study Behavior', *Annals of Human Biology, 11,* No. 5

Carr, E.G., Newsom, C.D. and Binkoff, J.A. (1976) 'Stimulus Control of Self-destructive Behavior in a Psychotic Child', *Journal of Abnormal Child Psychology, 4,* 139–53

Cronbach, L.J., Rajaratnam, N. and Gleser, G.C. (1963) 'Theory of Generalizability: A Liberalization of Reliability Theory', *British Journal of Statistical Psychology, 16,* 137–63

Dowdney, L., Mrazek, D., Quinton, D. and Rutter, M. (1984) 'Observation of Parent-Child Interaction with Two to Three Year Olds', *Journal of Child Psychology and Psychiatry, 25,* 379–408

Edelson, S.M., Taubman, M.T. and Lovaas, O.I. (1983) 'Some Social Contexts of Self-destructive Behavior', *Journal of Abnormal Child Psychology, 11,* 299–312

Favell, J.E., McGimsey, J.F., Jones, M.L. and Connon, P.R. (1981) 'Physical Restraint as Positive Reinforcement', *American Journal of Mental Deficiency, 85,* 425–32

Felce, D., de Kock, U. and Repp, A. (in press) 'An Ecological Comparison of Small Community-based Houses and Traditional Large Hospitals for Severely and Profoundly Mentally Handicapped Adults: The Provision of Opportunities for Staff and Client Engagement in Activity', *Applied Research in Mental Retardation* (in press)

Gould, J. (1976) 'Language Development and Non-verbal Skills in Severely Mentally Retarded Children: An Epidemiological Study', *Journal of Mental Deficiency Research, 20,* 129–46

Green, S.B. and Alverson, L.G. (1978) 'A Comparison of Indirect Measures for Long Duration Behaviors', *Journal of Applied Behavior Analysis, 11,* 530

Grimm, J.A., Parsons, J.A. and Bijou, S.W. (1972) 'A Technique for

Minimising Subject-Observer Looking Interactions in a Field Setting', *Journal of Experimental Child Psychology*, 14, 500–5

Hall, R.V., Axelrod, S., Tyler, L., Grief, E., Jones, F.C. and Robertson, R. (1972) 'Modification of Behavior Problems in the Home with a Parent as Observer and Experimenter', *Journal of Applied Behavior Analysis*, 5, 53–64

Harris, F.C. and Lahey, B.B. (1978) 'A Method for Combining Occurrence and Non-occurrence Agreement Scores', *Journal of Applied Behavior Analysis*, 11, 523–27

Harris, S.L. and Wolchik, S.A. (1979) 'Suppression of Self-stimulation: Three Alternative Strategies', *Journal of Applied Behavior Analysis*, 12, 185–98

Hartmann, D.P. (1977) 'Considerations in the Choice of Interobserver Reliability Estimates', *Journal of Applied Behavior Analysis*, 10, 103–16

Hartmann, D.P. (1984) 'Assessment Strategies' in D.H. Barlow and M. Hersen, (eds.), *Single Case Experimental Designs: Strategies for Studying Behaviour Change*, 2nd edn, Pergamon Press, Oxford and New York

Hawkins, R.P. and Dotson, V.A. (1975) 'Reliability Scores that Delude: An Alice in Wonderland Trip through the Misleading Characteristics of Interobserver Agreement Scores in Interval Recording' in E. Ramp and G. Semb (eds.), *Behavior Analysis: Areas of Research and Application*, Prentice Hall, Englewood Cliffs, New Jersey

Hersen, M. and Barlow, D.H. (1976) *Single Case Experimental Designs: Strategies for Studying Behaviour Change*, Pergamon Press, Oxford and New York

Hollenbeck, A.R. (1978) 'Problems of Reliability in Observational Research' in G.P. Sackett (ed.), *Observing Behavior. Vol. I: Data Collection and Analysis Methods*, University Park Press, Baltimore

Holmes, N., Shah, A. and Wing L. (1982) 'The Disability Assessment Schedule: A Brief Screening Device for Use with the Mentally Retarded', *Psychological Medicine*, 12, 879–90

Hopkins, B.L. and Hermann, J.A. (1977) 'Evaluating Interobserver Reliability of Interval Data', *Journal of Applied Behavior Analysis*, 10, 121–6

Hurlbut, B.I., Iwata, B.A. and Green, J.D. (1982) 'Non-vocal Language Acquisition in Adolescents with Severe Physical Disabilities: Blissymbol versus Iconic Stimulus Formats', *Journal of Applied Behavior Analysis*, 15, 241–58

Hutt, S.J. and Hutt, C. (1964) 'Hyperactivity in a Group of Epileptic (and some non-epileptic) Brain-damaged Children', *Epilepsia*, 5, 334–51

——— (1970) *Direct Observation and Measurement of Behaviour*, C.C. Thomas, Springfield, Illinois

Iwata, B.A., Dorsey, M.F., Slifer, K.J., Bauman, K.E. and Richman, G.S. (1982) 'Toward a Functional Analysis of Self-injury', *Analysis and Intervention in Developmental Disabilities*, 2, 3–20

———, Pace, G.M. Cataldo, M.F., Kalsher, M.J. and Edwards, G.L. (1984) 'A Center for the Study and Treatment of Self-Injury' in M.T. Stork, D.E. Williams, B.K. Almeyer, and H.K. Griffiths (eds.), *Advances in the Treatment of Self-Injurious Behavior*, Department of Health and Human Services, Texas Planning Council for Developmental Disabilities, Austin, Texas

Jones, M.C. (1983) *Behaviour Problems in Handicapped Children: The Beech*

Tree House Approach, Souvenir Press, London

Kalverboer, A.F. (1975) *A Neurobehavioural Study in Pre-School Children*, Clinics in Developmental Medicine No. 54, Heinemann, London

Kazdin, A.E. (1975) *Behavior Modification in Applied Settings*, Dorsey Press, Homewood, Illinois

Kelly, M.B. (1977) 'A Review of the Observational Data Collection and Reliability Procedures Reported in the Journal of Applied Behavior Analysis', *Journal of Applied Behavior Analysis*, 10, 97–101

Kent, R.N., Kanowitz, J., O'Leary, K.D. and Cheiken, M. (1977) 'Observer Reliability as a Function of Circumstances of Assessment', *Journal of Applied Behavior Analysis*, 10, 317–24

Kiernan, C. (1973) 'Functional Analysis' in P. Mittler (ed.), *Assessment for Learning in the Mentally Handicapped*, Churchill Livingstone, London

—— (1974) 'Behaviour Modification' in A.M. Clarke and A.D.B. Clarke (eds.), *Mental Deficiency: The Changing Outlook*, Methuen, London

King, R.D., Raynes, N.V. and Tizard, J. (1971) *Patterns of Residential Care: Sociological Studies in Institutions for Handicapped Children*, Routledge, London

Kleitsch, E.C., Whitman, T.L. and Santos, J. (1983) 'Increasing Verbal Interaction among Elderly Socially Isolated Mentally Retarded Adults: A Group Language Training Procedure', *Journal of Applied Behavior Analysis*, 16, 217–33

Landesman-Dwyer, S., Stein, J.G. and Sackett, G.P. (1976) 'Group Homes for the Developmentally Disabled: An Ecological and Behavior Study', *Technical Report*, Department of Social and Health Services, Olympia, Washington

Leitenberg, H. (1973) 'The Use of Single-case Methodology in Psychotherapy Research', *Journal of Abnormal Psychology*, 82, 87–101

Lobitz, W.C. and Johnson, S.M. (1975) 'Parental Manipulation of the Behavior of Normal and Deviant Children', *Child Development*, 46, 719–26

Lovaas, O.I. and Simmons, J.Q. (1969) 'Manipulation of Self-destruction in Three Retarded Children', *Journal of Applied Behavior Analysis*, 2, 143–57

Macoby, E.E. and Martin, J.A. (1983) 'Socialization in the Context of the Family: Parent-Child Interaction' in P.H. Mussen (ed.), *Handbook of Child Psychology*, vol. IV, John Wiley, Chichester and New York

Marholin, D., Touchette, P.E. and Stewart, R.M. (1979) 'Withdrawal of Chronic Chlorpromazine Medication: An Experimental Analysis', *Journal of Applied Behavior Analysis*, 12, 159–71

Maxwell, A.E. (1977) 'Coefficients of Agreement between Observers and their Interpretations', *British Journal of Psychiatry*, 130, 79–83

Melin, L. and Golestam, K.G. (1981) 'The Effects of Rearranging Ward Routines on Communication and Eating Behaviours of Psychogeriatric Patients', *Journal of Applied Behavior Analysis*, 14, 47–51

Morris, R.J. and Dolker, M. (1974) 'Developing Co-operative Play in Socially Withdrawn Retarded Children', *Mental Retardation*, 12, 24–6

Munoz, M. (1978) 'Changes in Ward Environment Related to Changes in Nurses' Behaviour', unpublished M. Phil. thesis, Institute of Psychiatry,

University of London

Murphy, G. (1980) 'Decreasing Undesirable Behaviour' in W. Yule and J. Carr (eds.), *Behaviour Modification for the Mentally Handicapped*, Croom Helm, London

——, Callias, M., and Carr, J. (1985) 'Increasing Toy Play in Profoundly Handicapped Children: I. Training to Play', *Journal of Autism and Developmental Disorders*, 15, 375–84

——, Carr, J. and Callias, M. (1986) 'Increasing Toy Play in Profoundly Handicapped Children: II Special Toys', *Journal of Autism and Developmental Disorders*, 16, 45–58

—— and Goodall, E. (1980) 'Measurement Error in Direct Observations: A Comparison of Common Recording Methods', *Behaviour Research and Therapy*, 18, 147–50

O'Leary, K.D., Kent, R.N. and Kanowitz, J. (1975) 'Shaping Data Collection Congruent with Experimental Hypotheses', *Journal of Applied Behavior Analysis*, 8, 43–51

Oliver, C., Corbett, J. and Murphy, G. (no date) 'Self-injurious Behaviour in People with Mental Handicap: A Total Population Survey', submitted to *Developmental Medicine and Child Psychology*

Patterson, G.R. (1982) 'Observations of Family Process', in *A Social Learning Approach to Family Intervention, vol. 3: Coercive Family Process*, Castalia Publishing Company, Oregon

Poole, A.D., Sanson-Fisher, R.W. and Lowe, I. (1982) 'An Electronic System for Recording Ongoing Behaviour in Real Time', *Behavioural Psychotherapy*, 10, 42–7

Powell, J., Martindale, A. and Kulp, S. (1975) 'An Evaluation of Time-sample Measures of Behavior', *Journal of Applied Behavior Analysis*, 8, 463–9

——, Martindale, B., Kulp, S., Martindale, A. and Bauman, R. (1977) 'Taking a Closer Look: Time-sampling and Measurement Error', *Journal of Applied Behavior Analysis*, 10, 325–32

—— and Rockinson, R. (1978) 'On the Inability of Interval Time-sampling to Reflect Frequency of Occurrence Data', *Journal of Applied Behavior Analysis*, 11, 531–2

Premack, D. (1959) 'Towards Empirical Behavior Laws: 1. Positive Reinforcement', *Psychological Review*, 66, 219–33

Rapport, M.D., Murphy, H.A. and Bailey, J.S. (1982) 'Ritalin vs. Response Cost in the Control of Hyperactive Children: A Within-subject Comparison', *Journal of Applied Behavior Analysis*, 15, 206–16

Raynes, N.V., Pratt, M.V. and Roses, S. (1979) *Organisational Structure and the Care of the Mentally Retarded*, Croom Helm, London/Praeger, New York

Reid, J.B. (1970) 'Reliability Assessment of Observational Data: A Possible Methodological Problem', *Child Development*, 41, 1143–50

—— (1978) *A Social Learning Approach to Family Intervention: Vol. 2: Observations in the Home Setting*, Castalia Publishing Company, Oregon

——, Taplin, P.S. and Lorber, R. (1981) 'A Social Interactional Approach to the Treatment of Abusive Families' in R. Stuart (ed.), *Violent Behavior: Social Learning Approaches to Prediction, Management and Treatment*, Bruner Mazel, New York

Repp, A.C., Roberts, D.M., Slack, D.J., Repp, C.R. and Berkler, M.S.

(1976) 'A Comparison of Frequency, Interval and Time-sampling Methods of Data Collection', *Journal of Applied Behavior Analysis, 9,* 501–8

Richman, N., Stevenson, J. and Graham, P.J. (1982) *Pre-school to School: A Behavioural Study,* Academic Press, New York and London

Rincover, A. and Devany, J. (1982) 'The Application of Sensory Extinction Procedures to Self-injury', *Analysis and Intervention in Developmental Disabilities, 2,* 67–81

Rojahn, J. (1984) 'Self-Injurious Behavior in Institutionalized, Severely Profoundly Retarded Adults — Prevalence Data and Staff Agreement', *Journal of Behavioral Assessment, 6, (1),* 13–27

——, Mulick, J.A., McCoy, D. and Schroeder, S.R. (1978) 'Setting Effects, Adaptive Clothing and the Modification of Head-banging and Self-restraint in Two Profoundly Retarded Adults', *Behavior Analysis and Modification, 2,* 185–96

Romanczyk, R.G., Diament, C., Goren, E.R., Trunell, G. and Harris, S.L. (1975) 'Increasing Social Isolate Play in Severely Disturbed Children: Intervention and Post-intervention Effectiveness', *Journal of Autism and Child Schizophrenia, 5,* 57–70

——, Kent, R.N., Diament, C. and O'Leary, K.D. (1973) 'Measuring the Reliability of Observational Data: A Reactive Process', *Journal of Applied Behavior Analysis, 6,* 175–84

Rosenthal, R. and Rosnow, R.L. (1969) *Artifact in Behavioural Research,* Academic Press, New York

Rusch, F.R. and Kazdin, A.E. (1981) 'Toward a Methodology of Withdrawal Designs for the Assessment of Response Maintenance', *Journal of Applied Behavior Analysis, 14,* 131–40

Russo, D.C., Cataldo, M.F. and Cushing, P.J. (1981) 'Compliance Training and Behavioral Covariation in the Treatment of Multiple Behaviour Problems', *Journal of Applied Behavior Analysis, 14,* 209–22

Sackett, G.P. (1978) 'Measurement in Observational Research' in G.P. Sackett (ed.), *Observing Behavior. Vol. II: Data Collection and Analysis Methods,* University Park Press, Baltimore

——, Stevenson, E. and Ruppenthal, G.G. (1973) 'Digital Acquisition Systems for Observing Behavior in Laboratory and Field Settings', *Behavior Research Methods and Instrumentation, 5,* 334–48

Singh, N.N., Manning, P.J. and Angell, M.J. (1982) 'The Effects of an Oral Hygiene Punishment Procedure on Chronic Rumination and Collateral Behaviors in Monozygous twins', *Journal of Applied Behavior Analysis, 15,* 309–14

Stephenson, G.R. and Roberts, T.W. (1977) 'The SRR System: A Generalized Encoding System with Computerized Transcription', *Behavior Research Methods and Instrumentation, 9,* 434–41

Sylva, K., Roy, C. and Painter, M. (1981) *Childwatching at Playgroup and Nursery School,* McIntyre, London

Swanson, H.L. and Watson, B.L. (1982) 'Behavioral Assessment' in *Educational and Psychological Assessment of Exceptional Children: Theories, Strategies and Applications,* C.V. Mosby, St Louis, Missouri

Taplin, P.S. and Reid, J.B. (1973) 'Effects of Instructional Set and Experimenter Influence on Observer Reliability', *Child Development, 44,* 547–54

Tizard, B., Cooperman, O., Joseph, A. and Tizard, J. (1972) 'Environmental Effects on Language Development: A Study of Young Children in Long-stay Residential Nurseries', *Child Development, 43,* 377–58

———, Philps, J. and Plewis, I. (1976) 'Play in Pre-school Centres: In Play Measures and Their Relation to Age, Sex and IQ', *Journal of Child Psychology and Psychiatry, 17,* 251–64

Weinrott, M.R., Jones, R.R. and Boler, G.R. (1981) 'Convergent and Discriminant Validity of Five Classroom Observation Systems: A Secondary Analysis', *Journal of Educational Psychology, 73,* 671–9

Wiggins, J.S. (1973) *Personality and Prediction: Principles of Personality Assessment,* Addison-Wesley, Massachusetts

Williams, J.A., Koegel, R.L. and Egel, A.L. (1981) 'Response Reinforcer Relationships and Improved Learning in Autistic Children', *Journal of Applied Behavior Analysis, 14,* 53–60

Wing, L. and Gould, J. (1978) 'Systematic Recording of Behaviours and Skills of Retarded and Psychotic Children', *Journal of Autism and Childhood Schizophrenia, 8,* 79–97

Yelton, A.R., Wildman, B.G. and Erickson, M.T. (1977) 'A Probability-based Formula for Calculating Interobserver Agreement', *Journal of Applied Behavior Analysis, 10,* 127–31

Young, J.A. and Wincze, J.P. (1974) 'The Effects of the Reinforcement of Compatible and Incompatible Behaviors on the Self-injurious and Related Behaviours of the Profoundly Retarded Female Adult', *Behaviour Therapy, 5,* 614–23

Yule, W. (1980) 'Evaluation of Treatment Programmes' in W. Yule and J. Carr (eds.), *Behaviour Modification for the Mentally Handicapped,* Croom Helm, London

Appendix

Details of Cited Test Instruments

In order to enable interested readers to follow up some of the tests, batteries and checklists described in this book, we list in this appendix most of those reported in Chapters 3 to 7 of the main text. These appear in alphabetical order. We wish to acknowledge the more detailed protocol that suggested presenting summary information of this sort, i.e. the 'Individualised Data Base (IDB) Project' prepared by the Neuropsychiatric Institute Research Group of the University of California, at Pacific State Hospital, Pomona, California, USA.

The psychometric tests described in Chapter 2 are not included in this appendix and the reader is referred to the standard text by Buros (1978) for full information on many of these, or to the manual accompanying the test material. Doucette and Freedman (1980) is also a useful resource. Chapter 8, of course, is not concerned with specific tests as such and the reader is referred to the original sources cited in the References of that chapter. We do not claim that this Appendix is comprehensive, and indeed for subjects like assessment of the home environment and of the family, a number of other assessment procedures exist which are beyond the scope of this volume.

REFERENCES

Buros, O. (1978) *The Eighth Mental Measurement Yearbook*, Gryphon Press, New York

Doucette, J. and Freedman, R. (1980) *Progress Tests for the Developmentally Disabled: An Evaluation*, Abt Books, Cambridge, MA (available exclusively from Brookline Books, Cambridge, MA)

AAMD — ADAPTIVE BEHAVIOR SCALE, PARTS I AND II

1. *Author(s):* K. Nihira, R. Foster, M. Shellhaas and H. Leland
2. *Date Initially Prepared:* — *Most Recent Revision:* 1974
3. *Distributor/Publisher/Key Source:* American Association on Mental Deficiency, 5201 Connecticut Avenue, N.W., Washington, D.C., 20015
   Source used: *AAMD Adaptive Behavior Scale Public School Version*, 1974 revision by Nadine Lambert, Myra Windmiller, Linda Cole and Richard Figueroa
4. *Availability:*
   Published
5. *Main Uses of the Instrument:*
   Assessment of client
   Planning for individual programmes and programme evaluation
   Research
6. *Chronological Age for which this Instrument is Appropriate:*
   Children to adults
7. *Disability Group for which this Instrument was Intended:*
   People with mental handicap
8. *Predominant Response Format for this Instrument:*
   Binary (e.g. yes/no, true/false)
   Rating (e.g. items are rated on a point scale, such as frequency of occurrence)
   Sequential (e.g. items ordered serially from low to high)
   Variable
9. *Who Completes the Instrument?*
   Parent
   Teacher
   Care-provider
10. *How is the Instrument Administered?*
    Rating scale or checklist completed by third-party informant
11. *Does the Instrument Require Special Training?*
    No
12. *The Standardisation Population Used to Develop and Test this Instrument:*
    Several studies using 900 and 2,000 subjects; both children and adults; varying in Mental Age from severe to mild handicap

ABERRANT BEHAVIOUR CHECKLIST

1. *Author(s):* M.G. Aman, N.N. Singh, A.W. Stewart and C.J. Field
2. *Date Initially Prepared:* 1985 *Most Recent Revision:* —
3. *Distributor/Publisher/Key Source:*
   M.G. Aman, Department of Psychiatry and Behaviour Sciences, University of Auckland, Auckland, New Zealand
4. *Availability:*
   Informally prepared for local use
5. *Main Uses of the Instrument:*
   Assessment of behaviour disturbance
   Research
6. *Chronological Age for which this Instrument is Appropriate:*
   Adolescents and adults
7. *Disability Group for which this Instrument was Intended:*
   Severely and moderately retarded individuals
8. *Predominant Response Format for this Instrument:*
   Rating
9. *Who Completes the Instrument?*
   Parent
   Teacher
   Care-provider
10. *How is the Instrument Administered?*
    Rating scale or checklist completed by third-party informant
11. *Does the Instrument Require Special Training?*
    No
12. *The Standardisation Population Used to Develop and Test this Instrument:*
    900 adolescents and adults in New Zealand who were either severely or moderately mentally retarded

ALBERT EINSTEIN SCALES OF SENSORIMOTOR DEVELOPMENT

1. *Author(s):* S.K. Escalona and H.H. Corman
2. *Date Initially Prepared:* 1966 *More Recent Revision:* Not known
3. Distributor/Publisher/Key Source:
   See S.K. Escalona and H.H. Corman (1969), see Chapter 3
4. *Availability:*
   Published

5. *Main Uses of the Instrument:*
   Assessment of a sensorimotor development in nonhandicapped infants
   Originally intended for use in longitudinal study of early ego development
6. *Chronological Age for which this Instrument is Appropriate:*
   0–24 months
7. *Disability Group for which this Instrument was Intended:*
   Not specifically intended for disability groups
8. *Predominant Response Format for this Instrument:*
   Binary
9. *Who Completes the Instrument?*
   Relevant professional
10. *How is the Instrument Administered?*
    Observation
11. *Does the Instrument Require Special Training?*
    Some
12. *The Standardisation Population Used to Develop and Test this Instrument:*
    292 infants (247 in cross-sectional and 45 in longitudinal studies) 0.9–26.5 months

ASSESSMENT IN INFANCY: ORDINAL SCALES OF PSYCHOLOGICAL DEVELOPMENT

1. *Author(s):* I.C. Uzgiris and J.McV. Hunt
2. *Date Initially Prepared:* 1963 *Most Recent Revision:* 1975
3. *Distributor/Publisher/Key Source:*
   University of Illinois Press, 54 E. Gregory Drive, Box 5081 Station A, Champaign, Illinois 61820
4. *Availability:*
   Published
5. *Main Uses of the Instrument:*
   Assessment of nonhandicapped infants 0–24 months
   Planning for programme development for people with developmental delays
   Has been extended to developmentally delayed individuals and can be employed with children and adults who are profoundly retarded
6. *Chronological Age for which this Instrument is Appropriate:*
   In nonhandicapped individuals 0–24 months; full age range of

people with mental handicap who are developmentally below 24 months
7. *Disability Group for which this Instrument was Intended:*
Not originally intended specifically for disabled groups but has been extended to these
8. *Predominant Response Format for this Instrument:*
Binary
9. *Who Completes the Instrument?*
Relevant professional
10. *How is the Instrument Administered?*
Observation
11. *Does the Instrument Require Special Training?*
Some
12. *The Standardisation Population Used to Develop and Test this Instrument:*
84 nonhandicapped infants, 1–24 months, both sexes

ASSESSMENT OF VISUAL ABILITY IN THE PROFOUNDLY HANDICAPPED

1. *Author(s):* J. Bell
2. *Date Initially Prepared:* 1983 *Most Recent Revision:* N/A
3. *Distributor/Publisher/Key Source:*
National Association of Deaf-Blind Rubella Handicapped Newsletter, Vol. 29, pp. 16–17, 311 Gray's Inn Road, London WC1X 8PT
4. *Avability:*
Published and informally prepared for local use
5. *Main Uses of the Instrument:*
Assessment of basic visual responses — how child uses vision
Planning for basic visual training
To identify conditions which lead to optimum use of vision
6. *Chronological Age for which this Instrument is Appropriate:*
Not stated, probably any individual with profound retardation
7. *Disability Group for which this Instrument was Intended:*
Children with severe and profound retardation, physical and sensory impairments
8. *Predominant Response Format for this Instrument:*
Open-ended, fill-in evaluation
Binary

APPENDIX

9. *Who Completes the Instrument?*
   Parent
   Teacher
   Care-provider
   Social worker
10. *How is the Instrument Administered?*
    Observation
11. *Does the Instrument Require Special Training?*
    No
12. *The Standardisation Population Used to Develop and Test this Instrument:*
    None, not intended to be a formal assessment, just guidelines for observation

AUDITORY ASSESSMENT AND PROGRAMMING MANUAL FOR SEVERELY HANDICAPPED AND DEAF-BLIND STUDENTS

1. *Author(s):* L. Goetz, B. Utley, K. Gee, M. Baldwin and W. Sailor
2. *Date Initially Prepared:* 1982 *Most Recent Revision:* 1982?
3. *Distributor/Publisher/Key Source:*
   The Association for the Severely Handicapped, Seattle, Washington
4. *Availability:*
   Published
5. *Main Uses of the Instrument:*
   Preparing students with severe multiple disabilities for audiological assessment by establishing reliable responding to an auditory cue
   Also to teach functional use of the auditory sensory channel
6. *Chronological Age for which this Instrument is Appropriate:*
   Any age. Describes use with 4–14 year olds
7. *Disability Group for which this Instrument was Intended:*
   Severely handicapped with multiple physical and sensory impairments
8. *Predominant Response Format for this Instrument:*
   Binary
9. *Who Completes the Instrument?*
   Teacher
   Care-provider
   Psychologist/audiologist

10. *How is the Instrument Administered?*
    Test or interview with individual being tested
11. *Does the Instrument Require Special Training?*
    No
12. *The Standardisation Population Used to Develop and Test this Instrument:*
    Not known

BALTHAZAR SCALES OF ADAPTIVE BEHAVIOR: (1) SCALES OF FUNCTIONAL INDEPENDENCE; (2) SCALES OF SOCIAL ADAPTATION

1. *Author(s):* E. Balthazar
2. *Date Initially Prepared:* BSAB-1 — 1971; 2 — 1973 *Most Recent Revision:* BSAB-1 — 1978
3. *Distributor/Publisher/Key Source:*
   (a) Consulting Psychologists Press, Incorporated, 577 College Avenue, Palo Alto, California 94306
   (b) NFER-Nelson, Darville House, 2 Oxford Road East, Windsor, Berkshire SL4 1DF
4. *Availability:*
   Published
5. *Main Uses of the Instrument:*
   Assessment of severely and profoundly retarded, emotionally disturbed
   Planning for programme development
   Individual assessment tool, research as well as clinical evaluation
6. *Chronological Age for which this Instrument is Appropriate*
   5–57 years
7. *Disability Group for which this Instrument was Intended:*
   Developmentally disabled, mentally retarded, and/or emotionally disturbed
8. *Predominant Response Format for this Instrument:*
   Rating
9. *Who Completes the Instrument?*
   Parent
   Teacher
   Care-provider
   Social worker
   Doctor
   Primarily a rater technician

10. *How is the Instrument Administered?*
    Observation
11. *Does the Instrument Require Special Training?*
    Some
12. *The Standardisation Population Used to Develop and Test this Instrument:*
    The population consisted of severely and profoundly, ambulant institutionalised residents; ages 5–57 ages (median 17.27 and semi-quartile range 8.39). BSAB-1: 122 subjects were tested on the Eating Scales; 200, Dressing Scale; and 129, Toileting Scale. BSAB-2: Original subjects (1964–69) 288; 100 subjects in 1970–71 study

BEHAVIOUR ASSESSMENT BATTERY

1. *Author(s):* C.C. Kiernan and M.C. Jones
2. *Date Initially Prepared:* 1977 *Most Recent Revision:* 1982
3. *Distributor/Publisher/Key Source:*
   Available worldwide from: NFER-Nelson, Darville House, 2 Oxford Road East, Windsor, Berkshire SL4 1DF
4. *Availability:*
   Published
5. *Main Uses of the Instrument:*
   Planning for severely and profoundly mentally handicapped
6. *Chronological Age for which this Instrument is Appropriate:*
   All ages, predominantly children and developmentally young
7. *Disability Group for which this Instrument was Intended:*
   Mentally and multiply handicapped
8. *Predominant Response Format for this Instrument:*
   Sequential
9. *Who Completes the Instrument?*
   Teacher
   Care-provider
   Doctor
   Psychologist
10. *How is the Instrument Administered?*
    Observation
    Test or interview with individual being tested
11. *Does the Instrument Require Special Training?*
    Some

12. *The Standardisation Population Used to Develop and Test this Instrument:*
    Mentally and multiply handicapped people, age range: infancy to adulthood of people with profound retardation

BEHAVIOR DEVELOPMENT SURVEY (AN ABBREVIATED VERSION OF THE ADAPTIVE BEHAVIOR SCALE)

1. *Author(s):* Individualized Data Base (IDB) Project
2. *Date Initially Prepared:* 1972 *Most Recent Revision:* 1975
3. *Distributor/Publisher/Key Source:*
   Individualized Data Base Project, UCLA, Neuropsychiatric Institute Research Group at Lanterman State Hospital, Pomona, California
4. *Availability:*
   For limited distribution (IDB affiliates and uses)
5. *Main Uses of the Instrument:*
   Assessment of the adaptive behaviour of developmentally disabled persons
   Planning for individual programmes
   Programme evaluation
6. *Chronological Age for which this Instrument is Appropriate:*
   Same as AAMD Adaptive Behavior Scale (ABS)
7. *Disability Group for which this Instrument was Intended:*
   Same as ABS
8. *Predominant Response Format for this Instrument:*
   II — Rating
   I — Sequential
   Variable: Part I has sequentially ordered levels within items and some checklist items. Items in Part II are rated on the frequency of occurrence, sometimes, occasionally, never
9. *Who Completes the Instrument?*
   Parent
   Teacher
   Care-provider
   Social worker
   Other knowledgeable about client
10. *How is the Instrument Administered?*
    Rating scale or checklist completed by third-party informant
11. *Does the Instrument Require Special Training?*
    No

12. *The Standardisation Population Used to Develop and Test this Instrument:*
    Same as ABS and see Chapter 4 of this volume

BEHAVIOUR DISTURBANCE SCALE

1. *Author(s):* I. Leudar, W.I. Fraser and M.A. Jeeves
2. *Date Initially Prepared:* 1981 *Most Recent Revision:* 1983
3. *Distributor/Publisher/Key Source:*
   Dr I. Leudar, Psychology Department, University of Manchester, Oxford Road, Manchester M13 9PL
4. *Availability:*
   Published
5. *Main Uses of the Instrument:*
   Assessment of behaviour disturbance
   Planning for rehabilitation
   Research, response to relocation, treatment and the changes with age
6. *Chronological Age for which this Instrument is Appropriate:*
   15–50 year olds
7. *Disability Group for which this Instrument was Intended:*
   Moderately and mildly handicapped individuals
8. *Predominant Response Format for this Instrument:*
   Rating
9. *Who Completes the Instrument?*
   Parent
   Teacher
   Care-provider
10. *How is the Instrument Administered?*
    Rating scale or checklist completed through interview with third-party informant
11. *Does the Instrument Require Special Training?*
    No
12. *The Standardisation Population Used to Develop and Test this Instrument:*
    The instrument was standardised with 600 Scottish mentally handicapped individuals, 15–50 years old, moderately and mildly handicapped, male and female

THE BEREWEEKE SKILL-TEACHING SYSTEM

1. *Author(s):* D. Dell, D. Felce, C. Flight, J. Jenkins and J. Mansell
2. *Date Initially Prepared:* 1983 *Most Recent Revision:* 1983
3. *Distributor/Publisher/Key Source:*
   Available worldwide from: NFER-Nelson, Darville House, 2 Oxford Road East, Windsor, Berkshire SL4 1DF
4. *Availability:*
   Published
5. *Main Uses of the Instrument:*
   Planning for remedial programmes
6. *Chronological Age for which this Instrument is Appropriate:*
   Adults and children (alternative forms)
7. *Disability Group for which this Instrument was Intended:*
   People with mental handicap
8. *Predominant Response Format for this Instrument:*
   Binary
9. *Who Completes the Instrument?*
   Teacher
   Care-provider
   Social worker
   Psychologist
10. *How is the Instrument Administered?*
    Observation
    Test or interview with individual being tested
11. *Does the Instrument Require Special Training?*
    Some
12. *The Standardisation Population Used to Develop and Test this Instrument:*
    Unspecified

CAIN-LEVINE SOCIAL COMPETENCY SCALE

1. *Author(s):* L.F. Cain, S. Levine and F.F. Elzey
2. *Date Initially Prepared:* 1963 *Most Recent Revision:*
3. *Distributor/Publisher/Key Source:*
   Consulting Psychologists Press, 577 College Avenue, Palo Alto, California 94306
4. *Availability:*
   Published

5. *Main Uses of the Instrument:*
   Assessment
   Planning
6. *Chronological Age for which this Instrument is Appropriate:*
   5–13 year olds
7. *Disability Group for which this Instrument was Intended:*
   Moderately mentally handicapped people
8. *Predominant Response Format for this Instrument:*
   Sequential
9. *Who Completes the Instrument?*
   Parent
   Teacher
   Care-provider
   Social worker
10. *How is the Instrument Administered?*
    Rating scale or checklist completed by third-party informant
11. *Does the Instrument Require Special Training?*
    Some
12. *The Standardisation Population Used to Develop and Test this Instrument:*
    716 trainable mentally retarded children aged 5–13 years

CLINICAL AND EDUCATIONAL MANUAL FOR USE WITH THE UZGIRIS AND HUNT SCALES OF INFANT DEVELOPMENT

1. *Author(s):* C.J. Dunst
2. *Date Initially Prepared:* 1980 *Most Recent Revision:* 1980
3. *Distributor/Publisher/Key Source:*
   Pro-ed, 5341 Industrial Oak Boulevard, Austin, Texas 78735
4. *Availability:*
   Published
5. *Main Uses of the Instrument:*
   Assessment of children requiring psychoeducational intervention
   Planning for early cognitive curriculum
   Explicitly this instrument is directed to children with special educational needs but could also be employed with adults who are profoundly retarded. Guidelines for developing intervention programmes are given (pp. 50–5)
6. *Chronological Age for which this Instrument is Appropriate:*
   Dependent on degree of development delay but assumes Mental

Age below two years
7. *Disability Group for which this Instrument was Intended:*
All special needs may be considered, Dunst providing data on individual's with Down's Syndrome, brain damage, spina bifida, cerebral palsy, mental retardation and others 'at risk'
8. *Predominant Response Format for this Instrument:*
Binary
9. *Who Completes the Instrument?*
Relevant professional
10. *How is the Instrument Administered?*
Observation
Test
11. *Does the Instrument Require Special Training?*
Some
12. *The Standardisation Population Used to Develop and Test this Instrument:*
No standardisation — see original manual

THE DEVELOPMENT TEAM FOR THE MENTALLY HANDICAPPED ASSESSMENT FORM

1. *Author(s):* Development Team for the Mentally Handicapped
2. *Date Initially Prepared:* 1979 *Most Recent Revision:* 1981
3. *Distributor/Publisher/Key Source:*
Development Team for the Mentally Handicapped, Department of Health and Social Security, Alexander Fleming House, Elephant and Castle, London SE1
4. *Availability:*
Published
5. *Main Uses of the Instrument:*
Assessment of mentally handicapped people
Planning for services
6. *Chronological Age for which this Instrument is Appropriate:*
All over age of five
7. *Disability Group for which this Instrument was Intended:*
Mentally handicapped people
8. *Predominant Response Format for this Instrument:*
Rating
Sequential
9. *Who Completes the Instrument?*
Parent

APPENDIX

      Teacher
      Care-provider
      Social worker
10. *How is the Instrument Administered?*
    Rating scale or checklist completed by third-party informant
11. *Does the Instrument Require Special Training?*
    No
12. *The Standardisation Population Used to Develop and Test this Instrument:*
    10,000 residents of hospitals and social service facilities

THE DISABILITY ASSESSMENT SCHEDULE

1. *Author(s):* L. Wing and J. Gould
2. *Date Initially Prepared:* 1981 *Most Recent Revision:* 1982
3. *Distributor/Publisher/Key Source:*
   L. Wing, Social Psychiatry Research Unit, Institute of Psychiatry, De Crespigny Park, London SE5 8AF
4. *Availability:*
   For limited distribution
5. *Main Uses of the Instrument:*
   Assessment of behaviour skills and behaviour problems
   Planning for screening and planning of placements and management
6. *Chronological Age for which this Instrument is Appropriate:*
   Children, adolescents and adults
7. *Disability Group for which this Instrument was Intended:*
   People with mental handicap
8. *Predominant Response Format for this Instrument:*
   Rating
9. *Who Completes the Instrument?*
   Parent
   Teacher
   Care-provider
   Social worker
10. *How is the Instrument Administered?*
    Rating scale or checklist completed through interview with third-party informant
11. *Does the Instrument Require Special Training?*
    Yes — the training given by authors

12. *The Standardisation Population Used to Develop and Test this Instrument:*
    Institutionalised adults

THE FINE MOTOR SKILL ASSESSMENT BATTERY

1. *Author(s):* James Hogg
2. *Date Initially Prepared:* 1978 Most Recent Revision: —
3. *Distributor/Publisher/Key Source:*
   James Hogg, Hester Adrian Research Centre, University of Manchester, Oxford Road, Manchester M13 9PL
4. *Availability:*
   Informally prepared for local use
5. *Main Uses of the Instrument:*
   Assessment of fine motor skills in young handicapped and normal children
6. *Chronological Age for which this Instrument is Appropriate:*
   0–30 months
7. *Disability Group for which this Instrument was Intended:*
   Children with Down's Syndrome, or severely or profound retardation
8. *Predominant Response Format for this Instrument:*
   Sequential
9. *Who Completes the Instrument?*
   Teacher
   Possibly psychologist
10. *How is the Instrument Administered?*
    Observation
    Test
11. *Does the Instrument Require Special Training?*
    No
12. *The Standardisation Population Used to Develop and Test this Instrument:*
    The standardisation — 22 mentally handicapped children, mean Chronological Age 35.7 months, mean Mental Age 15.3 months, mean Psychomotor Age 15.2 months

APPENDIX

THE FORCED CHOICE PREFERENTIAL LOOKING PROCEDURES

1. *Author(s):* D.Y. Teller
2. *Date Initially Prepared:* 1974 *Most Recent Revision:* 1979
3. *Distributor/Publisher/Key Source:*
   'The Forced-Choice Preferential Looking Procedure: A Psychological Technique for Use with Human Infants', *Infant Behavior and Development*, (1979) 2, 135–53
4. *Availability:*
   Published
5. *Main Uses of the Instrument:*
   Assessment of visual activity, contrast sensitivity and colour discrimination in infants
   Research
6. *Chronological Age for which this Instrument is Appropriate:*
   0–12 months
7. *Disability Group for which this Instrument was Intended:*
   'Normal' children and children with mental retardation
8. *Predominant Response Format for this Instrument:*
   Binary
9. *Who Completes the Instrument?*
   Needs an observer, a holder and a presenter/experimenter
   Teacher
   Psychologist
10. *How is the Instrument Administered?*
    Observation
    Test or interview with individual being test
11. *Does the Instrument Require Special Training?*
    Some
12. *The Standardisation Population Used to Develop and Test this Instrument:*
    Details on technical aspects of the assessment can be found in Shepherd and Fagar (1981)

FROSTIG DEVELOPMENTAL TEST OF VISUAL PERCEPTION

1. *Author(s):* M. Frostig
2. *Date Initially Prepared:* 1959 *Most Recent Revision:* 1966
3. *Distributor/Publisher/Key Source:*
   (a) NFER-Nelson, Darville House, 2 Oxford Road East,

Windsor, Berkshire SL4 1DF
(b) Consulting Psychologists Press, Incorporated, California, 577 College Avenue, Palo Alto, California 94306
4. *Availability:*
Published
5. *Main Uses of the Instrument:*
Assessment of perceptual development
Planning for related training programme
6. *Chronological Age for which this Instrument is Appropriate:*
4–8 years or older children with learning disabilities
7. *Disability Group for which this Instrument was Intended:*
Learning disabilities, visual-perceptual disabilities, cerebral palsy
8. *Predominant Response Format for this Instrument:*
Binary
Sequential
9. *Who Completes the Instrument?*
Teacher
Psychologist, speech therapist
10. *How is the Instrument Administered?*
Test or interview with individual being tested
11. *Does the Instrument Require Special Training?*
No
12. *The Standardisation Population Used to Develop and Test this Instrument:*
2,116 aged 3–9 years, American middle-class white children

FUNCTIONAL VISION SCREENING FOR SEVERELY HANDICAPPED CHILDREN

1. *Author(s):* B. Langley and R. DuBose
2. *Date Initially Prepared:* 1976 *Most Recent Revision:* 1980?
3. *Distributor/Publisher/Key Source:*
The New Outlook for the Blind, October 1976, 346–50, American Foundation for the Blind, 15 West 16th Street, New York 10011
4. *Availability:*
Published
5. *Main Uses of the Instrument:*
Assessment of basic visual responses
Planning for basic educational programmes
6. *Chronological Age for which this Instrument is Appropriate:*
Any, if profound retardation exists

7. *Disability Group for which this Instrument was Intended:*
   Severe and profound retardation, sensory and physical impairments
8. *Predominant Response Format for this Instrument:*
   Binary
9. *Who Completes the Instrument?*
   Teacher
   Care-provider
10. *How is the Instrument Administered?*
    Observation
    Test
11. *Does the Instrument Require Special Training?*
    No
12. *The Standardisation Population Used to Develop and Test this Instrument:*
    None

GLENWOOD AWARENESS, MANIPULATION AND POSTURE SCALE

1. *Author(s):* R.C. Webb, B. Schultz an J. McMahill
2. *Date Initially Prepared:* 1968? *Most Recent Revision:* 1977
3. *Distributor/Publisher/Key Source:*
   Dr Ruth Webb, Glenwood State Hospital School, Glenwood, Iowa
4. *Availability:*
   For limited distribution
5. *Main Uses of the Instrument:*
   Assessment of sensorimotor functioning in children who are multiply impaired
6. *Chronological Age for which this Instrument is Appropriate:*
   0–18 months
7. *Disability Group for which this Instrument was Intended:*
   Children with profound retardation and multiple impairments
8. *Predominant Response Format for this Instrument:*
   Rating
   Sequential
9. *Who Completes the Instrument?*
   Requires two informants; and an observer and evaluator
   Teacher
   Care-provider

Therapist
10. *How is the Instrument Administered?*
    Observation
    Rating scale or checklist completed by third-party informant
11. *Does the Instrument Require Special Training?*
    Yes
12. *The Standardisation Population Used to Develop and Test this Instrument:*
    None

THE HAMPSHIRE ASSESSMENT FOR LIVING WITH OTHERS

1. *Author(s):* M.J. Shackleton-Bailey, B.E. Pidcock and Hampshire Social Services
2. *Date Initially Prepared: — Most Recent Revision:* 1983 (4th version)
3. *Distributor/Publisher/Key Source:*
   Hampshire Social Services, Trafalgar House, The Castle, Winchester, Hampshire SO23 8UQ
4. *Availability:*
   Published
5. *Main Uses of the Instrument:*
   Assessment of mentally handicapped people
   Planning for residential and other services
6. *Chronological Age for which this Instrument is Appropriate:*
   Children and adults
7. *Disability Group for which this Instrument was Intended:*
   All mentally handicapped people but reported as of limited use with 'profoundly physically and mentally handicapped people'
8. *Predominant Response Format for this Instrument:*
   Sequential
   Symbols to be used
9. *Who Completes the Instrument?*
   Parent
   Teacher
   Care-provider
   Social worker
10. *How is the Instrument Administered?*
    Observation
    Test or interview with individual being tested
    Rating scale or checklist completed by third-party informant

11. *Does the Instrument Require Special Training?*
    Some
12. *The Standardisation Population Used to Develop and Test this Instrument:*
    None

THE OBJECT-CONCEPT AND OBJECT-RELATIONS SCALES

1. *Author(s):* T. Gouin Décarie
2. *Date Initially Prepared:* 1962 Most Recent Revision: —
3. *Distributor/Publisher/Key Source:*
   T. Gouin Décarie (1962), *Intelligence and Affectivity in Early Childhood*, International Universities Press, New York
4. *Availability:*
   Published
5. *Main Uses of the Instrument:*
   Assessment of nonhandicapped children and those with physical impairments arising from thalidomide
   Can be used with children with other forms of physical impairment and some degree of mental retardation
6. *Chronological Age for which this Instrument is Appropriate:*
   3–20 months for nonhandicapped children and 5 months to 3 years 8 months in thalidomide study — but could be used at higher Chronological Age
7. *Disability Group for which this Instrument was Intended:*
   Thalidomide-damaged children
8. *Predominant Response Format for this Instrument:*
   Rating — nine-point scale
9. *Who Completes the Instrument?*
   Relevant professional
10. *How is the Instrument Administered?*
    Observation
    Test or interview with individual being tested
11. *Does the Instrument Require Special Training?*
    Some
12. *The Standardisation Population Used to Develop and Test this Instrument:*
    90 infants — 3–20 months

THE OBJECT RELATED SCHEME ASSESSMENT PROCEDURE

1. *Author(s):* J. Coupe and D. Levy
2. *Date Initially Prepared:* 1983 *Most Recent Revision:* 1985
3. *Distributor/Publisher/Key Source:*
   J. Coupe and D. Levy (1985) 'The Object Related Scheme Assessment Procedure: A Cognitive Assessment for Developmentally Young Children who may have Additional Physical or Sensory Handicaps', *Journal of the British Institute of Mental Handicap, 13*, 22–4
4. *Availability:*
   Published
5. *Main Uses of the Instrument:*
   Assessment of developmentally young children with additional physical and sensory handicaps, particularly those with profound retardation
   Specifically intended as an assessment leading in to curriculum activities
6. *Chronological Age for which this Instrument is Appropriate:*
   Infancy to adulthood depending on degree of retardation
7. *Disability Group for which this Instrument was Intended:*
   Severe and profound retardation with additional physical and sensory impairments
8. *Predominant Response Format for this Instrument:*
   Binary
9. *Who Completes the Instrument?*
   Parent
   Teacher
   Therapist
10. *How is the Instrument Administered?*
    Observation
    Test or interview with individual being tested
11. *Does the Instrument Require Special Training?*
    No
12. *The Standardisation Population Used to Develop and Test this Instrument:*
    None

APPENDIX

OBSERVATION SYSTEM TO ASSESS SPONTANEOUS INFANT BEHAVIOUR-ENVIRONMENT INTERACTIONS

1. *Author(s):* G. Chatelanat and M. Schoggen
2. *Date Initially Prepared:* 1975 *Most Recent Revision:* 1980
3. *Distributor/Publisher/Key Source:*
   G. Chatelanat and M. Schoggen (1980) 'Issues Encountered in Devising an Observation System to Assess Spontaneous Infant Behaviour-Environment Interactions' in J. Hogg and P.J. Mittler (eds.), *Advances in Mental Handicap Research*, vol. 1, Wiley, Chichester and New York
4. *Availability:*
   Published
5. *Main Uses of the Instrument:*
   Assessment of both handicapped and nonhandicapped infants
6. *Chronological Age for which this Instrument is Appropriate:*
   0–24 months in nonhandicapped children
7. *Disability Group for which this Instrument was Intended:*
   Developed in the context of work with preschool children some of whom were mentally handicapped
8. *Predominant Response Format for this Instrument:*
   Binary
9. *Who Completes the Instrument?*
   Relevant professional
   Teacher
10. *How is the Instrument Administered?*
    Observation
11. *Does the Instrument Require Special Training?*
    Some
12. *The Standardisation Population Used to Develop and Test this Instrument:*
    Eight infants 12–16 months

THE 'PATHS TO MOBILITY IN "SPECIAL CARE"' CHECKLIST

1. *Author(s):* John L. Presland
2. *Date Initially Prepared:* 1982 *Most Recent Revision:* 1982
3. *Distributor/Publisher/Key Source:*
   Publication Department, British Institute of Mental Handicap, Wolverhampton Road, Kidderminster, Worcestershire DY10 3PP

4. *Availability:*
   Published
5. *Main Uses of the Instrument:*
   Assessment of gross motor skills in 'special care' children
   Planning for selection of teaching objectives
6. *Chronological Age for which this Instrument is Appropriate:*
   0–18 months, but possibly higher for wheelchair items
7. *Disability Group for which this Instrument was Intended:*
   Children with profound retardation and additional impairments of physical or sensory functioning
8. *Predominant Response Format for this Instrument:*
   Binary
   Sequential
   Other — must enter own criteria for success on each item
9. *Who Completes the Instrument?*
   Parent
   Teacher
   Care-provider
   Social worker
10. *How is the Instrument Administered?*
    Observation
    Checklist completed by third-party informant
11. *Does the Instrument Require Special Training?*
    No
12. *The Standardisation Population Used to Develop and Test this Instrument:*
    None

PLAY OBJECT SCHEMAS PROGRESS ASSESSMENT

1. *Author(s):* T. Foxen
2. *Date Initially Prepared:* 1975 *Most Recent Revision:* 1977
3. *Distributor/Publisher/Key Source:*
   Hester Adrian Research Centre, University of Manchester, Manchester M13 9PL
4. *Availability:*
   For limited distribution
5. *Main Uses of the Instrument:*
   Assessment of people with profound retardation and multiple impairments
   Planning for people with profound retardation and multiple

impairments
6. *Chronological Age for which this Instrument is Appropriate:*
Infancy-adulthood where profoundly retarded multiply impaired people are involved
7. *Disability Group for which this Instrument was Intended:*
Profoundly mentally handicapped people with additional sensory and physical impairments
8. *Predominant Response Format for this Instrument:*
Binary
9. *Who Completes the Instrument?*
Parent
Teacher
Therapist
10. *How is the Instrument Administered?*
Observation
Test with individual being assessed
11. *Does the Instrument Require Special Training?*
No
12. *The Standardisation Population Used to Develop and Test this Instrument:*
None — but developed with children who were profoundly retarded and multiply impaired

PORTAGE GUIDE TO EARLY EDUCATION

1. *Author(s):* S. Bluma, J. Shearer, A. Frohman and J. Hilliard
2. *Date Initially Prepared:* 1972 *Most Recent Revision:* —
3. *Distributor/Publisher/Key Source:*
   (a) The Portage Project, Caesar Twelve, P.O. Box 564, Portage, Wisconsin 53901
   (b) NFER-Nelson, Darville House, 2 Oxford Road East, Windsor, Berkshire SL4 1DF
4. *Availability:*
Published
5. *Main Uses of the Instrument:*
Planning for home intervention
6. *Chronological Age for which this Instrument is Appropriate:*
Children and developmentally delayed adults
7. *Disability Group for which this Instrument was Intended:*
Delayed development due to social reasons, people with mental handicap

8. *Predominant Response Format for this Instrument:*
   Binary
9. *Who Completes the Instrument?*
   Parent
   Teacher
   Care-provider
   Social worker
   Portage home visitor
10. *How is the Instrument Administered?*
    Rating scale or checklist completed through interview with third-party informant
11. *Does the Instrument Require Special Training?*
    Some
12. *The Standardisation Population Used to Develop and Test this Instrument:*
    None specified

PREOPERATIONAL ASSESSMENT (FROM 'A STUDY OF MENTAL GROWTH IN YOUNG SEVERELY SUBNORMAL CHILDREN')

1. *Author(s):* B. Smith
2. *Date Initially Prepared:* 1973 *Most Recent Revision:* 1982
3. *Distributor/Publisher/Key Source:*
   Thesis, 'A Study of Mental Growth in Young Severely Subnormal Children', from which assessment is taken is available from the University Library, University of Birmingham, PO Box 363, Birmingham B15 2TT
4. *Availability:*
   See 3
5. *Main Uses of the Instrument:*
   Assessment of children with mental handicap
   Can be used to suggest curriculum activities appropriate to developmental level
6. *Chronological Age for which this Instrument is Appropriate:*
   For children and adults with mental handicap from approximate Chronological Age three years upwards
7. *Disability Group for which this Instrument was Intended:*
   Children with severe mental handicap
8. *Predominant Response Format for this Instrument:*
   Open-ended, fill-in evaluation

Other — emphasis on analysis of strategic behaviour
9. *Who Completes the Instrument?*
Relevant professional
Teacher
Psychologist
10. *How is the Instrument Administered?*
Test with individual being assessed
11. *Does the Instrument Require Special Training?*
Some
12. *The Standardisation Population Used to Develop and Test this Instrument:*
N = 209, aged 7–13 years, male and female, attending ESN(S) schools (i.e. educationally sub-normal, severe)

PROGRESS ASSESSMENT CHART OF SOCIAL AND PERSONAL DEVELOPMENT

1. *Author(s):* H.C. Gunzberg
2. *Date Initially Prepared:* 1963 *Most Recent Revision:* 1977
3. *Distributor/Publisher/Key Source:*
   (a) In UK only from: The Book Shop, Royal Society for Mentally Handicapped Children and Adults (MENCAP), 123 Golden Lane, London EC1V 0RT
   (b) No current distributor in the USA
   (c) In Canada available from: Michener Centre, PAC Department, Box 502, Red Deer, Alberta T4N 5Y5
4. *Availability:*
Published
5. *Main Uses of the Instrument:*
Assessment of mentally handicapped children
Planning for services
6. *Chronological Age for which this Instrument is Appropriate:*
6–16 years
7. *Disability Group for which this Instrument was Intended:*
Mentally handicapped children
8. *Predominant Response Format for this Instrument:*
Binary
9. *Who Completes the Instrument?*
Teacher
Care-provider
Social worker

Psychologist
10. *How is the Instrument Administered?*
    Observation
    Rating scale or checklist completed by third-party informant
11. *Does the Instrument Require Special Training?*
    Some
12. *The Standardisation Population Used to Develop and Test this Instrument:*
    Children in training centres in England

PSYCHOPATHOLOGY INSTRUMENT FOR MENTALLY RETARDED ADULTS

1. *Author(s):* V. Senatore, J.L. Matson and A.E. Kazdin
2. *Date Initially Prepared:* 1985 *Most Recent Revision:* 1985
3. *Distributor/Publisher/Key Source:*
   Vincent Senatore, Department of Psychiatry, Western Psychiatric Institute and Clinic, University of Pittsburg School of Medicine, 3811 O'Hara Street, Pittsburg, Pennsylvania 15213
4. *Availability:*
   Published
5. *Main Uses of the Instrument:*
   Assessment of psychiatric problems in mentally retarded adults
   Research
6. *Chronological Age for which this Instrument is Appropriate:*
   18–71 years
7. *Disability Group for which this Instrument was Intended:*
   Severely, moderately, mildly and borderline retarded individuals
8. *Predominant Response Format for this Instrument:*
   Binary
9. *Who Completes the Instrument?*
   The client, subject, student
   Parent
   Teacher
   Care-provider
   Social worker
10. *How is the Instrument Administered?*
    Rating scale or checklist compared by third-party informant
11. *Does the Instrument Require Special Training?*
    No

12. *The Standardisation Population Used to Develop and Test this Instrument:*
The standardisation was 110 retarded adults (9 borderline, 51 mildly, 46 moderately and 4 severely); age 18–71, average 46 years old, 56 females, 54 males

THE SCALE FOR ASSESSING COPING SKILLS

1. *Author(s):* E. Whelan and B. Speake
2. *Date Initially Prepared:* 1979 *Most Recent Revision:* —
3. *Distributor/Publisher/Key Source:*
   Copewell Publications, 29 Worcester Road, Altrington, Middleton, Manchester M24 1PA
4. *Availability:*
   Published
5. *Main Uses of the Instrument:*
   Assessment
   Planning
6. *Chronological Age for which this Instrument is Appropriate:*
   Adolescents and adults
7. *Disability Group for which this Instrument was Intended:*
   Mentally handicapped people
8. *Predominant Response Format for this Instrument:*
   Rating
9. *Who Completes the Instrument?*
   Parent
   Teacher
   Care-provider
   Social worker
10. *How is the Instrument Administered?*
    Rating scale or checklist completed by third-party informant
11. *Does the Instrument Require Special Training?*
    Some
12. *The Standardisation Population Used to Develop and Test this Instrument:*
    People in Adult Training Centres

APPENDIX

STANDARDIZED PSYCHIATRIC INTERVIEW

1. *Author(s):* D.B. Goldberg, B. Cooper, M.R. Eastwood, H.B. Kedward and M. Shepherd
2. *Date Initially Prepared:* 1970 *Most Recent Revision:* 1980
3. *Distributor/Publisher/Key Source:*
   General Practice Research Unit, Institute of Psychiatry, De Crespigny Park, Denmark Hill, London SE5 8AF
4. *Availability:*
   Published
5. *Main Uses of the Instrument:*
   Assessment of mental and psychiatric disturbances
   A standardised psychiatric interview for use in community surveys
6. *Chronological Age for which this Instrument is Appropriate:*
   Adults
7. *Disability Group for which this Instrument was Intended:*
   Nonretarded subjects but with minor adjustments the scale is applicable to mentally retarded
8. *Predominant Response Format for this Instrument:*
   Rating
9. *Who Completes the Instrument?*
   Psychiatrist with training
10. *How is the Instrument Administered?*
    Observation
    Test or interview with individual being tested
11. *Does the Instrument Require Special Training?*
    Yes — a short induction course
12. *The Standardisation Population Used to Develop and Test this Instrument:*
    See Goldberg, Cooper, Eastwood, Edward and Shepherd (1970) 'A Standardised Psychiatric Interview for Use in Community Surveys', *British Journal of Social and Preventive Medicine,* 24, 18–23

STYCAR HEARING TEST

1. *Author(s):* Mary Sheridan
2. *Date Initially Prepared:* 1976 *Most Recent Revision:* —
3. *Distributor/Publisher/Key Source:*
   Available worldwide from: NFER/Nelson, Darville House, 2 Oxford Road East, Windsor, Berkshire SL4 1DF

4. *Availability:*
   Published
5. *Main Uses of the Instrument:*
   Assessment of children's ability to hear with comprehension
6. *Chronological Age for which this Instrument is Appropriate:*
   6 months–7 years
7. *Disability Group for which this Instrument was Intended:*
   Very young children (defined as above) with a mental handicap
8. *Predominant Response Format for this Instrument:*
   Binary
   Sequential
9. *Who Completes the Instrument?*
   Specialist teacher
   Doctor
   Psychologist
10. *How is the Instrument Administered?*
    Test or interview with individual being tested
11. *Does the Instrument Require Special Training?*
    Some
12. *The Standardisation Population Used to Develop and Test this Instrument:*
    Was undertaken, but numbers of children involved not specified. Done on 'normal' and retarded children

THE SYMBOLIC PLAY TEST

1. *Author(s):* M. Lowe and A.J. Costello
2. *Date Initially Prepared:* 1973 *Most Recent Revision:* —
3. *Distributor/Publisher/Key Source:*
   Available worldwide from: NFER-Nelson, Darville House, 2 Oxford Road East, Windsor, Berkshire SL4 1DF
4. *Availability:*
   Published
5. *Main Uses of the Instrument:*
   Assessment of children's cognition with respect to symbolic play
   Has potential for suggesting curriculum activities for developing play
6. *Chronological Age for which this Instrument is Appropriate:*
   12–36 months (or 12–36 months developmentally)
7. *Disability Group for which this Instrument was Intended:*
   Intended for communication disabled groups and has been

employed with children with mental handicap
8. *Predominant Response Format for this Instrument:*
   Binary
9. *Who Completes the Instrument?*
   Teacher
   Psychologist or therapist
10. *How is the Instrument Administered?*
    Observation
11. *Does the Instrument Require Special Training?*
    Some
12. *The Standardisation Population Used to Develop and Test this Instrument:*
    137 children of 12–36 months. Some tested two to five times at different age levels

SYSTEMATIC PROCEDURES FOR ELICITING AND RECORDING RESPONSES TO SOUND STIMULI

1. *Author(s):* Susan M. Kershman and Deborah Napier
2. *Date Initially Prepared:* 1982 *Most Recent Revision:* —
3. *Distributor/Publisher/Key Source:*
   The Volta Review, vol. 84, pp. 226–37
4. *Availability:*
   Published in article
5. *Main Uses of the Instrument:*
   Assessment of auditory activity levels
   Planning for individualised auditory training programme
6. *Chronological Age for which this Instrument is Appropriate:*
   Any age but article describes application to 11 months–6 years
7. *Disability Group for which this Instrument was Intended:*
   Deaf-blind, multihandicapped (defined as low functioning with physical impairments)
8. *Predominant Response Format for this Instrument:*
   Open-ended, fill-in evaluation, response to environmental sounds
   Binary
   Rating
9. *Who Completes the Instrument?*
   Parent
   Teacher
   Care-provider

10. *How is the Instrument Administered?*
    Observation
    Test or interview with individual being tested
11. *Does the Instrument Require Special Training?*
    No
12. *The Standardisation Population Used to Develop and Test this Instrument:*
    None — only reported on seven children or 11 months–6 years

TECHNIQUES OF ASSESSMENT OF SEVERELY SUBNORMAL AND YOUNG NORMAL CHILDREN

1. *Author(s):* W.M. Woodward
2. *Date Initially Prepared:* 1959 *Most Recent Revision:* 1967
3. *Distributor/Publisher/Key Source:*
   W.M. Woodward, Psychology Department, University College of Swansea, Singleton Park, Swansea SA2 8PP, UK
4. *Availability:*
   Not available in 1967 note form but details of material and procedure in Woodward (1959), cited in Chapter 3 of this volume
5. *Main Uses of the Instrument:*
   Research only
   Can be used as an assessment device with nonhandicapped children and individuals who are severely or profoundly mentally handicapped
6. *Chronological Age for which this Instrument is Appropriate:*
   For children not mentally handicapped Chronological Age approximately 24 months down; for individuals with mental handicaps, dependent on Mental Age around 24 months or less
7. *Disability Group for which this Instrument was Intended:*
   Specifically intended for individuals with severe or profound mental handicap, including some with neurological damage and additional impairments
8. *Predominant Response Format for this Instrument:*
   Binary
   Other — observational
9. *Who Completes the Instrument?*
   Professional assessor
10. *How is the Instrument Administered?*
    Observation
    Test or interview with individual being tested

11. *Does the Instrument Require Special Training?*
    Some
12. *The Standardisation Population Used to Develop and Test this Instrument:*
    Experimental sample from institution with age ranges 7–9 and 14–16 years. Included Down's Syndrome, phenylketonuric, tuberose sclerosis, microcephalic, spina bifida and epileptic children

VINELAND SOCIAL MATURITY SCALE

1. *Author(s):* E.A. Doll
2. *Date Initially Prepared:* 1935 *Most Recent Revision:* 1965
3. *Distributor/Publisher/Key Source:*
   American Guidance Service Incorporated, Publishers' Building, Circle Pines, Minnesota
4. *Availability:*
   Published
5. *Main Uses of the Instrument:*
   Assessment of client
   Planning for individual programmes
   Research also
6. *Chronological Age for which this Instrument is Appropriate:*
   Birth–30 years
7. *Disability Group for which this Instrument was Intended:*
   Mentally retarded and other handicapped people, such as blind, deaf, physically handicapped, health-impaired, emotionally handicapped, normal individuals
8. *Predominant Response Format for this Instrument:*
   Sequential
   Other — five-category rating system
9. *Who Completes the Instrument?*
   Informant or interviewer
10. *How is the Instrument Administered?*
    Rating scale or checklist completed through interview with third-party informant
    Recall by someone familiar with the client on a day to day basis
11. *Does the Instrument Require Special Training?*
    Some

12. *The Standardisation Population Used to Develop and Test this Instrument:*
    620 normal subjects — 20 subjects (ten male; ten female) per age group, ages birth–30 years

VISUAL CHECKLIST

1. *Author(s):* J. Sebba
2. *Date Initially Prepared:* 1978 *Most Recent Revision:* —
3. *Distributor/Publisher/Key Source:*
   Hester Adrian Research Centre, University of Manchester, Oxford Road, Manchester M13 9PL
4. *Availability:*
   Informally prepared for local use
5. *Main Uses of the Instrument:*
   Assessment of basic visual responses in people with profound retardation and multiple impairments
   Use (1) as evidence of need for specialist assessment; (2) to identify possible areas for visual training; (3) to identify conditions which lead to optimal use of vision
6. *Chronological Age for which this Instrument is Appropriate:*
   Any age if profound retardation exists
7. *Disability Group for which this Instrument was Intended:*
   People with profound retardation and multiple impairments
8. *Predominant Response Format for this Instrument:*
   Binary
   Sequential
9. *Who Completes the Instrument?*
   Parent
   Teacher
   Care-provider
   Social worker — residential
   Nurse
10. *How is the Instrument Administered?*
    Test of individual being assessed
11. *Does the Instrument Require Special Training?*
    No
12. *The Standardisation Population Used to Develop and Test this Instrument:*
    Not standardised, but developed with seven preschool-age profoundly retarded multiply impaired children

WESSEX BEHAVIOUR RATING SCALE

1. *Author(s):* A. Kushlick and G. Cox
2. *Date Initially Prepared:* 1963 *Most Recent Revision:* 1982
3. *Distributor/Publisher/Key Source:*
   John Palmer, Wessex Regional Health Authority, High Croft, Romsey Road, Winchester, Hampshire
4. *Availability:*
   Published
5. *Main Uses of the Instrument:*
   Assessment of mentally handicapped people
   Planning for services
   Research
6. *Chronological Age for which this Instrument is Appropriate:*
   All
7. *Disability Group for which this Instrument was Intended:*
   Mentally handicapped people
8. *Predominant Response Format for this Instrument:*
   Rating
9. *Who Completes the Instrument?*
   Teacher
   Care-provider
   Social worker
10. *How is the Instrument Administered?*
    Rating scale or checklist completed by third-party informant
11. *Does the Instrument Require Special Training?*
    No
12. *The Standardisation Population Used to Develop and Test this Instrument:*
    Mentally handicapped people in Wessex

THE WESSEX REVISED PORTAGE LANGUAGE CHECKLIST

1. *Author(s):* M. White and K. East
2. *Date Initially Prepared:* 1983 *Most Recent Revision:* 1983
3. *Distributor/Publisher/Key Source:*
   Available worldwide from: NFER-Nelson, Darville House, 2 Oxford Road East, Windsor, Berkshire SL4 1DF
4. *Availability:*
   Published

5. *Main Uses of the Instrument:*
   Planning for language and communication reading
6. *Chronological Age for which this Instrument is Appropriate:*
   Children and developmentally delayed adults
7. *Disability Group for which this Instrument was Intended:*
   Mental handicap
8. *Predominant Response Format for this Instrument:*
   Binary
9. *Who Completes the Instrument?*
   Parent
   Teacher
   Care-provider
   Social worker
   Portage home visitor
10. *How is the Instrument Administered?*
    Rating scale or checklist completed through interview with third-party informant
11. *Does the Instrument Require Special Training?*
    Some
12. *The Standardisation Population Used to Develop and Test this Instrument:*
    None given

WOODWARD'S APPROACH TO PREOPERATIONAL ASSESSMENT

1. *Author(s):* W.M. Woodward
2. *Date Initially Prepared:* 1972 *Most Recent Revision:* —
3. *Distributor/Publisher/Key Source:*
   Described in journal articles cited in Chapter 3 (Woodward (1972) and Woodward and Hunt (1972))
4. *Availability:*
   Published
5. *Main Uses of the Instrument:*
   Research only
   Readily adaptable to curriculum activities for nonhandicapped and handicapped children
6. *Chronological Age for which this Instrument is Appropriate:*
   18 months–5 years
7. *Disability Group for which this Instrument was Intended:*
   Nonhandicapped children and severely mentally handicapped

children included
8. *Predominant Response Format for this Instrument:*
   Analysis of strategy employed and products
9. *Who Completes the Instrument?*
   Research worker
10. *How is the Instrument Administered?*
    Observation
    Test
11. *Does the Instrument Require Special Training?*
    Some
12. *The Standardisation Population Used to Develop and Test this Instrument:*
    No formal standardisation but various items given to groups of nonhandicapped children (N = 20–40) and children with mental handicap (N = 23–96)

Author Index

Alexander, J. 133, *156*
Almeyer, B.K. *234*
Almond, S. 136, *155*
Altman, J. *233*
Alverson, L.J. 215, *234*
Aman, M.G. 116, *125*
Anastasi, A. 23, 33, *41*
Anderson, R.M. 144, *157*
Ando, H. 202, *233*
Angell, M.J. 201, *237*
Arick, J.R. 119, *127*
Armstrong, J. 114, *125*
Arnold, R. 40, *41*
Atkinson, J. 146, 147, *154*
Atkinson, M. *188*
Ault, M.H. 228, *233*
Axelrod, S. 218, *234*
Axworthy, D. 36, *44*

Baer, D.M. 227, 232, *233*
Bailey, J.S. 200, *236*
Bakeman, R. 212, 226, *233*
Baker, P. 222, *233*
Baldwin, M. 143, *155*
Ballinger, E.R. 114, 122, *125*, *127*
Balthazar, E.E. 92, 100, *103*, 111, 123, *125*
Bankes, J.L.K. 145, *154*
Barlow, D.H. 191, 199, *233*, *234*
Barratt, H. *154*
Barret, R.P. *127*
Bateman, B. 32, *41*
Bates, E. 175, *188*
Batt, R. 109, *126*
Battenburg, A.M. 146, *155*
Bauman, K.E. 196, *234*
Bauman, R. 215, *236*
Bax, M. *43*, 146, 152, *155*
Bayley, N. 23, *41*, 48, *78*, 160, *188*
Bell, C. 169, *189*

Bell, J. 148, 149, *155*
Benaroya, S. 73, *79*
Bendall, S. 168, *188*
Berg, J.M. 40, *41*, 42, *188*
Berger, M. 3, 4, 8, 9, 12, 14, 31, 32, 34, *41*, *44*, 160
Berkler, M.S. 215, *236*
Bernsen, A.H. *233*
Bijou, S.W. *108*, 159, *188*, 202, 228, *233*, *234*
Binet, A. 13
Binkoff, J.A. *233*
Bishop, D.V.M. 38, *41*
Blinkhorn, S. 37, *41*
Bluma, S. 163, 167, 173, *188*, *189*
Blunden, R. 86, 100, *105*
Bobath, B. 133, *155*
Bobath, K. 133, *155*
Boler, G.R. 202, *238*
Borthwick, S.A. 122, *126*
Bost, L. 109, *126*
Bowders, T. 109, *128*
Bower, T. 150, *155*
Boyd, R.D. 173, *189*
Braddick, O. 147, *154*
Bradley, V.J. 101, *104*
Braithwaite, A. 36, *44*
Breton, M.E. 147, *156*
Bricker, W.A. 45, *78*, 159, 160, *188*
Brierly, L.M. 74, *80*
Brown, J. 169, *189*
Browne, K. 222, 226, *233*
Bruininks, R.H. 96, *105*
Bruner, J. 175, *188*
Buros, D. 26, 33, *41*
Busch, C. 25, 34, *44*
Butler, S. *44*
Butterfield, E.C. 141, *155*

Cain, L.F. 94, 101, *103*
Cairns, G.F. 141, *155*

AUTHOR INDEX

Call, T. 100, *104*, 107, 120, 121, *126*
Callias, M. 197, 214, *235*, *236*
Cameron, J. 25, *42*
Cameron, R.J. *188*
Campbell, I. 110, *126*
Carr, E.G. 197, *233*, *238*
Carr, J. 23, 31, *41*, 214, *235*, *236*
Cataldo, M.F. 197, 200, *234*, *237*
Catford, G.V. 145, *155*
Chatelanat, G. 66, *78*
Cheiken, M. 229, *235*
Chomsky, N. 160
Cirrin, F.M. 175, *188*
Clarke, A.D.B. 23, 25, 40, *41*, *42*, *188*, *235*
Clarke, A.M. 23, 25, 40, *41*, *42*, *188*, *235*
Clements, P. 109, *126*
Cobb, H.V. 103, *104*
Cockburn, J. 37, *42*
Cohen, J. 228
Colvin, G.T. 164, *188*
Conners, C.K. 118, 119, *126*
Connolly, K. *42*
Connon, P.R. 207, *233*
Conroy, J.W. 100, 101, *104*
Cooper, B. 114, *126*
Cooperman, O. 200, *237*
Corbett, J. 231, *236*
Corman, H.H. 65, 66, *78*
Costello, A.J. 71, 72, *79*
Coupe, J. *78*
Cox, G.R. 86, 90, *105*
Cronbach, L.J. 231, 232, *233*
Cronin, J. *78*
Crystal, D. 39, *42*
Cunningham, C.C. 31, *42*, 136, 138, *155*
Cushing, P.J. 200, *237*

Dangel, R.F. *43*
Das, J.P. *79*
de Kock, U. 100, *104*, *233*
Dell, D. 163, 167, 177, *188*

DeRemer, P. 77, *80*
Dessent, A. *189*
Deutsch, M.R. 107, *128*
Devany, J. *237*
DeVries, R. 74, *78*
Diament, C. 216, 229, *237*
Dolker, M. 207, *235*
Doll, E. 82, 95, *104*
Dore, J. 175, *188*
Dorsey, M.F. 196, *234*
Dotson, V.A. 227, 228, *234*
Dowdney, L. 210, 224, *233*
Dubois, Y. 109, *126*
DuBose, R.F. 144, 146, 149, 150, 151, 152, 153, *155*, *156*
Dudek, F.J. 28, *42*
Dunn, L.M. 36, *42*
Dunn, L.M. 36, *42*
Dunst, C. 5, 49, 50, 60, 61, 63, 64 73, *78*

Eagle, E. 103, *104*
East, K. 167, 173, 174, 175, *189*
Eastwood, M.R. 114, *126*
Edelson, S.M. 196, 224, 225, *233*
Edwards, A.L. 181, *188*
Edwards, G.L. 197, *234*
Egel, A.L. 197, *238*
Elliot, C. 36, *42*
Elliot, R. 98, *104*
Ellis, D. *154*, *157*
Ellis, N.R. *80*, *125*, *127*, *156*
Elzey, F.F. 94, *103*
Erickson, M.T. 227, *238*
Escalona, S.K. 65, 66, *78*
Eyman, R.K. 100, *104*, 107, 120, 121, 122, *126*

Fagan, J.F. 147, *156*
Favell, J.E. 207, *233*
Feiber, N.M. 77, *78*
Felce, D. 100, *104*, 163, 167, 177, *188*, 200, 201, 203, 213, 222, 223, 224, 226, 229, *233*

AUTHOR INDEX

Fieber, N. 150, *155*
Field, C.J. 116, *125*
Fletcher, P. 39, *42*
Flight, L. 163, 167, 177, *188*
Fogelman, C.J. 100, *104*
Fontana, D. *188*
Foss, B.F. *78*
Foster, R. 83, *105*, 111, *127*
Foxon, T. 67, *78*
Francis, S.H. 120, *126*
Fraser, W.I. 6, 108, 110, 113, 118, 120, 121, 122, *126*, *127*, 201
Freedman, D.G. 139, *155*
Freeman, B.J. 121, *126*
Friedlander, B.Z. *105*
Friedman, M.P. *79*
Frohman, A. 163, 167, *188*
Frostig, M. 147, 152, *155*
Fryers, T. 129, *155*

Garman, M. 39, *42*
Gee, K. 143, *155*
Gesell, A. 5, 23, 33
Glaser, R. 159, *188*
Gleser, G.C. 231, *233*
Goetz, L. 143, *155*
Gold, R.D. 25, 34, *44*
Goldberg, D.P. 114, 115, *126*
Goldstein, H. 26, 33, *41*, *43*
Golestam, K.G. 200, *235*
Goodall, E. 215, 216, 220, 221, *236*
Goodman, J.F. 25, *42*
Goren, E.R. 216, *234*
Gouin Décarie, T. 65, *79*
Gould, J. 74, 80, 86, *106*, 109, 122, *128*, 202, 231, *233*, *238*
Graham, P.J. 29, *43*, 121, *127*, 202, *236*
Gray, J. 110, *126*
Green, B.F. 181, *188*
Green, J.D. 203, *234*
Green, S.B. 215, *234*
Grief, E. 218, *234*
Griffiths, H.K. *234*
Griffiths, R. 23, 33, *42*, 48, *78*, 160, *188*
Grimm, J.A. 202, *234*
Gunstone, C. *155*
Gunzberg, H.C. 88, 98, *104*
Guthrie, D. 121, *126*

Hall, R.V. 218, *234*
Halpern, A.S. 123, *126*
Hammill, D.A. 32, *42*
Harris, F.C. 227, *234*, 237
Harris, S.L. 207, 209, 216, *234*
Hart, A. 146, *155*
Hartmann, D.P. 227, 228, *234*
Hawkins, R.P. 227, 228, *234*
Heather, B.B. 114, *127*
Heber, R. 81, 82, 83, *104*
Hemming, J. 100, *105*
Herbert, M. 29, *42*
Hermann, J.A. 227, 228, *234*
Heron, A. 100, *105*
Hersen, M. 191, 199, *233*, *234*
Hersov, L. *41*
Hill, B. 96, *105*
Hill, P. 74, *79*
Hilliard, J. 163, 167, 173, *188*, *189*
Hindley, C.B. 25, *42*
Hisley, T. 149, *155*
Hof-van Duin, J. Van 146, *155*
Hogg, J. 5, 8, 25, *42*, 75, 76, 77, *78*, *79*, 135, 136, 137, *155*, *156*, *188*
Holle, B. 132, *156*
Hollenbeck, A.R. 227, *234*
Holmes, C. 109, *126*
Holmes, N. 87, 97, *105*, 109, 115, *126*, 231, *234*
Holt, K.S. 132, 133, *156*
Hopkins, B.L. 227, 228, *234*
Horner, R.H. 164, *188*
House, B.J. 41, *42*
Humphreys, S. 97, 100, *105*
Hunt, J.McV. 5, 50, 51, 53, 54, 57, 58, 59, 60, 62, 64, 67, 75, 78, *79*, *80*, 162, 184, *189*
Hunt, M.R. 67, 68, 69, *80*

Hurlbut, B.I. 203, 204, 206, 208, *234*
Hutt, C. 206, 215, *234*
Hutt, S.J. 206, 215, *234*
Huxley, R. *80*

Illingworth, R.S. 23, *42*
Ingram, E. *80*
Inhelder, B. 49, *79*
Irvin, L.K. 123, *126*
Iset, R. 109, 122, *126*, *128*
Iwata, B.A. 196, 197, 198, 203, *234*

Jacobson, J.W. 107, 109, 119, 120, 121, 123, *126*
Janicki, M.P. 120, *126*
Jeeves, M.A. 108, 113, 118, 120, *127*
Jeffree, D. 36, *44*
Jenkins, J. 99, *106*, 163, 167, 177, 178, *188*
Jenkins, R.L. 118, *127*
Jenkins, S. 146, *155*
Jesein, G.S. 173, *189*
Johnson, S.M. 202, *235*
Jones, F.C. 218, *234*
Jones, L. 143, *156*
Jones, L.M. 184, *188*
Jones, M.C. *156*, 163, 164, 165, 166, 167, 179, 180, 181, 183, *188*, 206, 220, *234*
Jones, M.L. *233*
Jones, R.R. 202, *238*
Joseph, A. 200, *237*

Kagin, E. 83, *105*
Kahn, J.V. 59, 75, 77, *79*
Kalsher, M.J. 197, *234*
Kalverboer, A.J. 220, *234*
Kanowitz, J. 229, 230, *235*, *236*
Katz, M. 107, 119, *126*
Kaufman, A.S. 14, 31, 32, 35, *42*
Kazdin, A.E. 116, 117, *128*, 191, 199, *234*, *237*
Kedward, H.B. 114, *126*

Kelly, M.B. 212, *234*
Kent, R.N. 229, 230, *235*, *236*, *237*
Kershman, S.M. 141, 142, 143, 153, 154, *156*
Kiernan, C. 3, 7, 8, 9, 22, 130, *156*, 159, 160, 163, 164, 165, 166, 167, 179, 180, 181, 183, 184, 186, *188*, 192, 197, *235*
King, R.D. 200, 207, 231, *235*
King, T. 122, *126*
Kirk, F.G.E. *155*
Kirk, S.A. 38, *42*
Kirk, W. 38, *42*
Klee, T.M. 39, *43*
Klein, L.S. 73, *79*
Kleitsch, E.C. 218, *235*
Knobloch, H. 23, *43*
Koegel, R.L. 197, *238*
Koller, H. 107, 119, 120, *126*
Krieder, J. 101, *106*
Kropka, B.I. 129, *156*
Krug, D.A. 119, *127*
Kulp, S. 215, *236*
Kushlick, A. 85, 86, 90, 99, *105*, 168, *188*

Lahey, B.B. 227, *234*
Lambert, N.M. 100, *105*, 118, *127*
Landesman-Dwyer, S. 212, *235*
Landman, J.T. 123, *126*
Langley, M.D. 144, 146, 149, 150, 151, 152, 153, *155*, *156*
Laurence, K.M. 25, *43*
Lavender, T. 100, *105*
Lawson, L.J. 144, *156*
Lefever, W. 147, *155*
Leitenberg, H. 199, *235*
Leland, H. 83, *105*, 111, *127*
Leudar, I. 6, 108, 110, 113, 118, 119, 120, 121, 122, 123, 124, *126*, *127*, 201
Levine, S. 94, 101, *103*
Levitt, S. 132, 133, *156*
Levy, D. *78*

279

AUTHOR INDEX

Levy, P. 26, 33, *41*, *43*
Lobitz, W.C. 202, *235*
Loftin, C.R. 32, *43*
Lorber, R. 203, *236*
Lorr, M. 118, *127*
Lovaas, O.I. 191, 196, 224, *233*, *235*
Lowe, I. 222, *236*
Lowe, K. 100, *105*
Lowe, M. 71, 72, 73, 78, *79*
Lunzer, E.A. 50, 68, *79*
Lynch, A. 36, *43*, *44*

McArthur, K. 136, 138, *155*
McCarthy, D.A. 36, *43*
McCarthy, J.J. 38, *42*
McCune-Nicholich, L. 74, *79*
Macdonald, L. 36, *43*
McLean, J.E. 176, *189*
McMahill, J. 135, *157*
Macoby, E.E. 224, 226, *235*
McCoy, D. 201, *237*
McDevitt, S. 113, *127*
McDevitt, S. 113, *127*
McGimsey, J.F. 207, *233*
McInnes, J.M. 144, *156*
MacKay, D.M. 98, *104*
McLaren, J. 107, 119, *126*
Madeley, R. 222, *233*
Madge, N. 23, 25, 40, *43*
Mann, L. *42*
Manning, P.J. 201, *237*
Mansell, J. 163, 167, 177, *188*
Marholin, D. 218, *235*
Markovits, A.S. 145, *156*
Marshall, A. 98, *105*
Martin, J.A. 224, 226, *235*
Martin, J.A.M. 40, *43*
Martin, N. *41*
Martindale, A. 215, *236*
Martindale, B. 215, *236*
Matson, J.L. 116, 117, *127*, *128*
Maxwell, A.E. 227, 229, *235*
Melin, L. 200, *235*
Meyers, C.E. 100, 120, *106*, *127*
Meyers, M. 100, *105*

Miller, C. 122, *126*
Miller, J.F. *43*
Miller, K.M. 40, *44*
Miller, M. 144, *156*
Mink, I.T. 100, 120, *106*, *127*
Mitchell, L.B. 36, *43*
Mittler, P.J. 1, *11*, 25, 31, 36, 38, *42*, *43*, 78, *105*, *156*, *188*, *235*
Mohn, G. 146, *155*
Molloy, J.S. 144, *156*
Molnar, G.E. 133, *156*
Morris, R.J. 207, *235*
Moss, S.C. 48, *79*
Mrazek, D. 210, *233*
Mulick, J.A. 109, *127*, 201, *237*
Muller, D.J. *188*, *189*
Munoz, M. 200, *235*
Murphy, G. 6, 8, 9, 10, 197, 214, 215, 216, 218, 219, 220, 221, 231, *235*, *336*
Murphy, H.A. 199, 200, *236*
Murray, D.J. 36, *42*
Mussen, P.H. *235*

Napier, D. 141, 142, 143, 153, 154, *156*
Neale, M.D. 39, *43*
Nelson, L.B. 147, *156*
Nettlebeck, T. 120, 123, *127*
Newnham, V. 34, *44*
Newsom, C.D. *233*
Nicholich, L.M. 73, *79*
Nicoll, R.C. 100, *105*, 118, *127*
Nihira, K. 83, 84, 91, 100, *105*, *106*, 111, 118, 120, 123, *127*
Nolan, M. 136, 139, *157*

O'Connor, N. *79*
O'Leary, K.D. 229, 230, *235*, *236*, *237*
Oliver, A. 145, *155*
Oliver, C. *236*
Ounstead, M. 37, *42*
Owen, C.F. 25, *43*

Pace, G.M. 197, *234*

Painter, M. 210, *237*
Palmer, J. 81, 99, *106*
Parsons, J.A. 202, *234*
Pasamanick, B. 23, *43*
Patterson, G.R. 202, 203, 210, 211, 212, 220, 224, 231, *236*
Paul, R. 39, *43*
Pearson, L.S. 36, *42*
Peterson, R.F. 228, *233*
Philips, J.L. 46, *79*
Phillips, I. 121, *127*
Phillips, J.L. 100, *103*
Philps, J. 206, *238*
Piaget, J. 5, 46, 47, 51, 52, 73, *79, 80*
Pidcock, B.E. 87, 88, 97, 98, *106*
Pill, R. 100, *105*
Plewis, I. 206, *238*
Polster, R.A. *43*
Poole, A.D. 222, *236*
Powell, J. 215, 216, *236*
Pratt, M.V. 200, *236*
Prechtl, H.V. *42*
Premack, D. 197, *236*
Presland, J. 133, 134, 152, *156*
Presley, A.S. 114, *125*

Quinton, D. 210, *233*

Rajaratnam, N. 231, *233*
Ramp, E. *234*
Rapport, M.D. 200, 203, 216, 217, *236*
Ratcliffe, S.G. 36, *44*
Rawlings, S. 97, *106*
Raynes, N.V. 5, 6, 101, *106*, 200, 207, 231, *235, 236*
Reid, A.H. 114, *125, 127*
Reid, B.D. 184, *188*
Reid, J.B. 203, 210, 211, 229, *236, 237*
Reiter, S. 109, *126*
Repp, A.C. 200, 215, 216, *233, 236*
Repp, C.R. 215, *236*
Reynell, J. 38, *43*

Reynolds, C.R. 14, 35 *42*
Richardson, S.A. 107, 119, *126*
Richman, G.S. 202, *234*
Richman, N. 196, *236*
Riguet, C.B. 73, *79*
Rincover, A. *237*
Ritvo, E.R. 121, *126*
Roberts, D.M. 215, *236*
Roberts, T.W. 222, *237*
Robertson, R. 218, *234*
Rockinson, R. 216, *236*
Rojahn, J. 201, 231, *237*
Ronanczyk, R.G. 216, 229, 230, *237*
Rondal, J.A. 38, *43*
Rosen, M. 113, *127*
Rosenbloom, L. 38, *41*
Rosenthal, R. 200, 230, *237*
Roses, S. *236*
Rosnow, R.L. 230, *237*
Roszkowski, M. 109, *126*
Rowland, C.M. 175, *188*
Roy, G. 210, *237*
Rubin, S.E. 147, *156*
Ruppenthal, G.G. 222, *237*
Rusch, F.R. 199, *237*
Russo, D.C. 200, *237*
Rutter, M. 24, 29, *41, 43*, 121, *127*, 210, *233*

Sabrotino, D. *42*
Sackett, G.P. 212, 222, 226, *233, 234, 235, 237*
Sailor, W. 143, *155*
Salagaras, S. 120, 123, *127*
Sanson, Fisher, R.W. 222, *236*
Santos, J. 218, *235*
Sattler, J.M. 29, 32, *43*
Saxby, H. 100, *104*
Scanlon, C.A. 119, *127*
Schoggen, M. 66, *78*
Schortinghaus, N.E. 173, *189*
Schroeder, C.S. 109, *127*
Schroeder, S.R. 109, *127*, 201, *237*
Schroth, P.C. 121, *126*
Schultz, B. 135, *157*

AUTHOR INDEX

Schwartz, A.A. 120, *126*
Searles, E. 109, *128*
Sebba, J. 7, 10, 75, 76, 77, *79*, 132, 136, 143, 149, 151, *155*, *156*
Semba, G. *234*
Semmel, M.I. 101, *106*
Senatore, V. 116, 117, 121, 122, *128*
Shackleton-Bailey, M.J. 87, 88, 97, 98, *106*
Shah, A. 87, 97, *105*, 109, 115, *126*, 231, *234*
Shearer, D.E. 32, *43*, 168, 173, *189*
Shearer, M.S. 163, 167, 168, 173, *183*, *189*
Shelhaas, M. 23, *105*, 111, *127*
Shepherd, M. 114, *126*
Shepherd, P.A. 147, *156*
Sheridan, M.D. 74, *80*, 140, 144, 146, *157*
Shiefelbusch, R.L. *188*
Silverstein, A.B. 25, 31, *43*
Simmons, J.Q. 191, *235*
Simon, T. 13
Sinclair, H. 73, *80*
Singh, N.N. 116, *125*, 201, *237*
Sitko, M. 101, *106*
Slack, D.J. 215, *236*
Slifer, K.J. 196, *234*
Smith, B. 68, 69, 70, 71, 75, 78, *80*
Smith, J. 168, *188*
Smith, L. 36, *44*
Snyder-McLean, L.K. 176, *189*
Sontag, E. *80*
Soucar, E. 122, *126*
Spache, G.D. 148, *157*
Speake, B. 89, 90, *106*
Spreat, S. 109, *126*
Stein, J.G. 212, *235*
Stephens, B. 77, *80*
Stephenson, G.R. 222, *237*
Steritt, G.M. *155*
Stern, D.J. 76, *80*
Sternlich, M. 107, *128*

Stevenson, E. 202, *237*
Stevenson, J. 222, *236*
Stewart, A.W. 116, *125*
Stewart, R.M. 218, *235*
Stork, M.T. *234*
Stuart, R. *236*
Stutsman, R. 37, *43*
Sumpton, R.C. 101, *106*
Swanson, H.L. 193, 195, 201, *237*
Sylva, K. *237*

Taplin, P.S. 203, *236*, *237*
Tarnopol, L. *41*
Taubman, M.T. 196, 224, *233*
Taylor, J.R. 119, *128*
Taylor, N.D. 73, *79*
Teller, D.Y. 147, *157*
Tew, B.J. 25, *43*
Thiel, G.W. 120, *128*
Thomas, M. 100, *104*
Thornburn, M.J. 169, *189*
Tierney, I. 36, *44*
Tizard, B. 200, 206, 216, *237*, *238*
Tizard, J. 23, 24, 25, 34, 40, *43*, *44*, 121, *127*, 200, 207, 231, *235*, *237*
Tonick, I. 121, *126*
Touchette, P.E. 218, *235*
Treffry, J.A. 144, *156*
Truman, M. 36, *43*, *44*
Trunell, G. 216, *237*
Tucker, I. 136, 139, *157*
Turpin, W. 109, *126*
Tyler, L. 218, *234*

Utley, B. 143, *155*
Uzgiris, I. 5, 50, 51, 53, 54, 57, 58, 59, 60, 62, 64, 67, 75, 78, *79*, *80*, 162, 184, *189*

Vernon, P.E. 23, 25, 40, *44*
Vincent, E.M. 36, *43*

Wachs, T.D. 74, 77, *80*

Wagner, R.S. 147, *156*
Wake, L. 121, *126*
Ward, J. 38, *43*
Warner, J. 136, *155*
Warnock, M. 1
Watson, B.L. 193, 195, 201, *237*
Webb, R.C. 135, *157*
Weber, I. 173, *189*
Wechsler, D. 33, 34, 35, *44*
Weiner, I.B. *42*
Weinrott, M.R. 202, *238*
Whelan, E. 89, 90, 98, 99, *106*
Wheldall, K. 36, *44*
Whetton, C. 36, *42*
White, M. 167, 173, 174, 175, *189*
Whitman, T.L. 218, *235*
Whitmore, K. 24, *43* 121, *127*
Whittacker, C.A. 73, *80*
Whittlesey, J.R.B. 147, *155*
Wiederholt, J.L. 32, *42*
Wiggins, J.S. 227, 231, 232, *238*

Wildman, B.G. 227, *238*
Williams, C. 129, 136, *156, 157*
Williams, D.E. *234*
Williams, J.A. 197, *238*
Williams, N. 121, *127*
Wilson, R.S. 25, *44*
Wincze, J.P. 201, *238*
Windle, C. 103, *106*
Wing, L. 74, *80* 86, 87, 97, *105, 106*, 115, 122, *126, 128*, 231, *234, 238*
Wolchik, S.A. 207, 209, *234*
Wolf, J.M. 144, *157*
Woodward, W.M. 5, 46, 49, 64, 67, 68, 69, 76, 77, *80*

Yeates, S.R. 74, *80*
Yelton, A.R. 227, 228, *238*
Yoshimura, I. 202, *233*
Young, J.A. 201, *238*
Yule, W. 3, 4, 8, 9, 14, 25, 29, 31, 32, 34, 40, *41, 43, 44*, 121, *127*, 160, 199, *235, 238*

Subject Index

AAMD Adaptive Behavior Scale Parts I and II 84, 91-2, 99-100, 111-13, 118-20, 123, 240
Aberrant Behaviour Checklist 118, 241
adaptive behaviour 5-7, 8, 81-103
　behaviour problems *see* behaviour problems
　and cognitive development 76-7
　communication 82, 87, 89, 90-5, 135, 152-3, 175
　community orientation 82, 90-4
　concept of 81-2
　employment 88, 89
　and IQ 81
　item selection 84
　reliability 96-101, 103
　self help 82, 86, 87, 89, 90-5, 169-71, 173, 178, 180, 197
　social interaction 82, 86
　standardisation 97-101
　and symbolic activity 86
　validity 96-101, 103
　vocational skills 82
aggressive behaviour 92, 112, 114, 118, 119
　programme for 210-12
Albert Einstein Scales of Sensorimotor Development 65-6, 241-2
American Association on Mental Deficiency Classification System 6
Assessment of Visual Ability in the Profoundly Handicapped (Bell) 148-9, 243-4
auditory assessment *see* sensory assessment

Auditory Assessment and Programming Manual for Severely Handicapped and Deaf-Blind Students 143-4, 244-5
autism 73, 107, 108, 119

Balthazar Scales of Adaptive Behavior (BSAB — 1 & 2) 92-3, 100, 111, 113, 245-6
Bayley Scales of Infant Development 23-4, 48, 160
Behaviour Assessment Battery 164, 165-6, 167, 179-84, 246-7
　evaluation 181-4
　relation to teaching 184
　reliability 181
Behavior Development Survey 93-4, 100-1, 247-8
Behaviour Disturbance Scale (BDS) 113-14, 122, 125, 248
behaviour modification 45, 159, 199
　deceleration techniques 207, 209-10
　and recording 190-1
　see also behavioural theory, functional analysis and single case experimental design
behaviour problems 6-7, 107-25
　definition of 107-10
　dynamic properties of 122-3
　incidence of 119-21
　and institutionalisation 119-20
　and language development 201-2
　and level of disability 121
　measurement of 123-4
　organisation 118-19

SUBJECT INDEX

psychiatric problems 117, 121–2
types of 82, 86, 87, 90–4, 107–10, 112–13, 114, 115, 116, 117, 118–19
unit for 206
see also aggressive behaviour, hyperactivity, self-injurious behaviour and stereotypies
behavioural theory 2–3, 45
operant concepts 194–5
see also functional analysis
Bereweeke Skill-Teaching System 163, 167, 177–8, 249
evaluation 178–9
reliability 179
Bliss symbols 206–7
Bobath technique 133
brain damage 29–30, 108, 119
British Ability Scales 36–7

Cain-Levine Social Competency Scale 94–5, 101, 249–50
Children's Handicap Behaviour Skills Structured Interview Schedule 86
Clinical and Education Manual for use with the Uzgiris and Hunt Scales of Infant Development (Dunst) 5, 60–4, 250–1
development of 60
sample records 61, 63, 78
cognitive development 74–7, 169, 171, 174, 178, 180
see also developmental assessment, development and pre-operational development
communication 135, 152–3, 175, 180
and multiple handicap adaptive behaviour and
see also language assessment
community orientation *see* adaptive behaviour

criterion referenced testing 9, 22, 32, 130–1, 133, 152, 158–87
characteristics 162–7
definition 7–8, 158–9
reliability 161–2, 166, 181, 185–6
validity 165–6
curriculum development 45, 76–7, 159–62, 173, 176, 184, 186–7

deterioration
assessment of 30–2
Development Team for the Mentally Handicapped 85, 251–2
developmental assessment 4–5, 23–4, 45–78
fine motor 136–8
gross motor 132–6, 171, 178
reflex assessment 133
Developmental Quotient 3–4, 47–50
developmental theory
curriculum development 45–6, 159–62, 166
see also developmental assessment
deviation scores 17–19
Diagnostic and Statistical Manual of Mental Disorders 117, 216
Disability Assessment Schedule (DAS) 86–7, 97, 115–16, 252–3
Down's syndrome 23–4, 31–2, 73, 75
ageing in 120
hearing 136, 138–9

echolalia 87
ethological approaches 191

fine motor assessment *see* developmental assessment
Fine Motor Skill Assessment Battery 135–7, 153–4, 253

SUBJECT INDEX

Forced Choice Preferential Looking Procedures 147, 254
Frostig Developmental Test of Visual Perception 147–8, 152, 254–5
functional analysis 191–7
Functional Vision Screening for Severely Handicapped Children 149–51, 152, 153, 255–6

General Case Programming 164
Gesell and Amatruda's Developmental Diagnosis 23, 33
Glenwood Awareness, Manipulation and Posture (AMP) Scale 135, 153, 256–7
Graded Arithmetic Mathematics Test 40
Griffiths Mental Developmental Scales 23, 33, 48, 160
gross motor assessment *see* developmental assessment
Group Intelligence Tests 26

Hampshire Assessment for Living with Others (HALO) 87–8, 97–8, 257–8
HANC2 87
HANC-F 87
HANC-S 87
hyperactive behaviour 92, 112, 191, 200
treatment 216–17

Illinois Test of Psycholinguistic Abilities (ITPA) 38–9
incontinence 91
individual differences 12
Individual Programme Planning 91, 93, 102, 103
auditory assessment 143
see also behaviour modification

Intelligence Quotient 3–4, 16–19, 82–3
critique of 47–50
educational attainment 24
relation of adaptive behaviour 81
relevance to mental handicap 40–1
stability 25–6
Intelligence Testing *see* Intelligence Quotient, Norm referenced testing
inter-disciplinary assessment 130–1

language assessment 38–9, 82, 87, 89, 90, 169–70, 172–7, 178
Language Assessment, Remediation and Screening Procedure (LARSP) 39
Literacy assessment *see* reading assessment

McCarthy Scales of Children's Abilities 36
manipulation — assessment of 64–5
measurement 9, 16–22
mental age (MA) 13–14, 16–17, 47–50
behaviour problems 121, 124
Mental Handicap Assessment, Development Team for the Mentally Handicapped, Form 85–6
Mental Handicap Register 85
multiple impairment 74–5, 129, 132
assessment 132–54
language programme 206–7, 208

National Development Group 85–6
Neale Analysis of Reading

SUBJECT INDEX

Ability 39
non-verbal communication 87
Norm referenced testing 3–5, 8, 12–41

Object-Concept and Object-Relation Scale (Gouin Décarie) 65, 258
Object Related Scheme Assessment Procedure 67, 259
Observation System to Assess Spontaneous Infant Behaviour-Environment Interactions 66, 260
observational techniques 8–9, 66, 190–232
　category choice 200–2
　continuous observation 205–6
　continuous recording 210–12; analysis of 224
　data analysis 222–6; concurrent 226; sequential 226
　discontinuous methods 212–18; interval recording 212, 214–18; time sampling 212, 214–18
　duration recording 207–9, 224; analysis of 224
　event recording 206–7; analysis of 224
　generalisability 231–2
　length of observation period 203–4
　observer effects 202–3
　recording techniques 218–22; event recorder 220–1; microcomputer 221–2; videorecording 220–1
　reliability 226–30; Cohen's kappa 228; computational formulae 227–9; interobserver 227–30; observer drift 229–30
　situational factors 202–4
　validity 230–1

Ordinal Scales of Development 24–5, 242–3

Paths to Mobility in 'Special Care' Checklist 133–5, 152, 260–1
performance intelligence 29–30, 33–5
physical assessment 132–6, 152–4
　see also physical impairment
physical impairment 7, 12, 65, 75, 88, 90, 129
　prevalence 129
physiotherapy 132, 135
Piagetian assessment 5, 8, 45–78, 162
　and Behaviour Assessment Battery 165–6, 184
　relation to psychometric assessment 74
play
　assessment of 71–4, 169
　and stereotypies 218–19
Play Object Schemes Progress Assessment (Foxen) 67, 261–2
Portage Guide to Early Education 32, 163, 167, 168–73, 177, 262–3
　checklist 169–72
　evaluation 172–3
　programme approach 168–9
precision, of test scores 19–20
Premack principle 197
Preoperational Assessment (Smith) 68–71, 78, 263–4
preoperational development
　assessment of 67–74, 171–2
　theoretical account 47
pre-senile dementia 110
profile analysis 32
Progress Assessment Chart of Social and Personal Development 88–9, 97–8, 264–5
Progress Evaluation Index 89

SUBJECT INDEX

psychometric assessment 4–5, 8, 12–21, 26–37, 40–1, 47–50, 66, 130
   relation to Piagetian assessment 74
Psychopathology Instrument for Mentally Retarded Adults 116–17, 265–6

Reading Assessment 39, 87, 90–1
reliability 9, 20, 96, 161–2, 166, 179, 181, 185–6
   of observational techniques 226–30
relocation shock 124
Reynell Sccales of Language Development 38, 160

Scale for Assessing Coping Skills (SACS) 89–90, 98–9, 266
self-help *see* adaptive behaviour
self-injurious behaviour 92, 112, 113, 114, 118, 191, 201
   functional analysis of 196–7, 224–5
sensorimotor developmental assessment of 50–67, 171–2, 180–4
   awareness 135
   theoretical account 46–7
sensory assessment 7, 75, 86, 87, 129
   auditory assessment 136, 138–44
   distraction test 138
   electrical response audiometry (ERA) 139
   general considerations 151–4
   impedance bridge measurement 139
   nonspecialist 140–4
   prevalence 129
   visual assessment 144–5; Catford Drum 145–6; opthalmological 145; nonspecialist 143–51; Snellen Chart 145
sexual behaviour 92, 112, 116, 118
single case experimental design 191, 199
social age 81
social competence 81
social interaction *see* adaptive behaviour
social quotient 81
Spelling Tests 40
standardisation 9, 15, 97
Standardized Psychiatric Interview (Goldberg) 114–15, 267
Stanford Binet Intelligence Scale 13–14, 35, 40
stereotypies 87, 92, 112, 113, 114, 118, 119, 191, 207, 209–10
   and toy play 218–19
Stycar Hearing Tests 140–1, 153, 267–8
Stycar Vision Tests 146–7, 152, 153
symbolic activity *see* adaptive behaviour and symbolic play
symbolic play
   assessment of 71–4
Symbolic Play Test 71–3, 78, 268–9
Systematic Procedures for Eliciting and Recording Responses to Sound Stimuli 141–3, 153, 269–70

Techniques of Assessment of Severely Subnormal and Young Normal Children (Woodward) 64, 270–1
thalidomide-damaged children 65

Uzgiris and Hunt's Ordinal Scales of Infant Development 5, 50–9, 78, 162
   development of 51–3

sample records 54–8

validity 9, 20–2, 96–7, 165–6
  of observational techniques 230–1
verbal intelligence 29–30, 33–5
verbal-performance score difference 29–30
Vernon Graded Word Spelling Test 40
Vineland Social Maturity Scale 95, 101–2, 271–2
Visual Checklist (Sebba) 149–51, 272

Wechsler Adult Intelligence Scale (Revised) (WAIS-R) 35
Wechsler Intelligence Scale for Children (Revised) (WISC-R) 29–31, 34–5
Wechsler Pre-school and Primary Scale of Intelligence (WPPSI) 33–4
Wessex Behaviour Rating Scale 86, 90–1, 99, 273
  Social and Physical Incapacity Scale 90–1
  Speech, Self Help and Literacy Scale 90–1
Wessex Revised Portage Language Checklist 167, 173–7, 273–4
  evaluation 175–7
Woodward's Approach to Preoperational Assessment 67–8, 274